Best Practice Occupational Therapy

In Community Service with
Children and Families

Best Practice Occupational Therapy

In Community Service with Children and Families

Winnie Dunn, PhD, OTR, FAOTA

Professor and Chair
University of Kansas Medical Center
Kansas City, Kansas

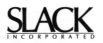

SLACK
INCORPORATED

6900 Grove Road • Thorofare, NJ 08086

Bay Shore

Publisher: John H. Bond
Editorial Director: Amy E. Drummond
Managing Editor: Debra Toulson
Design Editor: Lauren Biddle Plummer

Best practice occupational therapy: in community service with children and families/by Winnie Dunn.
    p. cm.
Includes bibliographical references and index.
ISBN 1-55642-456-6 (alk. paper)
1. Occupational therapy for children-- Standards. 2. Occupational therapy services-- Standards. I. Dunn, Winnie.

RJ53.O25 B47 2000
615.8'515'083--dc21   00-027243

Printed in the United States of America.

Published by: SLACK Incorporated
                   6900 Grove Road
                   Thorofare, NJ 08086-9447 USA
                   Telephone: 856-848-1000
                   Fax: 856-853-5991
                   World Wide Web: http://www.slackbooks.com

Contact SLACK Incorporated for more information about other books in this field or about the availability of our books from distributors outside the United States.

Authorization to photocopy items for internal or personal use, or the internal or personal use of specific clients, is granted by SLACK Incorporated, provided that the appropriate fee is paid directly to Copyright Clearance Center, 222 Rosewood Drive, Danvers, MA 01923 USA, 978-750-8400. Prior to photocopying items for educational classroom use, please contact the CCC at the address above. Please reference Account Number 9106324 for SLACK Incorporated's Professional Book Division.

For further information on CCC, check CCC Online at the following address: http://www.copyright.com.

Last digit is print number: 10   9   8   7   6   5   4   3   2   1

1/29/01

DEDICATION

I dedicate this book to my son Jim... my "Wizard of Oz"...
....who despite the occasional bluster, demonstrates through his passion that his
wisdom
courage
and heart

always prevail as he advocates on behalf of children and families in his work.

I deliver these "best ideas" of mine to nurture his soul on that journey.

CONTENTS

ACKNOWLEDGMENTS

Many people support my career activities. I want to acknowledge those who provided supports so that I could complete this book.

Beth Cada, Ellen Mellard, Gloria Clark, and Jean Linder provided wise counsel as I prepared this work. Their spirits and ideas reside in these pages with mine.

Jeannie Rigby supports me each day by tracking my work and anticipating what needs to be done. She makes me look good and I am eternally grateful.

Marguerite Green, Shelly Pyle, and Joan Delahunt prepared the bibliographies. Bonnie Danley compiled the files. Carol Hydeman made follow up phone calls. Because they completed these details, I could concentrate on thinking and planning; thank you.

The faculty and staff in Occupational Therapy Education at the University of Kansas take responsibility for our department along with me, making it possible for me to have professional accomplishments of my own. I honor all of you.

The graduate students in Occupational Therapy Education read early manuscripts and gave me invaluable feedback that improved this work. I thank all of you.

My practice and research colleagues and families who contacted me to ask questions, offer perspectives and challenge me to "think again"—prodding me to reconstruct my ideas. I appreciate their willingness to support my growth and my contributions.

ABOUT THE AUTHOR

Winnie Dunn is Professor and Chair of the Department of Occupational Therapy Education at the University of Kansas. Dr. Dunn holds a bachelor's degree in occupational therapy and a master of science degree in special education-learning disabilities from the University of Missouri. She earned her doctorate in applied neuroscience from the University of Kansas.

She is a fellow of the American Occupational Therapy Association (AOTA), has received the Award of Merit for outstanding service contributions to the profession, is a member of the Academy of Research of the American Occupational Therapy Foundation, and most recently was named the Eleanor Clark Slagle lecturer for her significant contributions to "conceptual and evidence-based neuroscience research and practice." She has served on the Commission on Practice, the Early Intervention and School Based Practice Task Forces of AOTA, has been the chair of the Research Development Committee of the AOTF, and just completed a decade of service on the National Board for Certification of Occupational Therapy (NBCOT). As Chair of the Research Advisory Committee of NBCOT, she directed the National Study of Occupational Therapy Practice, which led to the current test blueprint for the certification exam in occupational therapy.

Dr. Dunn has spoken and written extensively about service provision practices for children and families. Through her research, she has demonstrated the effectiveness of consultation and the use of theory to guide contextually relevant practice. Her line of research about sensory processing in daily life has been very fruitful, producing the *Sensory Profile* assessments that identify distinct patterns of sensory processing in various groups of infants, toddlers, children, youth, adults, and older adults.

CONTRIBUTING AUTHORS

Ellen Mellard, MS, OTR
Infant-Toddler Coordinator of Northeast Kansas Educational Service Center
Teaching Associate, University of Kansas Medical Center

Jean Linder, MA, OTR, FAOTA
State Consultant
Iowa Department of Education

Gloria Frolek Clark, MS, OTR
Occupational Therapist
Heartland Area Education Agency
Iowa Department of Education

PREFACE

How is it that a person comes to have strong beliefs about something? I suppose there are many ways. Sometimes it is our missteps that show us the edges, and the core of our beliefs; this is certainly true for me.

A very young mother taught me the importance of family-centered care. As I was serving her and her daughter, I determined that her daughter was ready to try self-feeding. The mother was quite reluctant about my suggestions and was not following my recommendations. The mother continued to feed her daughter.

I was quite put out by this mother's actions. I was giving her my best advice, the expertise that I spent many years learning, and the mother was being "passive-aggressive" with me by not following through. I spoke to others about this with frustration and disgust. Why would this mother neglect this opportunity to support her daughter's development?

It is fortunate for me (and for this mother and child) that I had a wise administrator at the time. He said "Winnie, why don't you go visit the mother in her home and see what you discover." I was not interested in investing that kind of time on this mother when she wouldn't even do what I had already told her to do. But each time I ranted and raved around the office, he would quietly suggest this same strategy over and over again until I felt pressure to comply.

So with little excitement, I scheduled a visit. I did have the insight to go close to a meal time since we were supposed to be working on feeding. It did not take long once I was immersed in this mother's life, to understand why I needed to be there. I needed to experience these two people's lives; only then could I know how to apply my knowledge and expertise in their service.

Although the mother had many appropriate toys around for her daughter, they were not interacting when I arrived. The daughter was sitting among the toys, but was not playing. This continued while the mother and I chatted. Then we began to move toward the kitchen for the meal, and everything changed. The mother and daughter began to interact with each other, using reciprocal eye contact and vocalizations; the mother played with her daughter, pulling the spoon in and out, and making her daughter move in anticipation toward the food.

In those moments, the clarity of my insight became so bright it was blinding me. I realized that with all her reluctance, comments, and behaviors, the mother had been trying to convey something very important. She somehow knew the essential nature of her intimacy with her daughter and only knew how to maintain this within the ritual of feeding time. I was so focused on my expertise that I failed to *listen*, observe, and derive meaning from her behaviors. My insight enabled me to see that she certainly could profit from my expertise, just not the part I was trying to wedge into her life. This mother and daughter needed me to teach them how to play together as an expanded form of intimacy.

It is for this mother and daughter and all the parents and children that have come into our professional lives since that defining moment that I am relentless about what constitutes best practice for children and families. Vulnerable children and families cannot afford the time it might take for service providers to discover the ideas in this book on their own. Perhaps having my best wisdom collected here will move us along to make these practices standard ways of working and provide the fertile ground for the next "best practices."

winnie dunn

CHAPTER 1

Best Practice Philosophy for Community Services for Children and Families

Winnie Dunn, PhD, OTR, FAOTA

Providing services in community-based settings is vital to the best application of occupational therapy principles and beliefs because occupational therapy professionals are concerned with individuals' daily lives. Community settings present life as it is, suggesting both a simplicity and a complexity that makes this practice have a potency that is unattainable elsewhere.

Best practices in early intervention and school-based services demand that occupational therapy professionals not only act in accordance with the knowledge, principles, and philosophies of their own profession, but also with a larger set of beliefs in mind. These beliefs and philosophies have grown out of collective experiences across disciplines and among families, as everyone has endeavored to find the best way to support children's growth when they have various challenges to their development and learning.

Professionals have a particular knowledge base that represents their profession and enables them to derive particular meaning from situations; individuals expect professionals to provide services that reflect the expertise of their discipline.

Individuals have the right to participate in daily life activities of their choosing; communities have the responsibility to provide reasonable access to these activities.

Professionals who serve children and families have the responsibility to provide family-centered care, i.e., to honor the family's priorities and style in designing and implementing intervention plans.

Professionals and families have the mutual and reciprocal right and responsibility to involve each other in the organization and structure of services within community-based systems.

Individuals have the right to consider options and choose interventions; professionals have the responsibility to provide information regarding the effectiveness of the options we offer as potential solutions.

We will discuss these statements in the subsequent sections of this chapter and offer examples of how occupational therapists construct and implement services while using these principles to guide their practice.

DEFINING BEST PRACTICE

Throughout this book, we use the term "best practice" when referring to various actions of the occupational therapist. We use this term to invite therapists to conduct their professional business in a particular way. *Best practices are a professional's decisions and actions based on knowledge and evidence that reflect the most current and innovative ideas available.* Many therapists, teams, and agencies engage in "standard practice", which is employing more traditional, routine, and established ways of providing services. This is a perfectly acceptable paradigm for conducting professional business, i.e., the routines or protocols are known and good enough; it is simply not the paradigm we are reflecting in this book.

It is not the location of practice that determines whether one engages in best practice; therapists can work in traditional or nontraditional settings and use standard or best practices. Best practice is a way of thinking about problems in imaginative ways, applying knowledge creatively to solve performance problems, and taking responsibility for evaluating the effectiveness of the innovations to inform future practices.

Let's consider an example: A therapist wishes to serve preschool aged children with disabilities. Using standard practice, this therapist would identify preschool programs that serve children with disabilities and seek employment in one of those preschools. Once employed, this therapist would set up routines or protocols for conducting occupational therapy assessments. The therapist would also participate with the team in designing intervention plans and provide direct therapy with selected children according to established protocols for addressing particular problems. The therapist would make suggestions to teachers and aides about ways to support these children in the curriculum when they ask the therapist for assistance.

Using best practice, the therapist would identify day care programs and preschool programs for children without disabilities that would be willing to support preschool children who have disabilities. The therapist would learn about the agency's philosophy and advocate both to be employed and for the agency to consider serving children with disabilities, pointing out the benefits of having an integrated program and the unique skills and perspectives of the discipline of occupational therapy that would enrich their programs. Once employed, this therapist would further explore the service philosophy of the community agency and the care providers, observe the preschool or day care programs, and interview staff and families to identify their goals and concerns. The therapist would also observe and evaluate the skills of particular children with disabilities in various settings (e.g., day care, home via videotapes if necessary) and use this information in concert with the agency information to identify supports and barriers to particular children's participation. In collaboration with service staff, the therapist would implement possible strategies, test their effectiveness (both for the child and for the staff), and make adjustments as needed.

In both cases, occupational therapy expertise is being applied to both the children's and families' needs. You see that the second example illustrates an emphasis on child-context interaction, a more integrated service pattern in which the therapist demonstrates responsiveness within the service system. In standard practice there is a stronger focus on addressing the child's skill development within a protocol that the team or agency has established.

In standard practice, it is more common to see separate attention to the child and the context/system, while in best practice the therapist is more likely to "stand in the space" between the child and the context and consider the impact of each part (i.e., the child and the context) on the other. We might say that best practice therapists are continuously seeking new ideas from evidence and dialogue in the profession; they are "early adopters" of new ideas and practices. Standard practice therapists are "late adopters" of new ideas and practices, i.e., they stay with demonstrated practices a longer time before changing routines (Rogers, 1978).

Remember: What is best practice today evolves into standard practice in the future. This is how knowledge advances in our discipline. The standard practices of today were best practices of the past that have influenced practice. When someone continues their standard practices across too long a time, we would say that their practice is out of date and would not stand up to standard practice scrutiny. As your career unfolds, watch for these transitions and recognize their contributions to our evolution as a discipline.

USING CORE KNOWLEDGE OF THE PROFESSION

Professionals have a particular knowledge base that represents their profession and enables them to derive particular meaning from situations; individuals expect professionals to provide services that reflect their discipline's expertise.

Each discipline and profession embraces a body of knowledge that reflects that discipline's perspectives. The background knowledge includes related subjects to the discipline as well as the core concepts of the discipline. For occupational therapy, we bring knowledge about development, neuroscience, psychology, and disability conditions to the table along with our discipline's core concepts about occupation and performance. This background forms our perspective about the importance of participation and the meaning people derive from various types of participation during their lives. Other disciplines combine knowledge to create another perspective.

When families engage with us related to their children's needs, they make an assumption that we are prepared with the background knowledge, have the perspective of occupational therapy, and are competent to apply that perspective (with its incumbent knowledge base) on behalf of their children. Our profession has mechanisms to ensure that entry-level professionals meet this expectation, such as the accreditation of educational programs, requirements for successful performance in school, and success on the certification from the National Board for Certification in Occupational Therapy (NBCOT).

The materials in this text are designed to support you to learn how to *apply* the background knowledge you have been acquiring to the practice challenges you face when serving children and families in community settings. You will need to refer to your other resources for the background knowledge (e.g., development books and notes, books and articles on models of practice) to solve the practice challenges set before you in this book and that you will encounter in practice. Be prepared to access those resources, because they will support your decisions in practice.

SUPPORTING PARTICIPATION

Individuals have the right to participate in daily life activities of their choosing; communities have the responsibility to provide reasonable access to these activities.

Pub. Law No. 94-142 (the Education for All Handicapped Act) and Section 504 of the Rehabilitation Act from previous decades (see Chapter 9) began a clear process of clarifying the ways that people obtain access to their environments for daily life. In the first half of the 20th century, our society focused on reducing the number of residents in large institutions (called *deinstitutionalization*).

As individuals who had various disabilities were more "present" in communities, the issues of how to involve them in living was on everyone's minds. The concept of "mainstreaming" was developed to address the need to provide access to natural environments for students in school. Pub. L. No. 94-142 stated that to the extent possible, children with disabilities would be placed with other children in the *"least restrictive environment"* for activities throughout the day. Many teams began placing children with disabilities in art, music, and physical education classes with peers who did not have disabilities for mainstreaming. The children continued to have the bulk of their academic days in separate special education classrooms.

During the 1970's and 1980's professionals began to see that children might be successful in more activities, and that professional expertise could be designed in new ways for children's benefit. The concept of mainstreaming evolved into "integrated" programming. This manner of combining programming invited best practice professionals to identify and implement creative ways to synthesize their knowledge; educational programs began to look very different for special education students. At this point, best practice involved a more collaborative effort on the professionals' parts, and children were spending more time with peers than in segregated classrooms. However, special education classrooms remained the home base for children with special education needs, and when children with disabilities were in regular education classrooms they were still "separate" in the sense that they had different work, sat in the periphery, or had an aide right there with them. During this period there was a lot of tension between the educators and the related service personnel (e.g., occupational therapists). There was pressure for therapists to participate in planning together rather than pull children out of their educational settings to provide therapy in isolation from the educational experience. Therapists were not as responsive as they needed to be during this period and continued isolated services.

During the 1990's the concept of daily life experiences and the "least restrictive environment" for children with disabilities reached a new level of intensity. The concept evolved to one called "inclusion", which urges professionals to do whatever it takes to make sure a child is successfully involved in the activities of peers in their natural settings. The Americans with Disabilities Act also outlined the responsibility of community members to make the world accessible to people. During this period, families and people with disabilities also had a greater voice in our society, making this evolution possible.

In a sense, this latest version of the principle of involvement acknowledges several things. First, inclusion invites us to acknowledge that everyone has the right to have access to what they want and need to do. Secondly, inclusion practices point out that disabilities are not the person's fault or responsibility any more than being short is. As a society, we have the opportunity to make some aspects of disability transparent, that is, to reduce or erase the impact of the disability on the person's performance and life options. When ALL bathroom stalls are big enough for a wheelchair, it won't matter how a person mobilizes to move about in the environment. Third, inclusion provides an opportunity for children without disabilities to experience the heterogeneity of the human experience, thus enabling them to keep disabilities in perspective (Salisbury & Dunst, 1997). When children grow up and learn together, disabilities are no more or less important or noticeable than other traits, such as "funniness", "shyness," or "thinness".

Inclusion practices are difficult to implement correctly. Just because a child is physically present in a regular classroom doesn't mean the child is "included". Inclusion means that the child is immersed and involved in the culture and learning of that setting; this might not mean that all the children will learn the same things, but it does mean that all children will participate to the extent possible in learning tasks. For inclusion to be implemented properly, schools will have to reconstruct themselves by shifting resources and conducting business differently. Teachers have not yet been prepared to conduct business this new way; special educators feel displaced when they don't have "classes" of children. Aides have to learn to support the whole class and not just the child with the disability. This will take time. Since occupational therapists are concerned with performance in daily life, they are the consummate professionals to take a leadership role in supporting inclusion practices. The American Occupational Therapy Association (AOTA) published an official paper stating our profession's firm commitment to inclusion practices and outlining our domain of concern related to this goal.

The International Classification of Impairments, Disabilities, and Handicaps-2 (ICIDH-2) outlines "disability", "activity", and "participation" as the levels of concern for health policy and research (see Appendix G). Participation involves the interaction between the person and the context, with the desired outcome of living a satisfying life. In the next millenium, I am confident that we will evolve as a society to the point that the human features we call disabilities today will just be human traits, nothing more and nothing less. Toward this outcome, a photographer, Rick Guidotti, published a photo essay in Life magazine (1998) showing the beauty of albinism. He shot young people in a glamorous venue, showing that what might have been considered a disability or limitation (e.g., lack of pigment) could be their signature feature of beauty that others might admire. Occupational therapists in the next millenium can also contribute forward thinking perspectives to our society with our emphasis on supporting persons to do and be what is relevant and satisfying for their lives.

FAMILY-CENTERED CARE PRINCIPLES

Professionals have the responsibility to provide family-centered care (i.e., to honor the family's priorities and style in designing and implementing intervention plans).

Family centered care means that professionals value, encourage and commit themselves to meaningful involvement of families in planning and implementation (Salisbury & Dunst, 1997). There has been a great evolution in our perspectives on family involvement in their children's care. We now know that children whose parents participate in programming are more successful than children whose parents do not (e.g., Epstein, 1993).

Parents and other family members are the most consistent people in a child's life. Therefore open communication is imperative among the various teams (not only within the team but also one team with another) and the family. Family-centered care dictates that professionals value and therefore create a successful communication strategy (Salisbury & Dunst, 1997), including providing interpreters, avoiding jargon, and using positive non-verbal strategies (e.g., eye contact, active listening).

Salisbury & Dunst (1997) outline several major barriers to family centered care. Sometimes professionals are insensitive to the unique features of families, and therefore interpret them as negative, difficult, or adversarial. For example, professionals might interpret a mother who has difficulty scheduling a time to come to school for a meeting as "non compliant", without considering factors that underlie this behavior, e.g., that she has two jobs to support her family and their schedules conflict with typical school hours. In best practice, we use family-centered care values and therefore we recognize and respect the mother for being resourceful as she endeavors to care for her children.

For every parent and family, there will be a preferred and optimal way to communicate; the professionals who practice family-centered care will take the time to identify these strategies and implement them in the interest of supporting the family's development as informed advocates for their child. Some families will want to meet more often, while others will request other ways to stay informed (e.g., phone messages and conversations, notes, audiotapes, videotapes, emails).

Another barrier occurs when professionals consider the parents less informed, insightful, or intelligent than the professionals. Regardless of their backgrounds, parents are the most knowledgeable about their own children. Practices such as constructing plans prior to the parents' involvement and disregarding the parents observations (particularly when they are in conflict with the professionals' findings) indicate lack of respect for parents as equal partners in the endeavor of serving their children and violates family-centered care principles. In fact, scholars have reported that parents are accurate assessors of their children's abilities and report information that the professionals cannot obtain through other means (e.g., Bricker & Squires, 1989; Dunn, 1999). For example, a parent might tell the team that the child eats successfully at home, when the team has reported difficulty with eating at school. Without family-centered care values, the professionals might dismiss the parents' comments as incorrect. From a family-centered care perspective, the professionals would invite the parents to describe eating at home so the team can identify how they have been successful (they might even have a video the team can view), and how eating at home and school differ so they can implement more successful interventions at school as well (Dunn, 1999).

A related issue in family centered care is the use of "person first language". **Person first language is the use of the person's name rather than other references such as the disability or disorder to identify the person.** We say "*Chris* needs a supported chair", rather than "*the cerebral palsied (CP) child* needs a supported chair". Or we say "When *a child who has cerebral palsy* needs to work at the table, we might design a supported chair", rather than "*a CP child* needs a supported chair to work at the table". In best practice, we are vigilant about using person first language because it is an ongoing way to demonstrate our respect for the child as a human being FIRST, regardless of whatever other characteristics might be relevant to the problem we are addressing.

In occupational therapy, there are many times when it is not even necessary to state the disability or disorder; our focus is on performance in daily life, so this needs to be our emphasis. Our knowledge about disorders is background for our problem-solving (i.e., scientific reasoning, see Chapter 3); we are not "curing" the disorder, we are addressing the performance need. Therefore, in best practice occupational therapy, professionals discuss the child and family in relation to what they want and need to do, e.g., "Chris wants to work with his peers at the table during social studies". It doesn't matter (except for our internal clinical reasoning processes to determine the best intervention) whether Chris has CP, a brain injury, muscular dystrophy, or attention deficit hyperactivity disorder; what matters is our ability to use our expertise to accomplish this desired performance outcome.

COLLABORATION PHILOSOPHY SUPPORTING FAMILIES

Professionals and families have the mutual and reciprocal right and responsibility to involve each other in the organization and structure of services within community-based systems.

Team Collaborations

There are many team structures and processes (see Chapter 2), but all teams have the goal of combining expertise and perspectives for the benefit of a child and family. The child's performance needs, the family's and other care providers needs, the contextual resources, and resources within a service system can influence which disciplines are represented on any team (Muhlenhaupt, 1991). School districts develop planning teams based on the regulations in IDEA 1997; these teams must include representatives from certain disciplines (i.e., psychology, speech therapy, and special education) and positions (i.e., parent of a child with an educational handicap who resides in the district).

Systems can involve other specialists or interested parties as they see fit to address the child's needs effectively. In some states, physician involvement in occupational therapy programs is mandatory under licensure statutes. It is appropriate for core team members to solicit input and feedback from specialists who might have insights to enhance the team planning processes. Core team members can use phone calls, copies of written documentation (including evaluations and notes), and email conversations to obtain current information. When employing best practice, these specialists are considered equal partners in the team planning process for community programming; it is always the team's responsibility together to make decisions about the best course of action.

Parents are also vital members of the teams that serve children. Parental concerns, goals, and resources (Dickman, 1985; Featherstone, 1980; Zins, Graden, & Ponti, 1988) are critical to the child's involvement in an intervention program. Additionally, federal mandates dictate that parents have the legal right to be an integral part of the planning teams for their children. The team can also include other family members and care providers as well if the parents believe it is important to planning. For example, siblings may want or need to participate in aspects of the child's at-home care and management (Muhlenhaupt, 1991). Certain family traditions or situations may necessitate that extended family members are the child's primary caregivers. Children with acute or chronic medical conditions may have nurses or other health care workers who attend to their needs at home or school. These persons have the potential to play an important role in planning and implementing the child's therapeutic and educational programs (Muhlenhaupt, 1991).

Interagency Collaborations

When serving families as part of the community, professionals must find effective strategies for communicating among each other on behalf of the child and family. Particularly when serving children with complex disabilities, communication is critical because these families will need service supports from a range of agencies. For example, a child with muscular dystrophy will need support from the physician, clinics that monitor the disease process and use of adaptive devices, community support groups (e.g., for family interactions and gatherings such as summer camps), school personnel, and pharmacists as part of comprehensive care. *Interagency collaboration, then, is the mechanism that professionals create in a particular community to engage with each other in service to a family.*

Occupational therapists are key members of the teams in any number of the community agencies that serve children and families, and therefore have an important role to play in interagency collaboration. Therapists can participate in the formal mechanisms of communication across agencies, but sometimes the more informal networks of communication are equally or even more important to overall collaborative efforts. The relationships among the actual service providers can sometimes be more powerful than formal agreements that focus on procedures. For example, families need the school-based occupational therapist and the children's hospital occupational therapist to collaborate so that their efforts are in concert with each other and families get consistent information about how to support their child at home. This relationship is more important to the family than whether the school and hospital have formal mechanisms for communication.

Quality interagency collaboration also requires members of the service teams to understand how and when to make referrals to each other. Each agency and each professional within a particular agency must have a clear awareness of the mission and purpose of the agency, which enables them to know what areas of service are inside and outside their purview as a community service agency. Additionally, each professional must recognize her or his own skills so that it is clear when to solicit another colleague within the same discipline or from another discipline to support the child and family. It is critical to successful interdisciplinary collaboration on behalf of families that professionals recognize the limits of their own and their agencies' capabilities. Families deserve the best services available in a community; making referrals to the most skilled community members demonstrates respect for families.

For example, if a school-based therapist determines that a child needs a resting hand splint based on the father's comments and her own observations, it is best for the school therapist to refer the family to a rehabilitation therapist who can make the splint efficiently for the family (e.g., the rehabilitation therapist has the tools and supplies, and constructs splints more regularly). Although splint construction is theoretically in the skill domain of all occupational therapists, it is not typically in the scope of public school practice. Therefore, it is most appropriate for the school therapist to make the referral.

Supporting Transitions in Programming and Agencies

A transition is a change from one situation to another. Occupational therapists participate in and support a number of transitions when serving children and families. The most frequent types of transitions are those that a child and family make as the child grows, and therefore becomes eligible for a different service system or agency. For example, infants at risk transition from hospital care to home and follow along care. Preschoolers transition from early childhood and day care programs to public schools. Adolescents transition to middle school and high school, and young adults transition to work and community living. Children and families can also transition from clinical therapy services to educationally-related services. Occupational therapists are involved with the service systems at all of these pre- and post-transition sites, and so will be intimately involved with the transition processes.

When participating in transitions, occupational therapists contribute in a number of ways. A therapist that serves in a pre-transition site has the responsibility to clearly document the child's current levels of performance, adaptations and supports that facilitate performance, other interventions that have been successful (and unsuccessful), and recommendations about goals and services for the future. A therapist that serves in a post-transition site has the responsibility to review materials about the child and prepare follow up questions that will provide clarity for planning.

Both therapists have a shared responsibility to collaborate with each other to ensure a smooth transition. It is of the utmost importance for the therapists to recognize the differences in their respective service systems and how each of these systems serves the children and their families. For example, when children transition from preschool services to the public schools, there are a number of issues to incorporate into planning and discussions with the families. Preschool services are frequently constructed to provide intense developmental interventions; the curriculum is developmentally-oriented and the therapy contributions have the same orientation. Professionals serve children in smaller groups or individually during the preschool years because this is developmentally appropriate for their cognitive abilities. As children move into the public schools, the focus is increasingly on cognitive and social development; children spend the whole day at school, work in larger groups, and the team works to incorporate the children's areas of therapeutic needs into the routines of this new kind of day.

Therapists providing best practice services make sure that families understand the meaning and importance of this transition; children who can function successfully in this more advanced environment are making the progress they need to make for independence in adulthood. Children who need the same level of support in grammar school as they did in preschool haven't profited from the preschool services. Therapists supporting this transition will collaborate to design the next setting plans and will communicate their optimism about the transition together. The preschool therapist will communicate enthusiasm about the child's growth and opportunities at school; both therapists can discuss how services are reformulated to support the child in public school with peers. This supports family-centered care as part of best practice.

EFFECTIVENESS OF PRACTICES

Individuals have the right to consider options and choose interventions; professionals have the responsibility to provide information regarding the effectiveness of the options we offer as potential solutions.

There has been an increasing call in professional circles for practice decisions and actions to be based on the evidence available about those practices (e.g., Jette, 1995; Lloyd-Smith, 1997; Sackett et al., 1991), rather than the background and experiences of a particular professional. Wennberg (1990) reported on several studies in which there was large variability in health care practices of experienced professionals, suggesting a need for guidelines to ensure the best quality care for everyone. Professionals agree that it is important to distinguish effective and ineffective practices, but there has not always been agreement about how to accomplish this goal. Additionally, as families have become more informed about their rights and responsibilities, they have wished to make informed decisions about the care they will receive.

In order for professions to determine which practices are effective, scholars and practitioners must participate together in research that discloses the impact of intervention practices on salient outcomes for the service recipient. Once we have data about particular interventions, professionals who employ best practice use this knowledge for two purposes. First, professionals use the knowledge gained from research to advance their problem-solving capabilities for practice decision making. Second, professionals relate effectiveness findings to families and other service recipients so they understand the potential risks and benefits of service options.

When professionals use outcomes of research to guide their practices, we call this evidence-based practice. *Evidence-based practice* is a systematic process of locating, evaluating, synthesizing, and incorporating research findings into one's internal resources to advance problem-solving and decision-making in practice (Rosenberg & Donald, 1995). This has not been the traditional way to train professionals in occupational therapy, but is becoming a more important feature of practice as payers and consumers demand verification for the practices they finance and select for themselves. Best practice requires professionals to engage in evidence-based practice.

There are several challenges to engaging in evidence-based practice. First, there is a scarcity of research literature that demonstrates the effectiveness of our practices. Occupational therapy is a relatively young field, and its history as an applied science (therefore creating a research base) is even shorter. The studies available are typically on very small samples and address discreet problems that certainly don't represent the scope of occupational therapy practice. We need more studies that are rigorous enough to reveal insights for practice.

This leads to the second challenge; some of the criteria that have been established for an acceptable study would eliminate valuable data available from consideration. In medicine they hold up the "randomized clinical trial" (RCT) as the gold standard for studies that inform practice decisions (Sackett, et al., 1996). An RCT requires an experimental and control group with matched samples of subjects; one search of occupational therapy literature revealed only six RCT studies (Dunn, McDowd, & Brown, 1999). This is not nearly enough evidence to guide practice. There are many other types of studies that can inform practice, and we need to recognize what these studies can inform us about and how to use the findings to advance knowledge for practice.

Finally, even with the outcomes research available, it is difficult for those in practice to locate it and translate it into meaningful information for practice decision-making. There are studies from both occupational therapy and other disciplines that can inform occupational therapy practice. We must consider it a priority for our profession to organize and synthesize knowledge from this range of studies in a way that makes it easy for those in practice to gain access, interpret properly, and inform themselves and families about the meaning of the findings for their service options.

Best practice means that we take the time to find out about the effectiveness of our intervention options for a particular child and family. We do not pass on "folklore", i.e., suggest an intervention because our teacher or supervisor told us about it or we saw another therapist trying it. We only consider options that we understand and can articulate a rationale for; if something is a newer, more experimental intervention option, we inform the family that this is true and include an extensive plan for data collection to determine its impact on the child. If the newer intervention (or any intervention for that matter) does not show effectiveness for the desired performance, we stop using it and design another option. We never continue an intervention based on beliefs without evidence, even if that evidence is from our data collection on this child only. Evidence-based practice requires us to step back from our lived experience with a child and family and evaluate the impact of our work on the desired performance outcome. In this book, we will demonstrate strategies for this aspect of best practice.

REFERENCES

Bricker, D., & Squires, J. (1989). The effectiveness of parental screening of at-risk infants: The monitoring questionnaires. *Topics in Early Childhood Special Education, 9*(3), 67-85.

Dickman, I. (1985). *One miracle at a time.* New York, NY: Simon and Schuster.

Dunn, W. (1999). T*he sensory profile.* San Antonio, TX: Psychological Corporation.

Dunn, W., McDowd, J., & Brown, C. (1999). *KUCORE: Exposing the seeds of truth for best practice occupational therapy. An outcomes research project of the department of occupational therapy education.* Kansas City, KS: University of Kansas.

Epstein, J. (1993, April). Make parents your partners. *Instructor, 19,* 119-136.

Featherstone, H. (1980). *A difference in the family: Living with a disabled child.* New York, NY: Basic Books.

Guidotti, R. (June, 1998). Rick Guidotti opens our eyes to the beauty of albinism. *Life,* 65-69.

Jette, A. (1995). Physical disablement concepts for physical therapy research and practice. *Physical Therapy, 74,* 380-386.

Lloyd-Smith, W. (1997). Evidence-based practice and occupational therapy. *British Journal of Occupation Therapy, 60,* 474-478.

Muhlenhaupt, M. (1991). Components of the program planning process. In W. Dunn (Ed.), *Pediatric Occupational Therapy: Facilitating effective service provision* (pp. 125-135). Thorofare, NJ: SLACK Incorporated.

Rosenberg, W., & Donald, A. (1995). Evidence-based medicine: An approach to clinical problem-solving. *British Medical Journal, 310,* 1122-1126.

Sackett, D., Rosenberg, W., Gray, J., Haynes, R., & Richardson, W. (1996). Evidence-based medicine: What it is and what it isn't. *British Medical Journal, 312,* 71-72.

Sackett, D., Haynes, R., Guyatt, G., & Tugwell, P. (1991). *Clinical epidemiology: A basic science for clinical medicine.* London, England: Little, Brown & Co.

Salisbury, C., & Dunst, C. (1997). *Homes, school, and community partnerships: Building inclusive teams. Collaborative Teams for Students with Severe Disabilities* (pp. 57-82). Baltimore, MD: Paul H. Brookes Publishing Co.

Wennberg, J. (1990). Outcomes research, cost containment, and the feat of health care rationing. *New England Journal of Medicine, 323,* 1202-1204.

Zins, J., Graden, J., & Ponti, C. (1988). Pre-referral intervention to improve special services delivery. *Services in the Schools, 4*(3/4), 109-130.

2

Structure of Best Practice Programs

Winnie Dunn, PhD, OTR, FAOTA

Now that we have the philosophy of best practice outlined (see Chapter 1), we need to consider how to structure services to facilitate the implementation of best practices in community-based settings. In this chapter, we will describe the structures for teams, occupational therapy services, and typical funding patterns for community-based services.

RECOGNIZING THE NATURE OF SERVICES AND PROFESSIONAL ACTIVITIES

Many agencies have different purposes when providing early intervention or special education and related services. The purpose of early intervention is to provide services designed to meet the developmental needs of children and the needs of families to enhance their children's development. Public education programs for children with disabilities are structured to provide education and related services necessary for children to benefit from education. Hospitals and other community agencies have as their missions to provide services for special purposes, such as medically-related health, financial assistance, work preparation and training, or mental health programs.

Occupational therapists may be employed in any number of settings by a wide variety of agencies. Occupational therapy services provided under that agency's administration and financing must be aligned with the purpose of the agency. For example, services provided in public education settings enable children to benefit from educational opportunities. Therefore, in the school setting it is only appropriate to address the concerns identified through assessment when those concerns negatively impact the child's participation in education. Areas of concern that do not influence a child's educational performance are addressed by other community agencies or resources.

Each occupational therapist has professional goals, with professional knowledge and application skills underlying these desired outcomes. It is important for therapists to define these goals clearly for themselves so that they choose professional activities that enhance goal attainment. Employment choices play a major role in either enhancing or blocking professional goal attainment, with the best outcomes occurring when the mission of the employing agency and one's professional goals are aligned.

Agency purposes often require professionals to play a variety of roles and have a wide range of responsibilities. For example, a role that occupational therapists may be required to play in early intervention programs is that of a case manager or service coordinator for specifically assigned families. Similarly, many therapists employed in school settings may be responsible for coordination of children's therapy services with those being provided by other community agencies or medical facilities. Traditional roles of occupational therapists are expanding as current practices with infants and children change to better reflect current public policy and legislation.

TEAM PROCESSES

All group members contribute to a team's operation (Lacoursiere, 1980). Their personal values, commitment, sense of professional identity, and comfort within the particular system influence the roles each member adopts and the dynamics used within the group.

Effective team communication facilitates members' understanding of their roles and functions (Losen & Losen, 1985). Formal and informal communications that take place during both group meetings and in casual contacts between members are important influences that generate an atmosphere of understanding and commitment toward program planning activities. At times it is difficult for team members with diverse backgrounds to communicate effectively with each other and with parents. Two critical communication strategies are for members to use jargon-free language and to describe behaviors in observable terms; these strategies equalize everyone's understanding and invite all members to participate in the dialogue. Since occupational therapists are trained in group process and communication skills, they can facilitate effective group behavior through their participation.

Some teams function with rotating roles and responsibilities. A teacher, therapist, social worker, or other staff member may lead the team in planning meetings and take responsibility for coordinating the necessary procedures required for the team to develop and implement the program. This approach allows members to experience different responsibilities in planning the child's program, broadening their understanding of various team member roles in the program planning process.

When a team experiences difficulty in working together to plan a child's program, they must assess the source of the problem and make a plan to resolve it. Team function can be impeded by problems with the team's evolution as a group, composition, or group process used (Bailey, 1984). In discussing factors that influence team function, Bennett (1982) has raised the issue of territoriality and "protection of turf" in relation to the increasing specialization in childhood services. This territoriality can occur within a team, across teams, and across agencies in interagency work. It is important for team members to avoid competition, and recognize and respect the varied backgrounds that form the resources for developing the child's service plan. When professionals tap expertise from diverse backgrounds, they can enhance the resulting plan, and members share an ownership and commitment toward the common goals and programs they have developed together (Maher & Bennett, 1984). Inservice training programs can be useful for the team to develop the group process skills, which are essential to effective team planning (Crisler, 1979).

TEAM STRUCTURES

There are several approaches to designing a team structure. Each approach focuses on developing programs to meet the child's need to participate in living. Systems select a particular team planning approach based on legal requirements, program philosophies, traditions, experience, or preference of staff members. **When engaging in best practice, only the interdisciplinary and transdisciplinary structures are compatible with collaboration and family-centered care.**

Multidisciplinary Team

Each professional evaluates the child and determines priorities, goals, and intervention strategies when serving on a multidisciplinary team. These persons do not come together to review initial assessment reports, or summarize the services recommended for the child (Muhlenhaupt, 1991). Their interventions tend to be implemented in isolation from each other (Bailey, 1984). Sparling (1980) describes the multidisciplinary team as one in which disciplines "co-exist". Programs using this model involve a number of persons working with one child. For example, a woman may visit an outpatient clinic for individual occupational and physical therapy sessions. A speech therapist may also visit her home and may be unaware of the occupational and physical therapy goals and intervention plans. For visits to the physician, the therapists might each send a report for the records.

The multidisciplinary model provides therapists and other team members with ample opportunity to plan and implement interventions that reflect their own perspectives and the philosophies of their chosen professions (Muhlenhaupt, 1991). This model is costly, time consuming, and inefficient in certain cases, i.e., when there is overlap between services. Since coordination between plans is not inherent in the model, interventions sometimes contradict each other. For example, the occupational therapist may recommend cursive writing as a strategy to improve a student's writing performance in the classroom (since cursive writing requires less starting and stopping of strokes drawn to form letters). In a multidisciplinary model, if the teacher opposes this plan because it conflicts with the classroom curriculum, the therapist and teacher's work could be at crossed purposes. Parents may feel confused by the various approaches, and receive mixed messages from the conflicting goals among services.

Interdisciplinary Team

An interdisciplinary team is also comprised of professionals from several disciplines. However, the team members of an interdisciplinary team collaborate with each other to interpret their findings and design intervention programs. Sometimes these professionals conduct evaluations together, as in a play-based assessment. They may also conduct separate evaluations. When designing the intervention program, it is typical for more than one discipline to be responsible for goals. For example, the speech pathologist, occupational therapist, and mother may work together to design and implement a feeding and eating program for a toddler. Team members negotiate about what the priorities are, and the intervention plan reflects the consensus of the group.

In a public school the educators frequently are the coordinators for the interdisciplinary activities. The regular and special education teachers might plan classroom goals that reflect the combined knowledge gained from the psychological, social work, educational, occupational, and speech therapy evaluations. The teacher's assistant reinforces the students, using strategies developed by the occupational therapist and special education teacher. Teachers and related service personnel (such as occupational therapists) can incorporate language goals into all daily and weekly routines. The music and art teachers might collaborate with the occupational therapist to incorporate postural control activities into their class sessions (e.g., movement activities, standing to work on projects).

Transdisciplinary Team

Transdisciplinary team members work together throughout assessment, diagnostic, planning, and implementation phases. The unique feature of the transdisciplinary approach is that the team members decide who is the logical person to implement services with the child and family, and that person acts on behalf of the team, representing all disciplines (Conner, et al., 1978; Sparling, 1980). Each discipline contributes information to the team assessment and goal setting process, then one person implements the program and becomes the child's primary provider or "program facilitator" (Sparling, 1980). In some cases, the parent serves in this role with a young infant. The primary service provider reports progress to the team, which meets to review and revise the program plan as appropriate. Team members may observe the primary service provider working with the child to gain additional data (Muhlenhaupt, 1991). Typically, the other professionals provide consultation to the primary provider, but any discipline specialist can provide periodic direct services (Orelove and Sobsey, 1987). The transdisciplinary model facilitates building rapport between parent, child, and service providers, and it is easier to implement consistent programming.

Classroom teachers serving children with physical disabilities frequently serve as the primary provider for the child on a transdisciplinary team. The school's occupational and physical therapists in these situations provide the teaching staff with ongoing training related to handling and positioning children with cerebral palsy during various school activities. They collaborate with each other and with the teachers, developing classroom interventions to facilitate performance during daily classroom activities. Specific interventions might include training in toilet transfer techniques and the use of adaptive equipment for snack and lunch periods. This is an excellent team model for classrooms, since the teachers are there every day and the related service personnel are not. The children's achievement of specific goals is reinforced through consistency and ample experience during activities within the natural school environment and class routine.

The transdisciplinary approach requires administrative support; parent and staff training (Sparling, 1980), which depend upon agency and program philosophies; parent and staff commitment; time; and financial resources. Professionals working within a transdisciplinary team have the opportunity to learn more about the child and about different approaches through the cross-disciplinary sharing that is essential in the model. However, the resulting role blurring (Conner et al., 1978) can be confusing to the new practitioner who is developing a professional role identity.

The transdisciplinary model reduces the staff time required for direct service provision; however, this does not translate to a large reduction in the staffing required. The other team members must be available to consult on cases; if an agency reduces the professional pool, the breadth of knowledge available for programming is reduced, and we do not create optimal programs for children.

Ottenbacher (1983) and Bennett (1982) cite obstacles in implementing this approach, including the fact that professionals continue to be trained in isolation from each other and sometimes have differing philosophical beliefs that are difficult to resolve in a model that requires trust. Some also express concern regarding professional liability related to training others to implement specific techniques that require specialized training (Ottenbacher, 1983).

ADDRESSING MANAGEMENT ISSUES

Supervision and Use of Others to Implement Services

Traditionally we think of supervision as the relationship between a worker and a boss. In practice with children and families, other patterns of supervision are more common. Occupational therapists who serve children and families engage in supervision when they oversee or guide activities that others implement with children for a therapeutic benefit. This can include the therapist supervising parents who are carrying out a feeding program, a teachers' assistant facilitating a toileting routine, a teacher supporting a cognitive development routine, or a job coach providing social supports for a young adult to stock shelves with coworkers. In these relationships, the occupational therapist is responsible for designing the programs (including collaborating as appropriate), training the direct service provider, checking the service provider's skill to carry out the program providing guidance about precautions, creating a documentation process, and constructing ongoing contact and feedback mechanisms. It is important for the occupational therapist to recognize overall accountability for these programs and their outcomes.

When occupational therapists supervise others to carry out programs, we extend our impact on the child's performance in daily life. Occupational therapists can never spend the time with the children themselves to provide enough practice; our time needs to be spent *designing* programs and *evaluating* progress. Service extenders imbed the therapeutic expertise into the daily routines.

More formal supervisory relationships can occur with paraprofessionals, COTAs, and less senior occupational therapists who are employed to support occupational therapy services, with COTA's and with less senior occupational therapists. The AOTA (1994) outlines three levels of supervision for these relationships. *Close supervision* means that the supervisor and supervisee have daily on-site, in sight contact. *Routine supervision* means that individuals have regular contact (by phone, email, fax) and meet together at least every 2 weeks. For these two types of supervision, there is an intention to provide developmental support and guidance for the evolving colleague (i.e., supervisee) in addition to establishing job competence. *General supervision* means that the individuals meet at least monthly, with access as needed at other times. This form of supervision is typically reserved for more advanced professionals who can anticipate the type of guidance they need.

Entry-level occupational therapists will be in close and routine supervision relationships moving toward general supervision as the therapist gains experience. In systems that serve children and families, occupational therapists are likely to have supervisors from other disciplines. Supervisors from other disciplines can provide mentoring and guidance related to collaborative practice and system level knowledge and functions. Entry-level therapists in these situations may design a strategy for obtaining occupational therapy mentoring during their initial years of practice to enhance their professional identification and development. Therapists can do this in a variety of ways. They can contract through their agency for time and resources to engage with a more experienced therapist, they can participate in study groups in the community, they can take graduate courses to provide a forum for formal learning and dialogue, or they can participate in data collection for research.

Determination of Workload

A critical aspect of best practice service provision is the determination of an appropriate workload. When there are too many children on a therapist's workload it interferes with effective service provision, because there is not sufficient time to give proper attention to individual needs. Therapists establish workloads that acknowledge the variety of tasks that are required within the service provision process and provide a mechanism for interacting with significant individuals such as family members, other team members, referral sources, and administrators.

There are three task categories when determining workload. The first category includes the non-service provision tasks, such as travel, lunch, and supervisory responsibilities. Novices need to include some time for mentoring/supervision for themselves to learn the system expectations and obtain guidance for the work. Calculate the non-service category by adding the actual time spent in each of these tasks.

The second category is comprised of associated service provision tasks, such as team meetings and assessments. An exact amount of time for these tasks is difficult to determine, due to variance from week to week or by time of year (e.g., more assessments at the beginning or end of the school year for school-based therapists). Estimate an average amount of time spent per week across the whole year. Add the non-service and the associated service tasks time together, and subtract the total from the total time available in the workweek.

i.e.:   Total time available per week: 40 hours
          – Total of categories one and two: (4 + 6 = 10 hours)
          = Time available for service provision: 30 hours

This third category is comprised of actual service provision tasks. Service provision includes both the time spent with the individual and the time needed to prepare for the intervention and document those interactions properly. Remember, your services are not complete until you have documented them in service to the child, the team, and the family. Documentation provides a written record of the actions taken and decisions made on behalf of the individual. Chapter 8 provides an informative discussion about effective documentation strategies.

A reasonable ratio between time spent providing services and time spent preparing and documenting is 80/20, that is, for every 4 minutes of providing service (i.e., direct, monitor or consult), you would set aside one additional minute for preparation and/or documentation. So, if you see a child for 30 minutes, you would add 7.5 minutes into the time allotted for a total of 37.5 minutes (0.625 of an hour). If seeing a child for 60 minutes, you would add 15 minutes, for a total of 1.25 hours.

Using the calculation above, there are 30 hours of time available after removing administrative and associated tasks. With the 80/20 ratio, this means that this therapist has 24 hours available for serving children (using all service models) and 6 hours to be used for preparation and documentation.

It is sometimes difficult for therapists to keep their documentation and preparation time in the schedules. Because we have selected a service profession, we want to make ourselves available to all the children who need support. Professionals must consider this situation very carefully. There is a point at which one's workload is so big that the children are not actually receiving quality occupational therapy services because the therapist is simply too busy to be effective.

When there are more children requiring services than the current therapists can handle, then we must join with administrators to solve the problem. The solution is NOT to take more and more children onto the workload, because the effectiveness of services will diminish. First, all the therapists in a system must examine their service patterns to make sure that they are providing the correct models and approaches for each child. A workload with all direct service models is inappropriate for most public school settings. Therapists typically have a mix of direct service, monitoring, and consultation, which indicates individualized decision-making. Therapists must also look for children who do not need the therapist's support, but who can flourish in the classroom with ideas from the building support team (the occupational therapist might be a member) or an after school community activity (e.g., tumbling, karate, scouts). On behalf of public schools, we must identify those children who cannot profit from their education without our support; these are the only children on our workloads. If all of this has been done, then we must solicit administrators to examine our other tasks to see if other duties can be changed to enable a higher concentration of service provision time. Finally, we can assist in finding additional therapists when there are still children needing services and there is no time available.

Scheduling and Time Management

Efficient scheduling and management of time is one mechanism that allows therapists to adequately address the needs of all children on a workload. Scheduling requires planning to increase efficiency. For example, therapists who schedule children in one classroom for services during a large time block will more efficiently accommodate for scheduling problems, such as student absences, than will the therapist who schedules children for individual time slots (e.g., Campbell, 1987). Scheduling all children receiving services in the same public school in one block of time (e.g., every Monday the therapist goes to Swinney elementary school) is another way of scheduling to manage time more efficiently. Similarly, scheduling home visits for all children in the same area of the city on the same day decreases the amount of time that may be required for travel.

Therapists can also consider creative plans for scheduling intervention with particular children. For example, a more intense direct service and supervised therapy schedule over a shorter period of time may enable a child to become successful more quickly in a regular education placement, than if that same child received those services spread out over the entire school year. Problems concerning scheduling and time management are challenging issues for occupational therapists. Creative solutions that are responsive to the organizational structure of the school or early intervention program are possible when therapists consider all options for service provision and maximally utilize available resource personnel.

Therapists also have the responsibility to keep administration informed about workloads in relation to one's schedule. The administrators need to know and understand the parameters for staffing their services; without information from the service providers, the administrator is at a disadvantage. For example, in a public school district there is a continuous flow of children into and out of services such as occupational therapy. The therapists in the district have the responsibility to find the most efficient ways to serve the children and to keep the administrator informed about their strategies. When therapists are using the most efficient ways (i.e., block scheduling, consultation with other team members, participation in pre-assessment- see Chapter 6) of serving children and their workloads are full, then they must collaborate with the administrator regarding how to handle new referrals and other duties. It is inappropriate for these therapists to continue to add children to their service workload and squeeze out times for planning, documentation, and meetings, because these are vital activities for the quality of services.

Therapists can agree that more children need occupational therapy services without feeling obliged to serve them themselves. The therapists might participate in locating another therapist to hire, they might sit together and review children's programs to see what alternatives they might implement to serve the children differently, or the administrator might have guidance about how to prioritize services. This negotiating process maintains the integrity of the services for the children. When a therapist has too many children to serve, there is a risk that none of them will receive quality services. This can lead administrators and other team members to conclude that occupational therapy is ineffective, and therefore unnecessary.

Use of Equipment and Materials to Enhance Intervention Outcomes

Therapists frequently use special types of equipment and materials to carry out intervention programs. We choose the equipment and materials because of the properties necessary to achieve functional outcomes. There are many cost-effective alternatives available from children's environments, and we always select low technology options first (e.g., use a communication board on the lap tray before purchasing a costly augmentative communication device). For example, equipment that provides an unstable surface to facilitate postural weight shifts may include not only a therapy ball, but also a high density foam block (available through furniture upholsterers), the cage ball from physical education class, or rocker boats and other elementary school gross motor and playground equipment. Skills are more likely to generalize to functional life tasks when the equipment is readily available during the day and week.

RESOURCES TO SUPPORT COMMUNITY PROGRAMS

There are a number of ways that community-based programs for children and families obtain funding to support their operations. Public and private agencies can submit grants from private, local, state, and federal initiatives. Agencies that conduct programs that are part of state and federal mandates receive money from governmental sources. Private agencies also operate with monies donated to them directly or through large campaigns such as the United Way. It is important for service providers, such as occupational therapy personnel, to know how their agencies are supported. This will have some impact on the scope of work for the agency (e.g., a grant will usually be for a specific project), on the types of services offered, and the kind of children that can be served.

The most common places for therapists to work are in early intervention and public school programs. These agencies obtain their operating funding from three primary sources: federal, state, and local funding. The ratio of these sources depends on the state, the population in each school district (called local education agency, or LEA), and the community in that LEA. Federal funding is typically a very small portion of an agencies' budget (est. 3 to 8%). Federal funds are currently available to LEAs based on their special education pupil count; this means that the districts must identify their criteria for all the special education diagnostic categories and submit a list of the children who meet those criteria. The LEA gets a set amount of money for each child, and this resulting pool of money passes from the federal government to the LEA (e.g., $500 per child) to support that LEA to implement the federal law (i.e., IDEA 97, see Chapter 9).

LEAs also have access to Medicaid funding. Several years ago, the schools and state departments of education began to tap Medicaid for some of the related services provided in the schools to children who were eligible for Medicaid. This was a particularly inviting option for more impoverished districts with a large population of children eligible for Medicaid. Some of the early work to obtain this funding was controversial because people disagreed about the appropriateness of providing "medically-related" funding for an "educationally-related" service. There were also some agencies that pressured therapists to "prefer" to include children who were eligible for Medicaid on their workloads (because the agency would have more access to this additional financial support for these children). Therapists also received pressure to provide direct services, because under Medicaid guidelines, only certain professional activities were "covered". However, to obtain Medicaid the therapists had to complete extensive paperwork, which took time away from services needed for children.

These pressures had the potential to erode best practices and the integrity of related services offered by occupational therapists and others. In educationally-related practice, our decisions must be based on what will support a child to benefit from educational experiences; this includes our selection of what service models to offer, as well as which children to serve. Therapists must *never* select (or reject) a child or a service pattern based on criteria other than the child's performance needs in a particular setting.

Agencies and the government have been trying to establish more effective ways to access appropriate Medicaid funding for schools. Paperwork requirements have been streamlined; some states have experimented with submitting "block" requests, listing all the children together rather than each separately. Only time will tell what strategies work best. Therapists must keep apprised of the developments in this aspect of service funding because the impact is greatest in the related service area. Programming decisions must always be separate from these considerations.

Each state designs its own methods for supporting its local agencies. A typical strategy is to provide a set amount of support *not* for the children, but for the personnel that the LEA employs to serve the children. For example, the LEA might get $20,000 for each professional, and $8,000 for each paraprofessional hired to support children in special education programs. For public schools, the Department of Education oversees this work; each state has selected its own particular agency to oversee early intervention (e.g., Department of Health, Department of Mental Health). These resources might account for 40% of the overall budget for a local agency.

The LEA also provides local tax money out of their general budgets to support services for children with special needs. As you can deduce, the monies from state and federal sources do not cover the salary and expenses for quality programming (e.g., it costs more than $20,000 for a teacher or therapist). This portion of an agency's budget can be highly dependent on the socioeconomic status of the area, with wealthier areas receiving more resources and more impoverished areas receiving very little local support. However, it is also important to remember that there are different pressures in different environments as well. In a wealthier district, there might be more pressure to provide other services and programs that would compete with special education for the resources (e.g., video conferencing, tennis program, intensive computer supports, debate, and academic scholar programs). All of this is part of the LEAs responsibility to serve a diverse population.

In the next decade there are likely to be very different patterns of funding for community programs for children. With the emphasis to include children with disabilities in every day life also comes a call to make funding "non-categorical", that is, that schools will get funded without amounts being based on children's disabilities or teachers' and therapists' credentials. This would mean that an LEA would have one pot of money for all services and programming for the entire district, and not have monies earmarked for special education. The positive aspect of this funding style is that it "normalizes" the view of all children. The negative aspect of this style is that it could reduce the protections for children with disabilities to receive the service supports they need. Occupational therapists must be active members of their agencies and communities so they can participate in these decisions on behalf of the children and families.

REFERENCES

AOTA. (1994). Guide for supervision of occupational therapy personnel. *American Journal of Occupational Therapy, 48,* 1045-1048.

Bailey, D. (1984). A triaxial model of the interdisciplinary team and group process. *Exceptional Children, 51*(1), 17-25.

Bennett, F. (1982). The pediatrician and the interdisciplinary process. *Exceptional Children, 48*(4), 306-314.

Campbell, P. (1987). The integrated programming team: An approach for coordinating professionals of various disciplines in programs for students with severe and multiple handicaps. *Journal of the Association for the Severely Handicapped, 12*(2), 107-116.

Conner, F., Williamson, G., & Siep, J. (1978). *Program guide for infants and toddlers with neuromotor and other developmental disabilities.* New York, NY: Teachers College Press.

Crisler, J. (1979). Utilization of a team approach in implementing Public Law 94-142. *Journal of Research and Development in Education, 12*(4), 101-108.

Lacoursiere, R. (1980). *The life cycle of groups.* New York, NY: Human Sciences Press.

Losen, S., & Losen, J. (1985). *The special education team.* Boston, MA: Allyn and Bacon, Inc.

Maher, C., & Bennett, R. (1984). *Planning and evaluating special education services.* Englewood, NJ: Prentice-Hall, Inc.

Muhlenhaupt, M. (1991). Components of the program planning process. In W. Dunn (Ed.), *Pediatric occupational therapy: Facilitating effective service provision* (pp. 125-135). Thorofare, NJ: SLACK Incorporated.

Orelove, F., & Sobsey, D. (1987). *Educating children with multiple disabilities – A transdisciplinary approach.* Baltimore, MD: Paul H. Brookes, Publishers.

Ottenbacher, K. (1983). Transdisciplinary service delivery in the school environment: Some limitations. *Physical and Occupational Therapy in Pediatrics, 3*(4), 9-16.

Sparling, J. (1980). The transdisciplinary approach with the developmentally delayed child. *Physical and Occupational Therapy in Pediatrics, 1*(2), 3-16.

3

Clinical Reasoning for Best Practice Services for Children and Families

Winnie Dunn, PhD, OTR, FAOTA

Clinical reasoning is a critical skill in artful implementation of practice. Clinical reasoning is a process that professionals use to tap knowledge, organize observations, plan and implement interventions, and reflect on what is happening to revise plans and possibilities for the future. A unique feature of clinical reasoning as a content area is that its focus is on the therapist: what the therapist observes, experiences, understands, and interprets. Most other knowledge and skills a therapist must acquire have a focus on children, their families, other professionals, the environments, and tasks of interest in performance. Therefore we might characterize clinical reasoning skills development as contributory to the evolution of "therapeutic use of self" because therapists gain insights about themselves as they reflect on their own reasoning processes.

CLINICAL REASONING CALLS UPON ALL FACETS OF INFORMATION PROCESSING

Sensorimotor

Schell (1998) describes clinical reasoning as a "whole body practice", or the process that therapists use to gather information about a situation. While on the surface, it may appear that the therapist is gathering concrete information from records and initial questions, in reality, skilled therapists take in a wealth of information through their own sensory systems. As part of the clinical reasoning process, these initial opportunities to use one's senses to "understand" the situation creates a baseline for gaining insights and making effective plans (Dunn, 1999).

For example, when a therapist meets a mother and toddler, she might engage in initial social interactions, such as greeting the mother and child, and inquiring about the mother's concerns. Whole body practice means that the therapist is also "recording" how the mother holds the child, whether they have eye contact with each other, and how the child expresses needs to the mother. The therapist might also touch the child to obtain information about muscle tone and listen to the quality of each of their voices (e.g., is the mother's voice strained?). The therapist can also smell whether the child needs diapers changed and hypothesize about the status of overall personal hygiene. **The purpose in gathering this additional information is not to judge this family, but to use it to aid in decisions about what other information might be needed and what supports this family might require.**

Cognitive

Clinical reasoning also activates several aspects of the therapist's cognitive processing (Bridge & Twible, 1997). At a very basic level, the therapist must pay attention, remember, organize thoughts, and match new ideas with previously gained knowledge. Additionally, clinical reasoning requires the therapist to use higher cognitive skills, such as problem-solving, to reconfigure the current problem in relation to potential solutions.

Experienced therapists also use metacognitive processes to evaluate activities and outcomes (Bridge & Twible, 1997; Schell, 1998). **Metacognition is the ability to analyze how you are thinking about something.** When a therapist can think about what she or he has done or planned, the therapist can evaluate the soundness of the action or plan, and ,hopefully, consider alternatives. Metacognition provides the method for bringing in other information, i.e., checking one's data bank (from both experiences and formal learning) and considering it's potential impact on the situation. There is also a time feature, in that one can project possible reactions to or outcomes with particular ideas and can change course if deemed necessary to improve outcomes.

In our example with the mother and toddler, the therapist might draw on her knowledge of development to determine what developmental level the toddler has mastered. The therapist might also demonstrate her attending and remembering by reflecting back on what the mother says as she expresses her concerns and needs. At the metacognitive level, having noticed tension in the mother's face and a strained sound in her voice, the therapist might reflect on the meaning of these observations and consider whether she ought to ask the mother if she is anxious and whether she wants to talk about it. During the metacognitive reflection, the therapist will recognize the possibility that a direct question might make the mother stop talking and perhaps end the interaction, but it might also bring relief to the mother to have the opportunity to discuss her concerns further. The therapist would then consider additional information that would assist in making a good decision about how to proceed.

Remember, this metacognitive process is occurring while the therapist, mother, and toddler continue to participate in their "getting to know you" interaction. Metacognition is a transparent filter that supports the therapist to make meaning out of the interaction while still participating with the mother and child.

ASPECTS OF THE CLINICAL REASONING PROCESS

Many authors have written about the clinical reasoning process (e.g., Schon, D. A., 1983; Schon, D. E., 1987; Mattingly & Fleming, 1994; Schell, 1998; Bridge & Twible, 1997) and each of them organize the components of clinical reasoning a little differently. I believe that for the novice professional embarking on the journey to become an artful practitioner, Schell's conceptualization is most accessible, and therefore I will use her structure to introduce the aspects of clinical reasoning.

Schell (1998) outlines 4 primary aspects of clinical reasoning: scientific reasoning, narrative reasoning, pragmatic reasoning, and ethical reasoning. Each aspect has a unique contribution to make to the therapist's thinking and planning processes, and they all interact to enable more complex problem-solving. In this section, we will discuss the 4 aspects of clinical reasoning, and in the subsequent section we will consider the power of their interactions for becoming an artful therapist. Figure 3.1 contains a list of questions relevant to each aspect of clinical reasoning.

Scientific Reasoning

Scientific reasoning is a logical process of gathering facts and information and linking this information to "what is known", just as one might do when planning an experiment. Scientific reasoning in practice enables therapists to

Primary Clinical Reasoning Concerns			
What are the person's occupational performance concens? What is the person's occupational performance status and potential? What will be done to improve occupational performance? How effective are interventions? When and how should interventions stop?			

Scientific Used to understand the nature of condition	Narrative Used to understand the meaning of condition to person	Pragmatic Used to understand the practical issues affecting clinical action	Ethical Used to choose morally defensible action, given competing interests
What is the nature of the illness, injury, or development problem?	What is this person's life story?	Who referred this person and why?	What are the benefits and risks to the person related to service provision and do the benefits warrant the risks?
What are common disabilities resulting from this condition?	What is the nature of this person as an occupational being?	Who is paying for services, and what are their expectations?	In the face of limited time and resources, what is the fairest way to prioritize care?
What are the typical performance components affected by this condition?	How has the health condition affected the person's life story or ability to continue his or her life story?	What family or caregiver resources are there to support intervention?	
What are typical contextual factors that affect performance?	What occupational activities are most important to this person?	What are the expectations of my supervisor and workplace?	How can I balance the goals of the person receiving services with those of the caregiver, when they don't agree?
What theories and research are available to guide assessment and intervention?	What occupational activities are both meaningful to this person and useful to meet therapy goals?	How much time is there to see this person?	To what degree should I customize documentation of services to improve reimbursement?
What intervention protocols are applicable to this person's condition?		What therapy space and equipment is available? What are my clinical competencies?	What should I do when other members of the treatment team are operating in ways that I feel conflict with the goals of the person receiving services?

Figure 3-1. Aspects and examples of clinical reasoning process. (Reprinted with permission from Schell, B. B. 1998. Clinical reasoning: The basis of practice. In *Willard & Spackman's Occupational Therapy,* 9th ed. pp. 90-99. Philadelphia, PA: Lippincott.)

understand the person's diagnosis or condition, the factors that might be affecting performance, and the possible interventions that are associated with those conditions and factors. Within the scientific reasoning process, therapists must identify and specify the problem (i.e., problem definition) and must decide what interventions are viable for the child and family (i.e., procedural reasoning) (Schell, 1998; Fleming, 1991; Rogers & Holm, 1991).

Problem Definition

Each profession has a particular perspective about the kinds of problems they can consider and address in intervention. For occupational therapists, the focus of the problem must be related to performance in daily life.

We review records and referral concerns and solicit information from family, the child, teachers, and other care providers to determine what the child and others need and want the child to do in daily life. For a very young child, the family might wish for the child to play with toys and assist with dressing in the morning. For a school-aged child, the professionals and family may be focused on schoolwork and socialization. An adolescent may want to participate with others in formal clubs or become a driver. In each example, the problem definition stage includes obtaining information about desired and required performance first. It is only then that the occupational therapist investigates contextual, task, or child features that might be contributing to or creating barriers to the primary focus: *performance in daily life.*

The problem definition process includes a variety of strategies. As discussed above, the therapist reviews records and other information available about the child. During these reviews, the occupational therapist is considering the concerns from an "occupational therapy" perspective. This means that the therapist is considering all the data through a particular set of filters to see what an occupational therapist would hypothesize about the situation. The occupational therapist is drawing from the "occupational therapy" body of knowledge to consider the possibilities. For example, with a referral about poor seatwork performance, occupational therapists consider WHY the child is having difficulty completing the task (e.g., poor attention, lack of cognitive skills to perform the work, busy environment, spaces too small on worksheet). This is the first step in scientific reasoning because it reflects the domain of concern of occupational therapy and demonstrates that the therapist is beginning to develop hypotheses based on background in the profession (including both experience and literature). This step also informs team members and families about the focus of occupational therapy as part of the interdisciplinary process.

Procedural Reasoning

The second aspect of scientific reasoning is procedural reasoning, which is the process that professionals use to reflect on the information available and consider which intervention possibilities are likely to resolve the performance problems. For this step the therapist engages in more formal activities (e.g., conduct interviews, skilled observations or assessments). These procedures are designed to test the original hypotheses with the hope of narrowing the possibilities; when we can focus in on the most precise aspect of the problem we can improve the effectiveness of the intervention planning process. Chapter 6 provides more detailed information about assessment processes.

Procedural reasoning continues as the therapist initiates intervention. With each activity, the therapist gathers more information, either from the child or from the professional or parent who is carrying out the recommendations. Because of an occupational therapist's perspective, he or she expects to have certain things happen as a result of the suggested activity. During procedural reasoning, the therapist discovers whether the expected outcomes occur, and this provides additional information about how to proceed. Chapter 8 discusses the process of "progress monitoring", which enables the team to determine the effectiveness of strategies.

In the previous example, the child was not completing seatwork. In the records, the therapist saw that the child tended to write bigger than other children, and so hypothesized that the child was having difficulty filling in answers on worksheets with a specified space. Acting on this hypothesis, the therapist suggested to the teacher that she enlarge some worksheets on the copy machine to make the spaces twice as big for the student. The therapist also designed a template with a transparency to make it easy for the teacher to evaluate the child's performance on the new worksheets. When checking back with the teacher, the therapist confirmed the hypothesis about size because the child got more answers completed and therefore got a higher score on several worksheets. The teacher continued to be concerned about the quality of letter and number construction, so they moved to that aspect of the seatwork performance next.

Both aspects of scientific reasoning address the factual aspects of the situation; this is necessary but not sufficient information for an artful occupational therapy practice. Narrative reasoning provides a means for considering the lived experience of persons, and not just their technical performance.

Narrative Reasoning

Narrative reasoning is a strategy for understanding the meaning of the experience from the child, family's, and other care provider's perspectives. People use the term "narrative" because this form of reasoning occurs in story form, i.e., the parent, teacher, and/or child tell you about their experience (Mattingly, 1994; Schell, 1998). Factual information from scientific reasoning does not inform us about the meaning of each experience for the persons who are living it. When serving children and families in practice, therapists must obtain narrative information from several sources (including the child and the providers), such as teachers and various family members. This is because in a real sense, all of these persons are receiving services from the therapist. Narrative reasoning enables the therapist to discover how everyone is coping with the situation, and this is critical to child and family practice.

For example, although many people have had experiences with the same child who has attention deficit hyperactivity disorder (ADHD) and all would tell you they care for the child, each of them would describe their experiences differently. Grandmother might find the child's high activity level charming, describing it as an "insatiable curiosity", while the teacher might describe the high activity level as "aggravating" during classroom instruction. Both of these persons are correct; they are describing the same behavior being manifested (i.e., high activity level—scientific reasoning). Narrative reasoning enables the therapist to consider each perspective when planning recommendations for both the grandmother and the teacher. When using narrative reasoning effectively, therapists make multiple plans so each individual experience can be effective and satisfying for everyone.

Narrative reasoning also provides a method for supporting families to imagine a new life path (Mattingly, 1994). Sometimes children's disabilities are so unfamiliar to families that they cannot imagine what will happen next and they have no way of considering a long-term future. In these cases, therapists can provide guidance because we have scientific reasoning to inform us about likely developmental and outcome patterns (from the literature and our experiences with other children with the same disabilities). We do not present our scientific knowledge, but rather use it to guide our narrative process with the family. Therapists first solicit stories from the family about their experience thus far; this often reveals how familiar the family is with the child's current capabilities and limitations. We might also find out if the family has been in touch with other families through church or other support groups, because this is a way for families to gather information for themselves.

Many times the family's awareness of their child's difficulties becomes clearer with the birth of a sibling who surpasses the first child's capabilities; the complicated feelings associated with this circumstance will affect the family's coping strategies. Through storytelling, the therapist can identify which aspects of the story are consoling (e.g., she has such a great temperament compared to her brother), and which are troubling (e.g., her brother is already walking and we still have to carry her, what will happen when we are too old to care for her). This information guides the therapist's clinical reasoning process by revealing what the family sees as strengths to build on and by suggesting an activity for the therapy process (i.e., life planning so the parents can reduce worrying about the future care needs and enjoy the present with their daughter and son).

Pragmatic Reasoning

Pragmatic reasoning is the form of reasoning that enables therapists to incorporate their knowledge about contexts into their decision making. Pragmatic reasoning moves the therapists' thinking beyond the child and family, to consider the features of the performance environment. In some cases environmental features can be enhancing to performance, while in other cases they can interfere or prevent performance. In either case, therapists must be aware of features that might affect outcomes in order to design effective interventions.

When therapists serve children and families in their homes, pragmatic reasoning includes consideration of the family's schedule, the arrangement of furniture and toys in the home, and the foods available during visits. For example, if the mother does not cook and therefore does not keep basic food supplies around, the therapist will have to investigate what eating rituals occur in order to support better feeding and eating skills for the toddler she is visiting. Perhaps the mom and therapist will agree on packaged foods to have on hand, or they will visit the nearby fast food restaurant and conduct their work there. Using pragmatic reasoning in this case means that the therapist recognizes that teaching this mother feeding and eating strategies that one would use when a family sits down to have a meal are not likely to be implemented, and therefore will not help the child and mother at all. Offering strategies that can actually be part of this family's mealtime experiences is more likely to be repeated, and therefore impact mealtime.

In public school practice, issues of teacher style and classroom organization become aspects of pragmatic reasoning. Teachers who like to have a clear schedule and expect a very clear set of behaviors from their students need to be dealt with differently than teachers who have a more casual organizational style. The interaction style of the team members affects the way the Individualized Educational Plan (IEP) is constructed, and therefore how the team will construct the intervention plans. For example, if the therapist recognizes that the team typically focuses on basic skills in reading and math, then the therapist can construct his information to make interpretations in relation to reading and math first, and then expand to other areas of concern. Pragmatic reasoning provides a means for anticipating the impact of options on the systems within which we work.

Ethical Reasoning

Ethical reasoning is the process that calls upon the therapist to use all the information gathered from the other aspects of clinical reasoning to decide what *ought* to be done (Schell, 1998). Ethical reasoning requires therapists to stand above the pressures of any particular stakeholder group to determine what is in the person's best interest, considering *all* factors. Other authors discuss the ethics of clinical reasoning in occupational therapy practice (e.g., Neuhaus, 1998; Fondiller, Rosage, & Neuhaus, 1990), and students are better served to use these references for more details.

When serving children and families, a central ethical reasoning issue is the implementation of family-centered care within various service systems (see Chapter 1). There is much discussion in the literature and in practice settings about the concept of family-centered care, which is a philosophy of intervention in which the family's wishes and perspectives are used to guide practice planning and decisions. However, many professionals were educated during a time when discipline expertise directed the decisions about what would happen with a child and family. This makes it difficult to practice family-centered care because these professionals do not have the background or skill development to implement this philosophy in day-to-day practice. Additionally, service systems have procedures in place that make it "less efficient" to take the time to invite the family to frame the problem. As new practitioners, you will have the opportunity to implement family-centered care as a "best practice", but you will face some barriers. Ethical reasoning directs you to identify the barriers and design solutions to ensure that everyone feels heard and included *and* that best practices, such as family-centered care, are implemented.

CLINICAL REASONING REQUIRES INTEGRATION AND FLEXIBILITY

An artful therapist using a best practice approach considers all four aspects of clinical reasoning throughout the therapy relationship. The insights gained from each type of clinical reasoning have an impact on the other aspects of clinical reasoning as well. In fact, some things cannot be understood without combining information from more than one form of reasoning.

For example, scientific reasoning enables the therapist to understand the possible movement restrictions for a child with cerebral palsy. However, the therapist can only understand what this means for the family when she learns that the parents are professional dancers. This enables the therapist to understand the meaning of movement as an essential feature of family life; the therapist can use this family feature to build therapeutic movement strategies into their home routines. By taking advantage of the family's unique skills and interests, the family members can feel important to their child's development and can include their child in more activities.

Situations change as children grow older and gain skills, and different possibilities and expectations emerge. Therapists must be able to modify their plans efficiently based on data suggesting that interventions are not working or based on changing circumstances. The clinical reasoning process provides a way to be responsive and to keep the therapy relationship relevant to the child and family's lives.

Clinical Reasoning Develops Over Time

Those entering practice in a profession watch expert practitioners in awe; they cannot imagine how the expert therapist figures out so many things in so little time. What the novice is experiencing is the contrast between beginning the process of learning clinical reasoning and mature, evolved clinical reasoning skills.

Novices are more likely to depend on rules and specific skills to guide practice (Schell, 1998). Because the novice is just trying out new information from theories and initial practice, the novice therapist is less likely to notice contextual cues, reducing the possibility of being quickly adaptable to subtle changes. The novice uses each aspect of clinical reasoning in a more narrow way; for example, conversation (i.e., narrative reasoning) is more likely to be used to establish rapport rather than to gather affective information. The novice focuses on the procedural nature of practice to establish the link between knowledge and intervention.

Within the first year, therapists become comfortable with the procedures necessary to practice, so now they can incorporate more cues from the context (e.g., tone of voice, structure of the physical environment, role of siblings and peers in an interaction). Therapists in this stage of development are beginning to establish a repertoire of experiences from which they can draw to make new interpretations. They also begin to understand the relationship between theoretical concepts and the implementation process.

The therapist's scope broadens in the first 5 years of practice, which also enables the therapist to take in more subtle features of each type of clinical reasoning. In time, therapists gain more and more information about practice from their therapeutic relationships and therefore can be more responsive to subtle changes in the child and family's needs. After about 10 years, therapists become more intuitive in their ability to process clinical reasoning information, making subtle changes efficiently and effectively.

This process takes a long time; it is not possible to enter the clinical reasoning process anywhere but at the beginning. I advise novices to find a mentor and develop a relationship with an experienced therapist to make this evolution successfully, and to participate in work or study groups to provide broader perspectives along the way.

REFERENCES

Bridge, C. F., & Twible, R. L. (1997). Clinical reasoning: Informed decision making for practice. In C. Christiansen & C. Baum (Eds.), *Occupational Therapy: Enabling function and well-being* (2nd ed.) (pp.159-177). Thorofare, NJ: SLACK Incorporated.

Dunn, W. (1999). *Sensory profile manual.* San Antonio, TX: The Psychological Corporation.

Fleming, M. H. (1991). The therapist with the three-track mind. *American Journal of Occupational Therapy, 45,* 1007-1015.

Fondiller, E. D., Rosage, L. J., & Neuhaus, B. E. (1990). Values influencing clinical reasoning in occupational therapy: An exploratory study. *Occupational Therapy Journal of Research, 10,* 41-55.

Mattingly, C. (1994). The narrative nature of clinical reasoning. In C. Mattingly & M.H. Fleming (Eds.), *Clinical reasoning: Forms of inquiry in a therapeutic practice* (pp. 239-269). Philadelphia, PA: F.A. Davis.

Mattingly, C., & Fleming, M. H. (1994). *Clinical reasoning: Forms of inquiry in a therapeutic practice.* Philadelphia, PA: F.A. Davis.

Neuhaus, B. E. (1998). Ethical considerations in clinical reasoning: The impact of technology and cost containment. *American Journal of Occupational Therapy, 42,* 288-294.

Rogers, J. C. & Holm, M. B. (1991). Occupational therapy diagnostic reasoning: A component of clinical reasoning. *American Journal of Occupational Therapy, 45,* 1045-1053.

Schell, B. B. (1998). Clinical reasoning: The basis of practice. In *Willard & Spackman's Occupational Therapy* (9th ed.) (pp. 90-99). Philadelphia, PA: Lippincott.

Schon, D. A. (1983). *The reflective practitioner: How professionals think in action.* New York, NY: Basic Books.

Schon, D. E. (1987). *Educating the reflective practitioner.* San Francisco, CA: Jossey-Bass.

4

Using Frames of Reference and Models of Practice to Guide Practice

Winnie Dunn, PhD, OTR, FAOTA

Practice dictates that professionals base their competent reasoning and decision-making on ideas that are consistent with the profession's philosophies. Although much of occupational therapy practice is based on common philosophy, sometimes it is difficult for others to see that consistency in our decision-making. This is most likely to occur when other professional colleagues and families cannot understand the links between what the occupational therapy professional says, writes about, and does.

For example, if the family expresses concern about their child developing friends, and the occupational therapist administers a gross motor assessment, the family might wonder if the therapist was listening. If a teacher discusses a child's inattention, and then sees the therapist spinning the child, the teacher may wonder what "magic therapy" is happening. Therapists have an obligation to not only be relevant, but to act in ways that demonstrate relevance to others.

That is why the various frames of reference in occupational therapy are so useful. They provide a systematic way to consider performance problems, and identify the priorities for intervention to address the problem. When used properly, they provide the therapist with the means to link the referral concern to the possible interfering factors and potential solutions. Therapists must study several frames of reference to appreciate the scope and limitations of each one. Frames of reference provide overarching guidance for professional practice, while models of practice provide more specific guidance for assessment and intervention planning.

OVERARCHING FRAMES OF REFERENCE FOR OCCUPATIONAL THERAPY PRACTICE

For this text, we will discuss three overarching frames of reference as most consistent with community-based models of practice, and most compatible with the philosophy of this book. Each of these conceptual frameworks describes an interactional relationship among persons, the tasks they wish to perform (i.e., occupations, activities), and the places in which they must perform (i.e., environment or context). The emphasis on context for performance makes them well-suited to community-based practice because daily life settings by their nature have constraints and supports within them. Settings ignoring context as a critical variable in per-

Figure 4-1. Person-environment-occupation relationship. (Adapted from Law, M., Cooper, B., Strong, S., Stewart, D. , Rigby, P., & Letts, L. (1996). A person-environment-occupation model: A transactive approach to occupational performance. *Canadian Journal of Occupational Therapy,* 63, 9-23.)

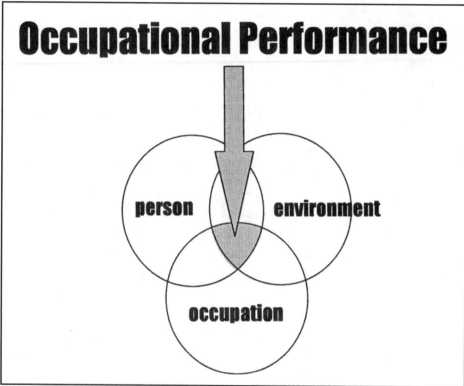

formance outcomes puts decision-making at risk. Therefore, by using one of these overarching frames of reference, occupational therapists ensure that they will consider the performance challenge in a manner consistent with community-based practice.

PERSON-ENVIRONMENT-OCCUPATION CONCEPTUAL FRAMEWORK

The Person-Environment-Occupation model (PEO) illustrates a transactive approach to understanding the person's occupational performance (Law, Cooper, Strong, Steward, Rigby, & Letts, 1996). These authors consider the relationships among the person, the environment, and the occupation dynamic ones, such that changes in one aspect can affect the others and in turn can affect overall occupational performance. Readers are encouraged to read the original work for more in-depth study of this conceptual framework. Figure 4.1 illustrates the proposed relationships among these factors.

In the PEO model, persons are individuals with unique physical, emotional, and spiritual characteristics, and who engage in various life roles such as student, friend, and family member. In this model, a person's values and beliefs affect the life-roles a person might select or feel satisfied with; values, beliefs, and skills might also contribute to group membership and participation as another way to manifest roles, skills, and interests.

The environment includes physical, social, political, economic, institutional, cultural, and situational contexts within which individuals act (Law, Cooper, Stewart, Letts, Rigby, & Strong, 1994). Each of these environments has inherent features that can enable or disable an individual's performance (Law, 1991), and this is the focus of occupational therapy in considering environmental variables. The environment can provide reminders about what to do or what is expected, and then the person interacts with these environmental cues to act in these environments. For example, when a child sees the personal hygiene products on the sink area, they remind the child about what to do (e.g., brush teeth, wash face), and can support the child to be successful in the personal hygiene rituals.

The feature of "occupation" refers to the activities and tasks that persons do to conduct their daily lives. Some occupations fulfill needs to be met, while others reflect the person's interests and desires. These authors characterize occupations as sets of tasks that are grouped in some meaningful way so that the person can carry out life-roles. For example, the role of parenting might be comprised of many tasks, such as feeding, diapering, playing, and nurturing the child.

These scholars characterize "occupational performance" as the transaction between the person, the environment, and the occupation. They state that the parts are inseparable if occupational therapists are to be successful in discovering the nature of the person's performance challenges and setting an effective course of action to improve occupational performance. Their model provides a way for occupational therapists to see that intervening with any of the features (i.e., the person, the environment, the occupation) can affect changes in the overall goal: improved occupational performance.

ECOLOGY OF HUMAN PERFORMANCE CONCEPTUAL FRAMEWORK

The Ecology of Human Performance (EHP) is based on very similar constructs as the PEO frame of reference. The EHP outlines "person", "task", and "context" variables, and states that the interaction among these variables determines one's performance range (Dunn, Brown, & McGuigan, 1994). Table 4.1 contains a listing of the definitions for the EHP framework.

In the EHP framework, the "person" variable is a product of the genetic endowment and the experiences that result in particular sensorimotor, cognitive, and psychosocial abilities and limitations. The "context" variable incorporates the physical (e.g., terrain, furniture), social (e.g., one's friends and family), cultural (e.g., expectations of certain groups) and temporal (e.g., demands related to age or stage of disability) aspects of the environment.

For these authors, "tasks" are objective sets of behaviors, which are generically available to anyone. Individuals select tasks based on their interests, skills, and available contexts; the tasks that fall within the individual's interests and skills and which are supported within a particular context are call the "performance range". Other tasks are available, but outside the performance range (Figure 4.2). When individuals have either limited personal skills or a restricted context, the performance range is narrowed. When occupational therapists provide intervention, they are working to expand the performance range to include more tasks. This can include a number of intervention strategies.

A unique feature of the EHP framework writings is that the authors offer specific therapeutic interventions to meet performance needs (see Dunn, Brown, McClain, & Westman, 1994). These are listed on Table 4.1 with definitions, and we will discuss them in relation to designing services in Chapter 7. The five interventions are: establish/restore (addressing person variable needs for performance), adapt/modify (addressing task and context changes that support performance), alter (finding new contexts for performance), prevent (anticipating performance difficulties and intervening to keep them from interfering with performance), and create (using therapeutic knowledge in the best interests of a community).

OCCUPATIONAL ADAPTATION CONCEPTUAL FRAMEWORK

The Occupational Adaptation (OA) framework is based on concepts of normal development, with a process-oriented depiction of how persons use occupation and adapt across their lives (Schkade & Schultz, 1992). This conceptual framework provides explicit explanations about the generic constructs that undergird occupational therapy.

These scholars discuss the person, the occupational environment, and the interaction among them as the elements of their model. The person has sensorimotor, cognitive, and psychosocial systems to support per-

Table 4-1.

Ecology of Human Performance: Definitions

Person: An individual with a unique configuration of abilities, experiences, and sensorimotor, cognitive, and psychosocial skills.
A. Persons are unique and complex and therefore precise predictability about their performance is impossible.
B. The meaning a person attaches to task and contextual variables strongly influences performance.

Task: An objective set of behaviors necessary to accomplish a goal.
A. An infinite variety of tasks exists around every person.
B. Constellations of tasks form a person's roles.

Performance: Performance is both the process and the result of the person interacting with context to engage in tasks.
A. The performance range is determined by the interaction between the person and the context.
B. Performance in natural contexts is different than performance in contrived contexts (ecological validity).

Context: The AOTA Uniform Terminology (3rd ed.) definition for context is as follows:
Temporal Aspects (Note: Although temporal aspects are determined by the person, they become contextual due to the social and cultural meaning attached to the temporal features):
    1. Chronological: Individual's age.
    2. Developmental: Stage or phase of maturation.
    3. Life cycle: Place in important life phases, such as career cycle, parenting cycle, educational process.
    4. Health status: Place in continuum of disability, such as acuteness of injury, chronicity of disability, or terminal nature of illness.

Environment:
    1. Physical: Nonhuman aspects of context (includes the natural terrain, buildings, furniture, objects, tools, and devices).
    2. Social: Availability and expectations of significant individuals, such as spouses, friends, and caregivers (also includes larger social groups which are influential in establishing norms, role expectations, and social routines).
    3. Cultural: Customs, beliefs, activity patterns, behavior standards, and expectations accepted by the society of which the individual is a member (i.e., political aspects or laws that shape access to resources and affirm personal rights; opportunities for education, employment, and economic support).

Therapeutic Intervention: Therapeutic intervention is a collaboration between the person/family and the occupational therapist, directed at meeting performance needs.
Therapeutic interventions in occupational therapy are multifaceted and can be designed to accomplish any or all of the following:

Establish/Restore a person's ability to perform in context.
    Therapeutic intervention can **establish** or **restore** a person's abilities to perform in context. This emphasis is on identifying the person's skills and barriers to performance and designing interventions that improve the person's skills or experiences.

Adapt contextual features and task demands so they support performance in context.
    Therapeutic interventions can **adapt** contextual features and task demands so they are more supportive of the person's performance. In this intervention, the therapist changes aspects of context and/or tasks so performance is more possible. This includes enhancing features to provide cues, or reducing other features to reduce distractibility.

Alter the actual context in which people perform.
    Therapeutic intervention can **alter** the context within which the person performs. This intervention emphasizes selecting a context that enables the person to perform with current skills and abilities. This can include placing the person in a different setting that more closely matches current skills and abilities, rather than changing the present setting to accommodate needs.

Prevent the occurrence or evolution of maladaptive performance in context.
    Therapeutic interventions can **prevent** the occurrence or evolution of barriers to performance in context. Sometimes, therapists can predict that certain negative outcomes are likely without interventions to change the course of events. Therapists can create interventions to change the course of events. Therapists can create interventions that address person, context, and task variables to change the course, thus enabling functional performance to emerge.

Create circumstances that promote more adaptable/complex performance in context.
    Therapeutic interventions can **create** circumstances that promote more adaptable performance in context. This therapeutic intervention does not assume a disability is present or has the potential to interfere with performance. This therapeutic choice focuses on providing enriched contextual and task experiences that will enhance performance.

(Reprinted with permission from Dunn, W., Brown, C., & McGuigan, A. (1994). The ecology of human performance: A framework for considering the effect of context. *American Journal of Occupational Therapy, 48,* 600.)

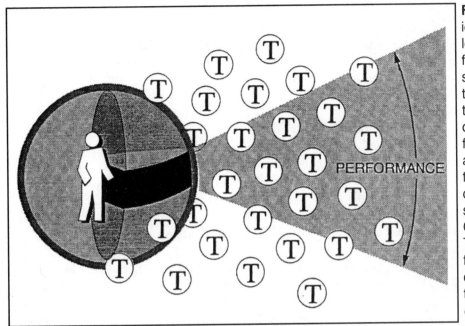

Figure 4-2. Schema of a typical person within the Ecology of Human Performance framework. People use their skills and abilities to "look through" the context at the tasks they need or want to do. People derive meaning from this process. Performance range is the configuration of tasks that people execute. (Reprinted with permission from Dunn, W., Brown, C., & McGuigan, A. (1994). The ecology of human performance: A framework for considering the effect of context. *American Journal of Occupational Therapy, 48,* 600.)

formance. Additionally, issues related to motivation and adaptation are included as a way to link the person's skills with occupational performance.

Occupational environments are the contexts in which persons engage in occupations. Unlike the PEO and EHP frameworks, they organize the environmental variables by the actual places in which persons perform; the other frames of reference discuss more general characteristics of environments, such as "physical" and "social" features. These authors also identify a "demand for mastery" feature in the occupational environment, which creates the link to the motivation, or "desire for mastery" from the person.

They have also described "occupations" more explicitly. As with the other frames of reference included in this discussion, they describe work, play, leisure, and self-maintenance as the performance areas of interest. However, they go on to discuss three properties of occupations: active participation, meaning, and a product (Law, Cooper, Strong, Stewart, Rigby, Letts, 1997). It is helpful that they included these properties because their inclusion points out the importance of individuals as the "directors" of their own life, and therefore a critical source of information when making practice decisions.

An intriguing concept that the OA framework emphasizes is the process of occupational adaptation. When persons are faced with "occupational challenges", which can be generated from their own desires to perform or from cues in the environment, they must either demonstrate competence in participating or identifying adaptive strategies to enable performance. Individuals are considered "competent" when they are able to generate adaptations to support their occupational performance, evaluate the effectiveness of the adaptation, and when successful, integrate the adaptation into their performance schemas for the future.

These ideas about OA form the basis for constructing the interventions. Individuals who require occupational therapy are experiencing occupational performance challenges; the focus of intervention is to improve the internal adaptation process. Therapists can manipulate environmental variables and the person's skills, with the emphasis on satisfying active participation.

For example, if working with an adolescent who had difficulty with time management, the therapist would first identify the meaningful parts of the student's schedule and how those parts of the schedule are managed in comparison to the troublesome parts of the schedule. This would provide information about the current adaptive strategies that are successful, and which are ineffective. Within this information, the therapist might also identify person and environmental factors that are contributing to the occupational challenge. The therapist can then interpret the information in light of the student's adaptive and maladaptive strategies and can design interventions to enhance person and environmental elements that support more adaptive performance overall. Perhaps the student uses a list-making strategy that he learned in a business class, but has difficulty prioritizing the lists. The therapist and student might have a weekly planning session for several weeks in which they add deadlines, anticipated length of task, and level of interest to the list, and then together prioritize based on this additional information. Then the student can evaluate the effectiveness of the extra information and begin to integrate useful parts into future plans.

SUMMARY

There are a number of frames of reference to guide occupational therapy practice, and we have reviewed three contemporary frameworks here. As you can see, these three have many things in common: they all discuss the importance of the person, the environment, and occupational performance. They all have some way to characterize the interaction among these key variables as a means to understand performance and difficulties with performance. Each framework has some unique features as well, primarily in the way that the authors create an emphasis for intervention planning.

So what is a budding occupational therapy professional to do with all of this information? It can certainly be confusing to have many authors go on and on about what seems to be the same issues. First, by studying all of these frames of reference, you might derive the core concepts of the profession, e.g., that a person's performance in context is important to occupational therapy practice. Part of how any profession explicates its discipline's contribution is through "trying out" ways to characterize the ideas and the practice.

Secondly, by studying these frameworks you are participating in the evolution of thought in the profession. Just as different groups of authors have spent time discussing core concepts for the profession and have presented them with their scholarly writings, so must you think about core concepts of the profession and formulate an infrastructure for your own thinking. These authors are reflecting for you the various ways that we might all think about the core concepts of occupational therapy. You and your classmates think a little differently from each other, and scholars do the same. As your mentors we recognize that one of the frameworks will be easier for each of you to understand and is organized more consistently with your thinking style. It will be important to have a conceptual framework imbedded in your thinking as a way to ensure that your decisions are **occupational therapy** decisions and not good ideas that are outside the practice domain of occupational therapy.

Additionally, from this treasure chest of ways to characterize the core concepts of the profession come insights for all of us. Since each framework emphasizes one area a bit differently, or even raises an issue that the others do not, we all have the opportunity to think about that concept. If we only had one perspective, some salient issue would not be raised at all. These points of similarity and difference then must be tested in scholarly work and in practice, so that the ideas can evolve even more.

MODELS OF PRACTICE TO SUPPORT THE INTERVENTION PROCESS

While the overarching frames of reference provide a mechanism for transmitting the general philosophy of occupational therapy, they cannot provide specific guidance for intervention planning. There are other conceptual models that focus the therapist's thinking on what might be supporting or interfering with performance. For example, using an EHP framework, the therapist might determine that contextual features are interfering with seatwork completion. But without additional ways to understand the performance difficulty, the therapist would be offering a litany of suggestions without focus or specificity. The more focused conceptual models provide the means to specify aspects of the context that are interfering, thus narrowing the potentially successful intervention options.

In this section, we will introduce the basic concepts of the eight most frequently used conceptual models in child and family practice. There are many other sources for more detailed information about these models (see References at the end of this chapter). The purpose of this section is to summarize salient features of these models of practice for use in community practice settings.

Models of practice provide a perspective about how to think about a problem. Although there is some literature in our profession that suggests that certain models of practice apply to certain diagnoses, I believe that this is an incorrect application of this knowledge. Occupational therapists develop knowledge and learn about diagnoses so we can understand the person's condition and possible risks associated with the condition. Occupational therapists focus on performance in daily life, and at this level the diagnosis or condition is information for scientific reasoning and is less relevant to intervention planning. What takes on more importance for occupational therapy is the impact of the condition on this person and their family's lives. **We do not provide intervention to change the disease or disorder itself** (e.g., children will continue to have cerebral palsy during and after occupational therapy intervention); **occupational therapy provides intervention to make life more satisfying.** Satisfaction can occur with increased skill, increased ease of access, ability to abandon useless tasks, etc.

Therefore, my perspective here reflects my desire to mentor you to engage in *perspective-taking* through these models of practice. What options do you have to offer if you use one practice model or another? What might you be missing if you neglect to consider one of the models of practice? What practice model(s) might provide insights to broaden your thinking in solving a particular problem? The models of practice have increased utility when used for perspective-taking.

One reason why persons tend to limit the use of models of practice is related to the evidence available to guide practice. For some of the models of practice, research indicating usefulness is limited to certain groups; we cannot always generalize findings from one group to another. This cautiousness is necessary for ensuring appropriate use of knowledge. It does not mean that professionals must not use evolving knowledge to guide practice; it only points out the critical need for professionals to record their decisions and the results of their choices more carefully so that data on effectiveness can accumulate (see Chapter 8).

One more word of caution is necessary. It is very seductive in practice to say "I use an eclectic approach to practice". This has been a traditional way that therapists have explained their use of more than one model of practice in their thinking. The difficulty with the idea of using an eclectic approach is that it can interfere with evidence-based practice. Researchers do not typically test an "eclectic" approach; they test methods related to theory, frames of reference, and models of practice in the interest of expanding knowledge. It is important for therapists to develop the kind of thinking that enables them to say "using the _____ model of practice, I would use these specific assessment strategies and suggest these particular interventions".

This does not mean that therapists must limit their thinking to one model of practice with each child; it is always informative to consider a child's performance needs from multiple models of practice (i.e., multiple perspectives). When professionals require themselves to link each of their thoughts and hypotheses to particular "perspectives", then assessment and intervention options become clearer for the professionals and others. This way, professionals are following each line of thinking consistently with a model of practice and this reveals both logical hypotheses for action and evidence for future practice decisions.

THE DEVELOPMENTAL PRACTICE MODEL

The developmental perspective has a pervasive influence on occupational therapy practice with children and families. This practice model provides professionals with background and guidance about what typically evolves in the course of growing up. In many ways, developmental models have formed the gold standard for children's performance. There are many textbooks and assessment tools that provide detailed information about development, and so I will not review this material here.

One of the most valuable aspects of the developmental model is its universality. Every discipline that serves children and families studies the developmental model, and so it provides information that all team members share. With a common set of concepts and language for discussing the child, the team members can communicate their perspectives on shared ground.

I do have a word of caution about the application of the developmental model when serving children who have various disabilities. An incorrect assumption that has grown out of using the developmental perspective as the gold standard for performance is that our goals with children who have disabilities is to facilitate their development to reach these milestones. Many children who have disabilities will never demonstrate the evolution of movement skill that is represented on a developmental continuum. Furthermore, children who have disabilities are likely to have alternate strategies for task accomplishment that are useful for them. We must not interfere with increasing levels of functional performance because the child's patterns "don't look good", or aren't like others. For example, children who have cerebral palsy learn to grasp toys and eating and writing utensils, but their grasping patterns are dominated by spasticity (i.e., they will have a hyperflexed or hyperextended wrist, use a more primitive grasping pattern, and will hold the objects more tightly, providing less opportunity for adjustments). Most of these children will never use a tripod grasp, and it would be inappropriate to interfere with their writing, playing, or eating skill development until they have "better grasp". The developmental model provides a rich backdrop for our considerations of children's performance, and as such is available for perspective-taking and guidance, but not as a way to limit a child's exploration and discovery of unique and successful ways to do things.

THE SENSORY INTEGRATION PRACTICE MODEL

Sensory integration is a practice model developed by A. Jean Ayres and was originally based on her hypotheses about how to apply neuroscience knowledge within her practice with children who had "minimal brain dysfunction" (Ayres, 1972). Sometimes the term "sensory integration" is confusing when discussing these ideas with colleagues from other disciplines because sensory integration is also a term used in neuroscience to describe the generic principle of the brain organizing sensory input.

Neuroscientists describe sensory integration as a neurological process of organizing sensory information from the body and environment (see Kandell, Schwartz, & Jessell, 1997). Dr. Ayres went on to hypothesize about how children use that information to respond appropriately to environmental demands (i.e., the "adaptive response"), and termed this application of knowledge "sensory integration" also.

Authors in occupational therapy describe three basic concepts upon which sensory integration knowledge has been built (Ayres, 1972; Clark, Mailloux, & Parham, 1985; Fisher, Murray, & Bundy, 1991; Kimball, 1999). First, a person's ability to interact with the environment is related to that person's ability to receive and organize sensory input. Second, this organization of sensory input (i.e., sensory integration) provides the foundation for cognitive development and emotional regulation. Third, the sensory experiences that are part of one's daily routines create meaningful links between the input and the adaptive response; this link advances sensory integration and supports cognitive and emotional development.

As stated earlier, the theory of sensory integration was built upon sound neuroscience knowledge. This is important to remember; the foundations for sensory integration are based on well-established features of how the nervous system operates (see Kandel, Schwartz, & Jesell, 1997). Dr. Ayres did not create these features; she built applied science hypotheses on them. So what are these building block neuroscience concepts?

First, *sensory input is necessary for the brain to function.* Many types of studies have shown this to be true, including studies of sensory deprivation in which persons could not tolerate a condition with no input to the brain and studies of infants who fail to thrive without touch and movement. Second, *sensory information gets combined and reorganized as it travels to the cortex.* From the brain stem upward, information from more than one sensory system converges on the same nuclei and is integrated before being sent on to the next systems. Third, *the central nervous system (CNS) has many interdependent circuits* that enable brain areas to share information, but also create a reliance on each other for proper functioning. Fourth, *the nervous system demonstrates plasticity at the cellular, system, and organism level.* Neuroscientists have demonstrated that the brain cells and systems can reform themselves in response to environmental demands and cues in an effort to "survive" and "thrive". Fifth, *for the CNS, learning is represented by changes in cell structure and organization, changes in system connections, and changes in efficiency of operations.* From these facts about brain function out of the neuroscience literature, Dr. Ayres built her hypotheses about the impact of these operations on performance (Ayres, 1972; Clark, Mailloux, & Parham, 1985; Fisher, Bundy & Murray, 1991).

When people interact with their environments and respond to demands, they are receiving sensory input and using it to construct an appropriate response (she called it an adaptive response). The responses themselves generate more sensory input, providing another opportunity for designing an adaptive response. Ayres characterized this generative process as a developmental evolution that enabled the person to acquire increasingly complex adaptive responses, cognitive strategies, and emotional tone.

Another concept Ayres incorporated into her work, and that has become a hallmark of sensory integration, is the concept of inner drive. She combined her knowledge from neuroscience and social science to hypothesize about how people demonstrate their motivation. She proposed that people have an internal incentive to be active and explore their own cognitive, sensorimotor, and psychosocial capacities. She went on to link this concept of inner drive to the generative processes described above, to hypothesize that the actions that occur from inner drive also contribute to increasing neural development and organization and therefore improved sensory integration. Dunn (1991) contributed further to knowledge about the link between CNS motivation and performance by discussing the role of the hypothalamus in integrating sensorimotor and emotional processing for generating adaptive responses.

Dysfunction in the Sensory Integrative Practice Model

Considering the performance challenges in daily life that Dr. Ayres observed in children and adults with brain injury, she hypothesized what might be interfering with their performance using the above concepts. Her early hypotheses have been studied, written about, and refined (see Fisher, Bundy, & Murray, 1991; Baloueff; 1997). Factor analytic studies have revealed patterns of performance that are indicative of specific performance difficulties (Ayres, 1972; Ayres & Marr, 1991; Fisher, Bundy, & Murray, 1991; Kimball, 1993). Generally, the literature currently reflects three clusters of behaviors that authors associate with sensory integrative dysfunction:

Disorders in Sensory Modulation. Individuals who have poor sensory modulation display behaviors in the extremes of responsivity. Over-responsiveness is characterized by noticing every stimulus (e.g., environmental sounds, the texture of clothing), so often that this noticing interferes with the conduct of daily life. We might use words such as "distractible" or "irritable" to describe persons who are overly responsive. Under-responsiveness is characterized by a lack of noticing stimuli, such that the person seems oblivious to what is happening. We might use words such as "spaced out" or "dull" or "slow" to describe persons who are too unresponsive. Some persons tend to be at one extreme or the other, while others demonstrate both extremes at different times. In any case, these conditions represent poor balance of excitation and inhibition in the nervous system (i.e., poor modulation). When a person has poor modulation, it is difficult to be appropriately responsive to environmental demands, and this can interfere with development of adaptive responses, function in daily life, and overall learning capacity.

When a child has poor sensory modulation, the therapeutic process must be consistent with the types of responsiveness the child demonstrates. Therapists, teachers, caregivers, and friends become familiar with the indications of poor modulation and adjust activities to support the child to have a more functional response pattern (i.e., alert enough to notice what is going on and yet not distracted).

Dyspraxia. Individuals who have dyspraxia display difficulty with organizing movements to meet the demands of a task; we believe they have difficulty conceiving of and planning adaptive responses because they are receiving and interpreting sensory information incorrectly or inefficiently. Praxis is a cognitive function of organizing sensory input (particularly tactile) to design an adaptive response; it involves the same centers of the brain that support other cognitive functions, such as communication and problem-solving. Praxis is NOT a motor response (Ayres, 1989), although we observe motor behaviors when we watch children perform. If a child has only a movement problem, skill practice will improve performance very quickly; dyspraxia involves the sensory maps in the brain to organize a plan for responding (Ayres, 1989). With dyspraxia, the therapeutic process must be systematic in addressing the underlying sensory processing issues that are interfering with performance.

There seems to be two types of dyspraxia in children: difficulty in ideation and difficulty in planning (Ayres, 1989). When children have difficulty with ideation this means that they don't demonstrate the ability to generate new ideas for themselves. These children may appear dull or uninterested in a free-play situation; they cannot think of what to do with themselves or the objects in the environment as other children can. We believe that these children are not receiving and storing sensory information to learn about their bodies and the world (either from poor operations of the sensory input mechanisms or from poor ability to receive and store the information), and therefore do not have information to generate responses.

When children have difficulty with planning, they are receiving and storing information, but they have difficulty when they try to construct a plan for responding. These children have ideas; sometimes they will boss others around to get something done, or tell you what needs to be done. They also can evaluate the quality of their own performance because their comparison between the ideas and the outcomes don't match, so they tend to refuse to try after a while. For these children, we believe that the parts of the brain that are responsible for planning our movements are not effective (e.g., the cerebellum, the superior parietal lobe, the association motor cortices). Therapeutic interventions must be designed to encourage exploration while minimizing the opportunities for the child to make errors, because incorrect movements generate incorrect sensory patterns, maladaptive responses, and continued frustration.

Disorder in Vestibular Bilateral Integration. Individuals with poor vestibular bilateral integration display clumsiness, incoordination, and poor postural control. They have difficulty with tasks requiring stability in one part of the body while another body part moves in space, e.g., kicking a ball, reaching for a glass, handwriting, sewing). We believe that these persons are having difficulty processing information from the movement senses (i.e., vestibular and proprioceptive systems) to tell them about their body position in space. It is this lack of body awareness as the body interacts with the environment that seems to interfere with the development of muscle tone, postural control, and ultimately performance.

Therapeutic interventions have several facets. We must provide support for the child to reduce the interference of poor postural control on daily life activities such as sitting in the desk. We can also encourage the child and family to locate recreational options that emphasize bilateral organization such as karate, swimming, and gymnastics. Since most functional tasks require the use of stability and mobility patterns, engaging these children in all types of activities can be very beneficial.

Effectiveness

Of all the models of practice in occupational therapy, sensory integration has received the most attention (Kielhofner, 1992; Ottenbacher, 1991). I believe that this is partly due to the fact that an occupational therapist began this work, and it somehow holds a fascination for all of us. I also believe that as sensory integration ideas have evolved, the knowledge and insights from this practice model have become the most unique gifts we give to families and colleagues (along with our focus on performance in daily life). We share attention with other disciplines on all the other models of practice, but sensory integration has its roots and its evolution in the fabric of occupational therapy. This is a perspective about which others look to us for guidance; occupational therapy influences the evolution of thinking about individuals and about the human experience through our contributions regarding this practice model.

Intervention studies have reported both effective (e.g., Horowitz, Oosterveld, & Adrichem, 1993; Allen, 1997; Lockhart & Law, 1994; Soper & Thorley, 1996; Humphries, Wright, Snider, & McDougall, 1992; Kemmis & Dunn, 1995) and ineffective (e.g., Arendt, MacLean, & Baumeister, 1998) outcomes of sensory integrative therapy. Researchers have demonstrated improvements in eye movement patterns, behavior, level of responsiveness, and motor control. There have been more equivocal findings regarding improvements in school performance.

As stated earlier, colleagues from other disciplines have been critical about the usefulness of sensory integration (e.g., Arendt et al., 1998). As a profession matures, these criticisms are part of the evolution of the discipline's knowledge. When occupational therapy was younger and more obscure, there wasn't enough awareness about our ideas for people to be critical; now that we are having a more central role and impact, other colleagues have the opportunity to critique our work. I encourage you to read some of the articles which debate the utility of sensory integration so you can be prepared to respond and interact without seeming either defensive or naïve (e.g., the series of articles following Arendt et al., 1998, containing occupational therapy responses to criticisms).

Intervention

In the early writings about sensory integration, therapeutic interventions focused on improving sensory processing, praxis and bilateral integration within therapist-child dyadic interactions (Kimball, 1999; Bundy, 1991; Clark, Mailloux, & Parham, 1992). As public school practice, home-based interventions, and family-centered care have become more central to practice with children and families, therapists have recognized that the principles of sensory integration can be used within many daily life routines as a critical part of the therapeutic process (Dunn, 1999). When we remember that the basic principles underlying the sensory integration practice model are solid neuroscience principles, we recognize that the brain is active all the time, not just during "therapy". Therefore, as occupational therapists using a sensory integrative practice model perspective, we must analyze every task for its sensory processing features and opportunities and take advantage of each one. This empowers family members, teachers, and others to support the child in positive ways. Kemmis & Dunn (1995) demonstrated that teachers and therapists could collaborate to solve classroom performance problems using the sensory integration frame of reference.

For example, if a child is so lethargic in the morning that the family is frustrated about getting him to school, we might suspect poor sensory modulation. We can encourage the parents to add more sensory opportunities to the morning routine, such as bending over to tie or close shoes, placing personal hygiene supplies away from the sink to require more moving about, turning on the radio or a fan, and using cologne or air spray in the room. For this same child at school, we might put his books on the floor so he has to bend down to get them throughout the day. Using models of practice to view the possibilities in daily life keeps the link clear between our background knowledge and our central focus on daily life.

THE NEURODEVELOPMENTAL PRACTICE MODEL

The neurodevelopmental practice model (NDT) has evolved from work of medicine, physical therapy, human development, and brain injury literature. The original work evolved out of Karel and Berta Bobath's service to individuals who had brain injury similarly to Dr. Ayres' early work. NDT is a sensorimotor approach that serves to enhance the child's motor and postural capacities so that the child can participate more actively in tasks. This model incorporates attention to the developmental sequence that enables a child to gain mastery over primitive reflexes for purposeful movement and knowledge about how the sensorimotor system receives and interprets input for motor responses (Schoen & Anderson, 1993). There must be a good working knowledge of normal development to apply this practice model, because concepts of abnormal movement are judged in relation to "normal developmental milestones".

Normal development contains core principles related to sensory motor feedback patterns, movement components, and motor sequences (Schoen & Anderson, 1993; Bly, 1991). The *principles of normal development* include the ideas that movement control occurs from head to foot, from the center of the body to the limbs and hands or feet, and from large to small movements. *Sensory motor principles* address the fact that most movements, even reflexive ones, originate based on a sensory stimulus or sensory input. For example, in the rooting reflex, the child turns toward a touch stimulus on the cheek; in the grasping response, the child clutches an object touching the palm. Eventually, the child internalizes this information about the body and movement, and can gain control over the movement; but the sensory input paired with the movement is part of the memory of that movement pattern.

The child develops *components of movement* as building blocks for more complex movements later. The primary principle that guides development of movement components is the interaction between the need for stability and the desire for mobility. NDT and the biomechanical practice model share this concept and emphasis. Stability occurs when complementary muscle groups can contract in synchrony, thereby holding a body area or joints in place. We need stability to "ground" us and to mediate the effects of gravity on our control of body in space. It creates a base of support for movements required for interaction. Mobility occurs as the child attempts to explore and engage in the environment. Mobility requires stability, the ability to shift one's body mass, and the ability to separate movements of the trunk and limbs from the point of stability. For example, a child might establish stability in the shoulders by cocontracting the front and back chest muscles and pulling the clavicle and scapula down so that the child stays upright when reaching out for a cup.

Finally, the child must develop patterns of movement that support more complex interactions. There are movement patterns in each stage of motor development from lying on the ground, to sitting, kneeling, and standing. A key feature of the patterns of movement is the child's ability to engage in many combinations of movement and to demonstrate fluidity, i.e., an ability to move into and out of movement patterns easily. NDT has an assumption that these normal movement patterns are essential to all children's development, even children with movement disorders (i.e., cerebral palsy). From this perspective, competence is compromised when the child develops a reliance on compensatory patterns of movement to accomplish tasks in daily life (Schoen & Anderson, 1999); because normal movement patterns are most efficient, they must be preferred.

Dysfunction in the Neurodevelopmental Practice Model

Because this practice model was developed out of work with persons who had brain injury, it is essential for a therapist to understand abnormal motor development associated with brain injury in order to employ this practice model. Some believe the abnormal movements are the result of poor inhibitory control in the nervous system, while others characterize the difficulty as obstructions in particular sections of the trunk and postural control areas or persistence of primitive reflexes (e.g., Bobath, 1971; Bly, 1980).

From an NDT perspective, children have dysfunction when they do not have control over their own movements. Children can lack control in several ways. A child with very low muscle tone will have poor control because the effects of gravity are so powerful that the child does not have the power to move the body away from gravity. These children have a hard time being upright without supports from equipment or people, and movements can lead to the child falling over (i.e., towards gravity) because there is no stability to support the movement. Children with very high muscle tone (e.g., spasticity) also don't have control over their own movements, but their bodies tend to look "locked up". Any movement attempts move the whole body as a mass (e.g., whole body rolls over when the child was trying to reach for a toy); the child has a great deal of difficulty separating one body part from another for functional movements. Children create compensatory strategies to minimize the effects of these motor impairments. For example, a child with poor head and trunk control may stay curved over in sitting, but push the head and neck out to see others rather than work to obtain cocontraction in the trunk muscles for sitting upright.

Effectiveness

A number of research teams have investigated the effectiveness of NDT with varying results. In earlier work, researchers compared NDT to "no therapy", early intervention, motor learning, and other traditional therapies, with mixed results. Some findings indicated that there were no differences between NDT and other interventions (e.g., Wright & Nicholson, 1973; Scherzer, Mike, & Olson, 1976; Breslin, 1996; Jonsdottir, Fetter, & Kluzik, 1997), some supporting alternative interventions over NDT (e.g., d'Avignon, 1981; Palmer, Shapiro, Wachtel, Allen, Hiller, Harryman, Mosher, Meinert, & Capute, 1988), and one demonstrating the benefit of NDT (Carlsen, 1975). These studies used heterogeneous samples of children in relation to age and severity of disability.

In more recent work, Lilly & Powell (1990) found no differences in dressing skills after either NDT or play interventions with two children who had cerebral palsy. Law, Cadman, Rosenbaum, Walter, Russell, & Dematteo (1991) investigated the effects of upper extremity inhibitory casting and NDT on motor and performance skills, and found that casting and NDT together improved the quality of upper extremity movements and wrist extension in children with cerebral palsy. Additionally, more intensive NDT and NDT alone did not have an effect on these measures; hand function improvements were equivocal. Jonsdottir, Fetter, & Kluzik (1997) compared practice to NDT, and found no differences in head or shoulder displacement; there were some indications that postural alignment measures might show differences with NDT being preferred.

All of the evidence points out the difficulty in deciding the proper focus of measurement in intervention studies. Although we might see changes in motor component movements, we must question the utility of spending the child and family's resources for this type of intervention if those do not translate into functional outcomes. Work needs to be done to investigate possible links between NDT and daily life.

Intervention

The traditional application of the NDT practice model in intervention involves individual interactions between the therapist and the child. In this model, the therapist prepares the child by engaging the child's body in passive movements at first, and then increasingly provides sensory input and task demands to engage the child in more active movements. Patterns of engagement encourage cocontraction for stability with controlled movements of selected body parts as the child interacts with others and objects. Eventually, the child takes over more responsibility for stability and mobility with actions such as propping and other weight-bearing tasks; weight-bearing also provides intense sensory support for the stability (i.e., proprioception and touch pressure). Therapists also take advantage of supportive devices and equipment to reduce the child's load while learning new skills, as we would when using the biomechanical model. Therapists must have a working knowledge of the sensory inputs that facilitate and inhibit muscle activity, a clear picture of developmentally appropriate movement sequences, and specialized skill in the NDT techniques to provide this type of intervention.

This traditional form of providing NDT intervention may or may not be effective in particular circumstances (as summarized above); it is not useful in its traditional form for serving children and families in community settings. At home and in school, the focus is on the child's participation (see Appendix G). The principles of NDT intervention are very useful for other service models that are appropriate for community practice. The methods for reducing the negative effects of tone can be applied to caregiving routines. For example, when a child has high muscle tone, the legs are frequently pushed together in adduction, making it difficult to remove and insert diapers. We can teach parents and other care providers how to increase hip flexion and release this tightness, which enables them to complete diaper changing efficiently. We can also teach some of the handling strategies for carrying the children as care providers transport them throughout the day.

We must be cautious in applying the NDT model of practice; the current evidence does not support its broad use. As best practice therapists, we must convey the equivocal nature of the evidence when discussing options with families. For example, we might say "researchers have found some changes in the trunk when we activate the muscles evenly (i.e., postural activation study of Jonsdottir, Fetter, & Kluzik, 1997), but findings are not consistent, so we will need to collect data on your child to see if it is working with her". We would also need to be prepared with other options if the family does not select this more equivocal option.

THE BIOMECHANICAL PRACTICE MODEL

The biomechanical practice model is based on the application of physics principles to the human body. In applying physical science principles to the human experience as in the study of kinesiology, we make two assumptions. First, motor responses (i.e., the action of the physical object—the body) are based on sensory input that has created maps of the body. Second, there is a predictable pattern of development of the automatic responses that the person will use to move with and against gravity (i.e., postural control) (Colangelo, 1999). Biomechanical perspectives are like physics, in that the movements related to weight, gravity, mass ,etc. are going to be similar to the movements of inanimate objects. When using the biomechanical perspective, we must also consider the cognitive and emotional aspects of the human organism as the object of interest because the person has drives to interact with the world. Predictions about movement outcomes have to be mediated from a purely physics point of view. Just as physics will be different on an object that is imperfect (e.g., a sphere with a flat spot on it), variations in the human organism change the way that the biomechanical properties can manifest themselves.

Gravity is a major focus in the biomechanical practice model. Gravity is a constant force on the human body, and the individual's ability to move about in relation to gravity plays a large part in determining effectiveness. Therefore, there are primary areas of focus when using the biomechanical practice model for perspective-taking (Colangelo, 1999). First, we want to reduce the impact of gravity on the individual's ability to move. We can do this by getting the body aligned in relation to gravity. When the body is aligned, there is an equal pull on all the parts radiating from the center of the body's weight. Alternatively, we can reduce the impact of gravity by enhancing postural reactions; when individuals have better control over posture and position due to better muscle actions, they can reduce the power of gravity to pull them over. Second, we want to improve functional performance and skilled limb, hand, and foot use. We do this by finding ways to reduce the impact of gravity and associated postural reactions so that individuals can concentrate their efforts on skilled performance.

The biomechanical practice model also relies on knowledge from development literature. Colangelo (1999) provides an excellent discussion of the reflexive and motor development issues from the biomechanical perspective; I encourage you to obtain this reference for your files. In normal development, infants move reflexively at first and then gain control over those movements, enabling them to explore the environment in increasingly complex ways. The early reflexes provide predictable experiences for the infant, in which certain sensory stimuli (e.g., head movement and touch on a body surface) yield a consistent motor response (e.g., arm extension and grasping ,respectively). As the child acquires these sensorimotor experiences, the relationship between the sensory and motor maps in the brain begin to form, and the child can gain more control over movements. We also know from developmental literature that reflexes and other automatic responses to movement and gravity evolve in a predictable manner, increasingly supporting the child to move into upright postures against gravity.

Once the child gains control over these basic movements, the child begins a process of developing stability in one body area to support mobility in another body area. For example, when the child is propping the head up with the forearms in prone position, the forearms, trunk, and legs are providing stability so that eventually the child can shift weight to one side and reach with the "free" arm. At each stage of being more upright (e.g., sitting, kneeling, standing), this pattern of creating a stable base for movement occurs. These milestones of movement and control are related to the effects of gravity on the child as an object in the environment. Therefore, using a biomechanical perspective, we must be aware of children's abilities to control their mass in relation to the force of gravity in order to support their development.

Dysfunction in the Biomechanical Practice Model

The musculoskeletal system is the most common target for the biomechanical practice model. We tend to focus on children who have complex physical disabilities in relation to their disorders, such as cerebral palsy and muscular dystrophy. However, it is important to remember that many children do not have control over their postural mechanisms even though they don't have a frank disability, and the biomechanical practice model offers a useful perspective for these children as well.

The key issue that triggers therapists to take a biomechanical perspective is the child's difficulty with stability and mobility. Just as modulation is required to process sensory information in the sensory integration practice model, modulation between stability and mobility for successful performance is critical from the biomechanical perspective. Whenever modulation is the issue, we can conclude that children might have difficulty related to too much, too little, or high variability in their responses. For the biomechanical practice model, this translates into considerations of muscle tone (the building block of postural control and movement) and skeletal alignment.

Muscle tone is the ability of the muscle to contract when needed. Normal muscle tone reflects a balance of excitation and inhibition from the nervous system acting on the muscle. Excitation comes from the reflex arc (i.e., the sensory neuron, interneuron, and motor neuron—see your neuroscience text), inhibition comes from the descending motor neurons that serve that limb or muscle. When children have CNS disorders, such as cerebral palsy, muscle tone can be disrupted, resulting in high muscle tone (i.e., excess tension) or low muscle tone (i.e., lack of activation). This occurs because the balance of power in the system is upset; whenever the balance of power is disrupted, we can see either extreme as a result. In the case of high muscle tone (i.e., spasticity) the reflex arc is "released" from inhibitory control due to disruptions in the brain areas that send the descending motor messages. Without the inhibitory control, the reflex arc continues to generate activity in the muscle, so it contracts more and more often, makes the muscle very tense, and interferes with fluid movement. When tone is very low, we believe that the "release" phenomenon is related to lack of activation of the reflex arc, leading to a very unresponsive muscle. In this case, the inactive muscle makes the limb and joints very mobile and therefore unable to support either stability or active movement for function. It is the lack of control over the musculoskeletal movements that interferes with performance.

When children have more subtle difficulties with body control, we can still see the interference of poor postural stability and mobility in their daily life. These children may hang on furniture and other people for support, may lay on their desks during seatwork, and may tire more easily than children the same age. They may have difficulty learning skills even when motivated, such as riding a bike or climbing on the play equipment at school. The biomechanical practice model can be useful for these children as well, because it offers options for supporting these children's performance.

Effectiveness

Most of the literature related to the biomechanical practice model has addressed the issues of persons with severe and multiple disabilities. These persons are the most challenged by gravity, and their ability to engage in daily life is interfered with or prohibited by this lack of ability to master gravitational influences on movement and stability. Studies have shown that we can increase a person's engagement by adding purpose to repetitive movements (Riccio, Nelson, & Bush, 1990). Sharpe (1992) applied the biomechanical practice model to fabricate orthotic devices and showed that they were effective at reducing stereotypic behaviors and increasing toy contact in children who had Rett's syndrome. Children with severe disabilities perform better when the biomechanical practice model is used to design assistive technology support that provides multimodal stimuli (Daniels, Sparling, Reilly, & Humphry, 1995). Hainsworth, Harrison, Sheldon, & Roussounis (1997) showed that children with cerebral palsy have better gait and range when they used their lower extremity orthoses.

Studies are typically done with small numbers of participants and tend to use research designs that are more individualized, e.g., that chart the specific performance goals of the study subjects. This is appropriate for documenting changes in those persons, but sometimes it becomes hard to generalize from these small samples to the population at large as one can in a study with many subjects. Be careful to look for similarities and differences between individuals reported in the literature and the individuals you are serving when using this evidence to make practice decisions. You must also have a clear data collection plan to document the effectiveness or ineffectiveness of the intervention.

Intervention

The emphasis for intervention using a biomechanical practice model is to establish a useful relationship with gravity through positioning to support and facilitate functional movements. Therapists can establish useful relationships with gravity in two ways. First, we can engage the child in activities that will facilitate the child to have better postural control. Second, we can supply adaptive equipment and devices that provide external support for parts of the body, thereby reducing the load on the child to meet the constant challenge of gravity. Once the child has a stable relationship with the forces of gravity, it is possible to introduce skilled movements and interactions with the environment, including manipulation with hands, looking at toys and friends, reaching and grasping, and moving about in space.

It is important to gauge the therapeutic emphasis when using a biomechanical perspective. There are times when it is appropriate to emphasize increased postural control by requiring the child to exert personal effort to improve muscle control to hold the body up against gravity. At other times, this type of exertion may yield very little progress overall and exhaust the child, making the child unavailable for other interactions. In these cases, it is more useful to introduce adaptive devices that provide the postural support; the device "erases" the impact of gravity on the child without the child's effort and thereby reserves the child's personal resources for skilled movements that stimulate cognitive and emotional development.

Therapists must consider the cost-benefit analysis of each choice. It is inappropriate to set up situations in which the child has to "earn" the right to participate by improving postural control before participation is made available. Whenever a participation opportunity is available, best practice dictates that occupational therapists provide adaptations to make participation possible; these are not the times for the child to work on postural control. We ask ourselves: "what would I have to introduce here to erase the effects of gravity on this child's body so this child can participate with the others?" For example, we would supply a child who has a severe disability with a wedge when in prone position, so the child can see friends playing on the floor instead of making the child develop head control to see friends. This is one of the best features of the biomechanical practice model; it provides you with explicit information for giving the child access to living. The disability can become "transparent" for a bit of time so the child can learn the enjoyment of engaging in daily life activities.

Think about yourself. If you want to watch a movie with your friends, and your shoulders and neck are sore from a previous workout, you are likely to create a supported sitting spot with pillows, rather than make yourself "work on" these sore muscles while you watch the movie. You do not need to miss your time with your friends when there are ways to make it easy to participate in spite of your current difficulty.

The biomechanical practice model also informs us about how to use gravity to the child's benefit. When we position a child properly in relation to gravity, we can make it easier to generate active movement. For example, when a child is placed in a sidelying position, the child can move the arms along the lines of gravity, making the weight of the arms less troublesome. The ground can support one arm as the child reaches, and the child doesn't have to support the weight of the head to look at the hands as the child makes contact with toys in proximal space. In a prone support, the child's arms can move toward gravity to touch and manipulate objects. When children become more active with objects, they can develop the cognitive and perceptual skills they need for more complex activities.

These principles are also applicable to children with more subtle disabilities. Children who have poor trunk control may be squirmy in their desk chairs, or may fall out of them during class. Changing to a chair with arms and making sure the child's feet are firmly placed on the floor can be enough to support the child in the chair for seatwork. Sometimes turning a chair backwards so the child can lean on the backrest while working is enough support for successful school performance. To apply the biomechanical practice model during daily life, always think, "if I changed this child's relationship to gravity or reduced the power of gravity by supporting body parts, would performance improve?"

MOTOR CONTROL AND MOTOR LEARNING MODELS

The motor control and motor learning literature contains more contemporary views of movement acquisition. Shumway-Cook & Woollacott (1995) define motor control as "the study of the nature and cause of movement" (p. 3), and motor learning as "the study of the acquisition and or modification of movement" (p. 23). We might also view these areas of study as the basic science of movement (i.e., motor control) and the applied science of movement (i.e., motor learning).

There are many theories guiding knowledge development about motor control. Earlier theories of motor control focused on reflexive and hierarchical structures within the CNS (see Sherrington, 1947; Magnus, 1926; Weisz, 1938), while more recent theories have incorporated more complex hypotheses about the CNS (e.g., van Sant, 1987; Forssberg, Grillner, & Rossignol, 1975; Bernstein, 1967), models of action separate from the CNS in particular (e.g., Thelen, Kelso, & Fogel, 1987; Kugler & Turvey, 1987; Schmidt, 1988), and considerations of task and environmental influences (e.g., Greene, 1972; Gibson, 1966; Woollacott & Shumway-Cook, 1990). As with all emerging theoretical knowledge, each of the scholars have contributed particular information to our understanding of motor control mechanisms. As therapists, the information from the motor control literature provides us with scientific reasoning knowledge for our decision making; the more we understand the underlying mechanisms that support or create barriers to performance, the better our intervention planning options can be.

Complex concepts require many perspectives. Researchers in motor control are looking at an integrated model that acknowledges the need to understand the CNS, the mechanisms for actions, and the person-task-environment interface (Shumway-Cook & Woollacott, 1995). With this integrated view, it becomes necessary for motor control researchers to consider cognitive, sensorimotor, and ecological factors in their quest to fully understand motor control mechanisms. It is interesting that although this area of research has evolved from other disciplines, these researchers have also determined that they need to understand person-task-environment interactions to make progress in knowledge development.

The motor learning literature concerns itself with acquisition, practice, generalization, and adaptation of movements for action. There are four concepts that underlie the motor learning literature (Schmidt, 1988): learning is a process of acquiring skills, learning emerges from practice and experience, we surmise what learning has occurred from the behaviors we observe, and learning by its nature produces relatively permanent changes.

There are also several theories guiding the motor learning knowledge development. Some of the earlier theories emphasized the sensorimotor feedback loop and motor programs as the core building block to support motor learning (e.g., Adams, 1971; Schmidt, 1988); in these models the motor programs got stronger with practice. Newell (1991) proposes that persons must increase the coordinated efforts between perceptual information and one's actions to have motor learning occur. Newell also considers the task and context as factors that have an impact on motor learning. All of the motor learning theories address the hypothesized processes for persons to acquire skills; this is in contrast to the motor control theories that concerned themselves with the actual mechanisms that support movement. The motor learning literature is more directly applicable to practice decision-making.

Dysfunction in the Motor Learning Practice Model

Within the motor learning literature, some authors define dysfunction in relation to the skills the person cannot perform successfully (Kaplan & Bedell, 1999). Additionally, authors consider the aspects of learning that seem to be supporting or interfering with function (Shumway-Cook & Woollacott, 1995). Those who consider a more global view of the dysfunction will also look at task and environmental variables to see what might be interfering with the person's ability to learn; this information is very helpful for intervention planning (Held, 1987). For example, age is an important variable in recovery of task performance; there is a complex interaction between CNS areas and age, with some being vulnerable or invulnerable at different ages from infancy to adulthood (Shumway-Cook & Woollacott, 1995). The environmental variable of training conditions interacts with the state of the system (i.e., the CNS) to affect dysfunction and recovery. Dysfunction seems to be less with training that is more immediate to the injury and when there are forced-use conditions (i.e., we make the person use the more involved limbs to function) (Held, 1987).

Effectiveness

The research in motor learning has informed us about effective (and ineffective) ways to support people to learn. One critical factor to motor learning is feedback, which can be from internal mechanisms (i.e., body sensations) or from external sources (i.e., from the environment, including from other persons). Bilodeau, Bilodeau, & Schumsky (1959) showed that it is important to know the effectiveness of movement in order to learn. However, it is still unclear what parameters we must place on this feedback about the results of performance. For example, experimenters have been unable to identify the optimal time to wait between practice trials, or how long to wait (or not wait) to give the feedback about performance (also called "knowledge of results") (Schmidt, 1988). People also seem to profit most from a summary of their performance, rather than feedback after each trial; Schmidt (1988) hypothesizes that giving feedback after each trial may be too encumbering, and leads the person to rely on external feedback too much. Children and adults profit from feedback that is consistent with their information levels; adults may profit from more precision and detail because they understand the material (e.g., providing information about inches, pounds).

Motor learning researchers have also studied the aspects of practice that make learning more effective. Although people fatigue with repeated practice on a task and get worse when they get tired, this type of practice enables generalization of routine tasks (Schmidt, 1988). People also perform better when they have been able to practice variations of the task (Catalano & Kleiner, 1984), when they practice the whole task rather than isolated parts that are not explicitly part of the functional performance (see Kaplan & Bedell, 1999, for a discussion related to children), and when the practice and performance contexts are similar (Schmidt & Young, 1987). Rawlings, E., Rawlings, I., Chen, & Yilk (1972) showed that when individuals practice mentally, they perform almost as well as those that practice physically. Other studies have suggested (see Singer, 1980; Schmidt, 1988) that we must be careful in our use of guidance for learning; it seems that individuals profit from initial guidance for learning (i.e, physically supporting the movement or verbally directing the movement), but not as a long-term strategy.

There is a rich source of information about practice in the motor learning literature. Although the studies are not about occupational therapy practice, they are very informative regarding how we might construct effective interventions. This is a great place to keep current on reading for future developments.

Intervention

In the motor learning literature, researchers discuss the process of recovery of function. From a strict perspective, recovery means that the person returns to their abilities prior to their injury without any changes in the pattern of performance (Almli & Finger, 1988). Bach-y-Rita & Balliet (1987) discuss the "forced recovery" process in which we specifically design interventions to require movements that we believe are having an impact on reorganizing the neural mechanisms that support motor movements. These perspectives reflect the idea of "fixing" the person; more contemporary views acknowledge the person's interactions with the environment as an additional factor in function and recovery (Law, et al., 1997; Christiansen & Baum, 1997). With a broader view, it is possible to consider both restorative strategies and compensatory strategies to support motor learning and recovery of function.

The motor learning literature informs us that knowledge of results of performance and practice is important for positive functional outcomes. Practice must be variable to have the most lasting effects, including changing order and demands (Catalano & Kleiner, 1984). When people can practice in a natural setting, they do better than when we create isolated practice opportunities for them; this also facilitates generalization (Winstein, 1991; Winstein & Schmidt, 1990). People also improve with mental practice of movements, not just physical practice (e.g., Rawlings, E. , Rawlings, I., Chen, & Yilk, 1972). We must also balance skill acquisition with skill generalization (Singer, 1980) (i.e., when we make tasks more difficult at first, acquisition will be slower, but generalization might be better). We must also avoid the temptation to give feedback about performance continuously; data suggest that people perform better in the long run when they receive summary feedback (Schmidt, 1988).

THE COPING PRACTICE MODEL

The coping practice model is based on theoretical constructs from child development and psychology (e.g., Compas, 1987; Werner & Smith, 1982). Coping is defined as the "process of making adaptations to meet personal needs and respond to the demands of the environment" (p. 396) (Williamson, Szczepanski, & Zeitlin, 1993). There are two unique features of this practice model: coping addresses the adaptive features of a child's skills regardless of the child's background or type of disability, and coping is best used along with other models of practice (Williamson & Szczepanski, 1999).

Coping is a feature of the adaptive process. As such, coping can only occur as part of the interaction between the child and the context, which includes the persons, objects, and settings for performance. There is a level of stress that accompanies these interactions that stimulates the child to act; children learn coping strategies through these interactions. The stressors can be internal (e.g., anxiety, excitement, interest) or external (e.g., complexity of the physical surroundings, requests or demands for performance, changes in routines), and yet can have the same impact on the effectiveness of the coping strategies. It is through skilled observation and interviews that the therapist can uncover the features of the child, the environment, and the behavioral repertoire that relate to the coping process for the child.

The coping literature contains research about the construct of coping (e.g., Lazarus & Folkman, 1984; Zeitlin, Williamson, & Rosenblatt, 1987), but this work was not designed to address the application of these coping constructs to practice. Williamson, Szczepanski, & Zeitlin (1993) designed a model for applying the coping constructs to support better understanding of coping in children, and therefore make it possible for these ideas to impact practice for children with disabilities. The model proposes four steps in the coping process. The first step involves *determining the meaning of the event for the child* who has internal and external stressors to contend with, some demand for action, and some skills and ideas about how to perform. As we observe these aspects of the event and the child's behavior, we might determine that the event is upsetting, challenging or thrilling (i.e., the meaning or interpretation) for the child.

The second step is to *design an action plan.* This step is dependent upon the child's awareness and the actual availability of internal and external resources to support an action. Younger children tend to be more reactive related to immediate needs (e.g., I am very hungry), while older children can use their cognitive skills and life experiences to consider options for responding. The action plan that is developed is framed by the child's consideration of these resources as possible supports to solve the problem.

The third step in the coping process is to *implement a coping effort.* After developing a plan or options, the child must act. The authors state that the coping effort is focused on one of several intended impacts. The child might select an action that deals with the stressor directly (e.g., asks for help in getting the snack food), manages the emotions created by the stressor event (e.g., moves away from the kitchen to stop the frustration of not getting the snack food), or changes the associated physical tension (e.g., begins to play a tumbling activity to enable the body to "regroup"). Whatever actions the child takes, there will be corresponding internal feedback from the movements and external feedback from the impact of the action on the environment.

Therefore, the fourth step in the coping process is *evaluating effectiveness of the coping effort.* As stated above, the child receives feedback internally and externally from the coping effort. The child will tend to demonstrate positive behaviors if he or she determines that the intended outcome is reached (e.g., the stressor is reduced), or will demonstrate negative behaviors if the child perceives that the coping effort was unsuccessful (e.g., physical tension remains). When the child interprets the outcome as negative, this triggers another coping cycle. The authors point out that as more coping opportunities occur, the child accumulates information that influences his or her sense of self-efficacy and identity.

It is very important to remember that this model of coping is in relation to the child's perspective about the effectiveness of the coping effort. There are many situations in which the child's and an observing adult's decisions about the effectiveness of the coping effort will be different. A child may be delighted with the exploration of a new activity, while the adult may feel uncomfortable that the child is unable to participate "successfully" (i.e., according to some rule or standard). A child may be overwhelmed by a request deemed to be simple by the adult making the demand.

Dysfunction in the Coping Practice Model

From this practice model's perspective, children have difficulty with coping when there is a bad fit between their skills and resources and the demands of a particular situation. This condition is universal in the sense that every type of disorder or disability has the potential to acquire good or poor coping skills. Therefore, the behaviors that are indicative of dysfunction could be present in any child with mild to severe difficulties from other points of view.

We would identify a child as having coping dysfunction when the child is unable to meet the demands of daily life. This could manifest itself in many ways. A child could simply not be able to get ready for the day, or could demonstrate frustration over the requirements for getting ready (e.g., saying "the toothpaste is too hard to squeeze", or throwing it down). The child could appear active but be ineffectual in the morning routine or could express negativity regarding self or the ability to be successful (e.g., "I can't..."). The child could also demonstrate rigidity in behavior and performance as an indicator of poor coping skills.

Effectiveness

Scholars in related disciplines have studied the features of coping. Researchers have found a relationship between self-concept, academic achievement, and coping skills in children with and without disabilities (DiBuono, 1982; Kennedy, 1984). Zeitlin (1985) reported relationships between coping behaviors and a child's sense of personal mastery. Generally children with disabilities have inferior coping strategies when compared to their peers without disabilities (Lorch, 1981; Yeargan, 1982). Children in poor socioeconomic conditions also demonstrate less success in coping than do their peers with better socioeconomic conditions (Brooks-Gunn & Furstenberg, 1987). In a series of studies conducted by Williamson, Zeitlin, and Szczepanski (1989) and Williamson and Zeitlin (1990), they found consistent differences between infants and toddlers with and without disabilities. They comment that although both groups had wide ranges of performance capabilities, the children with disabilities seemed "...more vulnerable to the stress of daily living" (p. 406). This may be due to having less internal resources (e.g., because of the neuromuscular system working less effectively) or the reduced capacity of external resources due to high caregiving demands (Turnbull, A. & Turnbull, H., 1990).

Other authors have pointed out the critical role that families play in the coping process. Following up with at-risk populations, Zeitlin, Williamson, & Rosenblatt (1987) designed a counseling model to support families with children who had disabilities. They demonstrated success at infusing more adaptable coping strategies into these family constellations.

Intervention

The primary focus for intervention when using a coping practice model is to find the best match between the child's resources and the demands of the environment. When there is a better match, children can be available for learning (just as the biomechanical practice model provides external supports to reduce impact of gravity, enabling the child to interact). There must be a "just right" challenge before the child; when the challenge is too simple, a "stressor" is not created, and the child does not have to call upon coping resources. When the challenge is too great, the child becomes overwhelmed and cannot interact, or interacts inappropriately, creating more stress.

There are three categories of emphasis for intervention using the coping practice model (Williamson, Szczepanski, & Zeitlin, 1993). Other models of practice provide guidance about the many ways that therapists can design changes to support a child's work toward more effective coping.

We can *modify the demands placed on the child*. The environment has many features that can be adjusted to become more consistent with a particular child's abilities. We can remove extra objects that might be distracting or emotionally upsetting, or we can create and demonstrate more simplified directions. The cognitive practice model offers ways to adjust strategies for children with varying cognitive abilities.

Secondly, we can *improve the child's resources for coping*. This can include the child establishing more skills or redesigning the environment to make possibilities more available. The sensory integrative practice model provides guidance about how to enhance a child's sensory processing abilities to be able to notice salient stimuli and screen out other stimuli; both strategies would enhance coping.

Third, we can *ensure the child receives and interprets feedback*. In order for coping to improve, the child must be able to derive meaning from the changes in self and environment that occur with coping efforts. First, we must attend to the child recognizing the feedback, then to interpreting it, and, finally, to generalizing the feedback for new events. The behavioral practice model offers insights about how to create more salience in feedback.

THE BEHAVIORAL PRACTICE MODEL

The behavioral practice model has emerged from social sciences and includes cognitive learning and social interaction theoretical constructs. A core concept in the behavioral perspective is that all behavior is learned; this learning is based on the child's capacities (including developmental level, skill development, cognitive ability), the child's drive to engage or perform, the situation or environment, the demands for learning and performance, and the feedback or support for the behavior or performance (Bruce & Borg, 1987). Like the developmental model, many disciplines study the behavioral model, so this model provides another common ground for understanding children's needs and potential interventions.

The behavioral literature is concerned with learning and what supports learning to occur. From a behavioral point of view, we consider the characteristics of the desired behavior, the stimulus for the desired behavior (sometimes called the "antecedent behavior" or "cue"), and the reinforcement for the desired behavior (sometimes called the "subsequent event"). We want the cue to trigger the desired behavior, and we want to provide a reinforcer just after the desired behavior to encourage this desired behavior to occur more often. We also want to reduce undesirable behaviors or inappropriate uses of the desired behavior; in this case, we ignore the behavior (called "extinguishing") (Bruce & Borg, 1993). Both reinforcing and extinguishing are ways to provide feedback. For example, if the teacher wishes for children to be quiet when she turns off the lights, she would turn the lights off (cue), watch for some children to be quiet (desired behavior) and say "I am so proud of Thomas and Marsha for being quiet when I turn the lights off" (reinforcer), while also ignoring children who continue to talk (extinguishing).

We must be aware of the *features of the cue or stimulus,* and which of these features are salient to the desired behavior. In the above example, the teacher wishes for the lights going off to be the salient cue; however, in order for the lights to go off, she must be standing in a particular location in the room (e.g., by the door where the light switch is located). One arm is probably going to be in an upward bending pattern to reach the switch. If a child focuses in on these features, the child may get quiet every time the teacher goes toward the door, or raises her hand to point, thereby missing the cue of interest to the teacher (i.e., the lights off). Another child may be oblivious to the teacher's behavior and may only get quiet when a peer pokes him or her (the peer notices the correct cues). In this case, the child would begin to pair being quiet with the peer behavior; therefore, if the peer is moved or absent the child's behavior will be inappropriate.

Second, we must *understand what is reinforcing to the person* whose behavior we wish to change. In our classroom example, the teacher is counting on her positive attention to be desirable to the children (and therefore "reinforcing"). For a child that does not care about the teacher's approval, her praise will have no affect on being quiet. If there is a shy child in the room, the child may not wish to be "singled out" by the teacher, and therefore may find ways to avoid this attention. We must take the time to find out what is reinforcing to the person we are serving and construct our reinforcement to meet that person's needs and desires if we want a behavioral approach to improve behavior.

Dysfunction in the Behavioral Practice Model

The behavioral and coping models of practice both consider dysfunction in relation to the person's behavioral repertoire, rather than based on more traditional diagnosis or condition factors. Therefore anyone can be a candidate for the behavioral practice model if they have behaviors that interfere with successful performance, or if they lack needed behaviors to participate. Because of the intimate relationship between behaviors and the context for performance, most applications of the behavioral model will be environmentally specific, i.e., the dysfunctional behavior may only be present in certain environments. Behaviorism is not concerned with the internal or past reasons for a person's dysfunctional behavior; unlike psychoanalytic approaches that might address one's earlier experiences or one's feelings about what is happening. The behavioral practice model considers dysfunction is in relation to the environment, e.g., poor cues for behavior or lack of reinforcement for the precise behavior of interest.

Effectiveness

During the 1970's there was a period of rapid expansion of behavioral practice model ideas. A corresponding number of authors in occupational therapy reported on the effective application of behavioral principles to improve outcomes in persons who have disabilities (e.g., Ford, 1975; Jodrell & Sanson-Fisher, 1975; Leibowitz & Holcer, 1974; Lemke & Mitchell, 1972; Ogburn, Fast, & Tiffany, 1972; Weber, 1978; Wehman & Marchant, 1978). These studies investigated the effectiveness of behavioral applications for work outcomes, learning, play, socialization, and skill development. Stein (1982) provides a review of the application of the behavioral strategies within occupational therapy as well. In recent years, there has been less emphasis on studying the impact of behaviorism within occupational therapy practice, but the application of behaviorism within intervention programming is prevalent (Bruce & Borg, 1993). Behaviorism has grown as a discipline in the last two decades, and much of the current work comes out of behavioral psychology and interdisciplinary research entities. Odom & Karnes (1988) provide an excellent resource for some of the seminal work; if you anticipate working on an interdisciplinary team with a behavioral paradigm, I recommend you become familiar with this and other related work.

Intervention

Behaviorism is concerned with getting rid of behaviors that interfere with successful performance and increasing the number and complexity of behaviors that are functional for the child and family in daily life (Bruce & Borg, 1993). The behavior and coping models of practice share an intervention feature also; both are appropriate models of practice to use as complementary models with other perspectives. This is helpful when we work on interdisciplinary teams. Other team members may be familiar with the behavioral model but not with a more traditional occupational therapy practice model, such as sensory integration. When we can converse in a language that is familiar to our colleagues, we create common ground for more refined intervention planning.

We must *recognize ways to build behavioral schemas*. Many times children do not have the behaviors they need in their repertoire, and so we must find ways to reinforce the child along the way to learning the desired skill. One strategy is to "shape" the behavior; this means that we reinforce behaviors that are approximations of the desired behavior, and systematically increase the preciseness needed for reinforcement. For example, if we want a child to wash her face, we may initially praise her for getting water on her face, then for rubbing over the whole face, and, finally, for using soap in the routine. Another strategy is called "chaining". In this procedure, we recognize the smaller steps in a complex task and construct reinforcers for each part. For young children, it is often best to begin with the last step so the child can feel the sense of accomplishment, and then move to involvement with earlier parts. For example, when learning to tie shoes, children get discouraged by the complexity, and give up before their shoes are tied; when parents have to finish the job, the children have no sense of having participated. If, however, the parent does all the early steps and involves the child in pulling the loops at the end, the reinforcement can be paired with "tying your shoes". The parent then slowly involves the child in earlier steps until the child is doing the whole job alone.

We must also recognize *ways to sustain desirable behaviors*. It is unreasonable to think of constructing a child's life so that the child will receive reinforcement from you each time a task, or portion of a task, is completed. Additionally, with an "every time" reinforcement schedule, the child's behavior can deteriorate very quickly without the reinforcer. Less frequent reinforcement, and unpredictable (i.e., "intermittent") reinforcement schedules actually lead to more sustained behavioral patterns. When a child does not know when he will get a sticker for his homework, he will do it more often than if he knows he will get one every time. Intermittent reinforcement provides a mechanism for the child to internalize the behavior and sense of accomplishment.

THE COGNITIVE PRACTICE MODEL

The cognitive practice model originates from work in psychology, education, medicine, and neuroscience. In all of these fields, professionals have been fascinated with the way the brain is organized and how it receives, interprets, and uses information. There are a number of theories about how the cognitive processes work; they are not so much conflicting with each other as emphasizing different aspects of the evolution and use of cognitive abilities (Bruce & Borg, 1993). From an information processing perspective, the person receives input from sensory channels, processes this information (and stores aspects in memory), and produces a response based on the interpretation. You will notice that this way of describing processing is similar to the way that the sensory integration practice model describes it; this is because both of these models of practice are based in neuroscience. The difference between these models of practice lies in their chosen emphasis of interest, which also leads to different ideas for intervention planning. The information processing perspective leads us toward a consideration of knowledge, memory, problem-solving, and methods of processing, while the sensory integration perspective leads us toward a consideration of the receipt and meaning of sensory events for developing responses. Occupational therapy, psychology, and education are the team disciplines most likely to have studied the cognitive model, and therefore can use this common ground for intervention planning.

Within information processing models, scholars discuss the content of knowledge as *declarative* (facts, concepts, ideas) and *procedural* (processes, actions). Persons use declarative knowledge as content for their procedural knowledge; procedural knowledge advances an interest or cause. When the person faces a problem, the person must call upon the relationships developed among the declarative and procedural information available to organize thinking and identify possible strategies. Each person finds particular strategies more (or less) helpful. For example, some people use post-it notes as a cueing strategy for tasks, while others might find all those "flags" on their work distracting.

As persons gain insight about what works for them, their problem-solving improves because they do not spend effort considering or trying ineffectual approaches. In the last decade, cognitive psychologists termed this process of gaining insights *metacognition*. Metacognition is the ability to think about what you are or have thought about; it is a process of considering your own perspective and deciding about the wisdom of it. The reflective nature of metacognition facilitates growth and enables persons to consider others' points of view. It also enables individuals learning new knowledge and skills to receive explicit guidance about their own learning from a teacher, coach, or therapist.

A complementary perspective on the cognitive practice model is the structural perspective (Bruce & Borg, 1993). You are probably familiar with the work of Jean Piaget; he describes an evolutionary process that supports the development of cognitive skills. He discusses *assimilation* (i.e., the process of taking new information into the current cognitive structures) and *accommodations* (i.e., the process of revising and advancing one's cognitive structures due to increasing awareness of differences and complexities that will not fit into the current way of thinking). Throughout the developmental period, individuals use assimilation and accommodation to incorporate information into their cognitive structures. The developmental nature of this perspective enriches the cognitive practice model application options because it points out the discovery aspects of cognitive development. Bruce & Borg (1993) provides a very good summary of cognitive development.

Dysfunction in the Cognitive Practice Model

Within the cognitive practice model, dysfunction can be related to frank disruption in the brain structures making cognitive centers of the brain inaccessible or inoperative (as with brain injury), more subtle brain dysfunction (e.g., learning disability or attention deficit hyperactivity disorder), or environmental demands that are so great that they surpass the person's ability. Occupational therapy researchers have developed cognitive assessments for adults (e.g., Abreu & Toglia, 1987), but it is more common to have formal cognitive assessments for children from interdisciplinary team members (e.g., measures of intelligence and psychoeducational abilities); therapists can derive insights from these findings. However, as occupational therapists, we identify cognitive dysfunction most frequently as we observe and interact with children in daily life activities. This is vital information for the team because it represents the "operationalizing" of cognitive abilities. Sometimes children can demonstrate isolated cognitive skills, but cannot use those skills when needed. This must be part of the team's information for planning.

For example, the therapist observes an adolescent in home economics class and sees that the student can clean up after cooking but places objects in the wrong places (e.g., puts the cups in the refrigerator, bowls with ingredients with the clean dishes). The therapist might also report that the student can follow single directions, but cannot put them in the right order (e.g., puts the cheese on the griddle and then butters the bread). These observations can shed light on the student's ability to use cognitive abilities in a daily routine. These are applied cognition errors in performance that indicate the adolescent's difficulty with perceptual skills, organization and sequencing—all cognitive processes.

Effectiveness

Studies in occupational therapy intervention indicate that there is a relationship between cognitive capacity and self-care performance in adults who have had a stroke (Bernspang, Viitanen, & Ericksson, 1989; Carter et al., 1988). However, we don't know whether a self-care performance approach or a cognitive approach would be most effective in intervention.

For those of us who work with children and families, the literature has provided us with data validating the relationship between cognitive and perceptual difficulties and various disabilities (Goodgold-Edwards & Cermak, 1990; Menken, Cermak, & Fisher, 1987; O'Brien, Cermak, & Murray, 1988), but there also is a paucity of literature on effectiveness of cognitive interventions. Cognitive effectiveness literature is more commonly found in the education and psychology arenas. Educators are particularly likely to use cognitive models of practice in their styles of teaching along with other models of practice (e.g., behavioral, developmental). For example, Spence (1994) reported that younger children benefit less from cognitive approaches than older children, perhaps due to evolving cognitive ability. A confounding variable in these studies is that cognitive and behavioral strategies are used together, making it difficult to identify the effects of each model to the outcomes (Spence, 1994). Prout, S. & Prout, H. (1998) conducted a meta-analysis of cognitive approaches used in counseling in public schools and found that these interventions were more effective in groups. When combined with behavioral strategies, the best effects were found on the children's reporting of their improved internal state.

Intervention

The cognitive approach to intervention in occupational therapy is multifaceted and based on the premises that the brain is plastic, engagement in occupational performance can enhance brain organization, and adaptations can minimize the effects of cognitive impairments (Kielhofner, 1992). Authors also discuss the need to consider perception, attention, memory, problem-solving, and generalization (e.g., Todd, 1993; Abreu & Toglia, 1987).

Since the occupational therapist's unique contribution to the team is an awareness of performance in daily life, intervention to change the impact of cognitive difficulties on performance is critical (Kielhofner, 1992). The occupational therapist can design adaptations to minimize the effects of cognitive limitations (e.g., placing cues around the bedroom about the morning routine to minimize the effects of memory loss on efficiency), design restorative interventions to improve cognitive abilities (e.g., working on alternating attention in the kitchen by making the person prepare lunch and fold the laundry), or find activities or environments with demands that are more congruent with the person's current cognitive abilities (e.g., working with the teacher to select a better matched reading group). It is our expertise at translating cognitive data about a person into the impact on his or her life that is extremely valuable to families and educators.

REFERENCES

Abreu, B., & Toglia, J. (1987). Cognitive rehabilitation: A model for occupational therapy. *American Journal of Occupational Therapy, 41,* 439.

Adams, J. (1971). A closed loop theory of motor learning. *Journal of Motor Behavior, 3,* 110-150.

Allen, C. (1997). Cognitive disabilities: How to make clinical judgments. In N. Katz (Ed.), *Cognitive rehabilitation: Models for intervention in occupational therapy.* Rockville, MD: American Occupational Therapy Association.

Almli, R., & Finger, S. (1988). Toward a definition of recovery of function. In T. LeVere, R. Almli, & D. Stein (Eds.), *Brain injury and recovery: Theoretical and controversial issues* (pp. 1-4). New York, NY: Plenum Press.

Arendt, R., MacLean, W., & Baumeister, A. (1998). Critique of sensory integration therapy and its application in mental retardation. *American Journal on Mental Retardation, 92,* 401.

Ayres, A. (1972). *Sensory integration and learning disorders.* Los Angeles, CA: Western Psychological Services.

Ayres, J. (1989). *Sensory integration and praxis tests.* Los Angeles, CA: Western Psychological Services.

Ayres, A. & Marr, D. (1991). Sensory integration and praxis tests. In A. Fisher, E. Murray, & A. Bundy (Eds.), *Sensory integration: Theory and practice* (p. 203). Philadelphia, PA: F. A. Davis.

Baloueff, O. (1997). Sensory Integration. In *Willard & Spackman's Occupational Therapy* (9th ed.) (pp. 546-549). Philadelphia, PA: Lippincott.

Bach-y-Rita, P. & Balliet, R. (1987). Recovery from stroke. in P. Duncan & M. Badke (Eds.), Stroke rehabilitation: The recovery of motor control (pp. 79-107). Chicago, IL: Yearbook Medical Publishers.

Bernspang, B., Viitanen, M., & Ericksson, S. (1989). Impairments of perceptual and motor functions: Their influence on self-care ability 4 to 6 years after stroke. *Occupational Therapy Journal of Research, 9,* 27.

Bernstein, N. (1967). *The coordination and regulation of movement.* London, England: Pergamon Press.

Bilodeau, E., Bilodeau, I., & Schumsky, D. (1959). Some effects of introducing and withdrawing knowledge of results early and late in practice. *Journal of Experimental Psychology,* 142-144.

Bly, L. (1980). Abnormal motor development. In D. Slaton (Ed.), *Development of movement in infancy.* Chapel Hill, NC: University of North Carolina at Chapel Hill.

Bly, L. (1991). A historical and current view of the basis of NDT Pediatric. *Physical Therapy, 3,* 131-135.

Bobath, B. (1971). Motor development, its effect on general development and application to the treatment of cerebral palsy. *Physiotherapy, 57,* 526-532.

Breslin, D. (1996). Motor learning theory and the neurodevelopmental treatment approach: A comparative analysis. *Occupational Therapy in Health Care, 10*(1), 25-40.

Brooks-Gunn, J., & Furstenberg, F. (1987). Continuity and change in the context of poverty: Adolescent mothers and their children. In J. Gallagher & C. Ramsey (Eds.), *The malleability of children* (pp. 171-188). Baltimore, MD: Paul H Brookes Publishing.

Bruce, M., & Borg, B. (1987). *Frames of reference in psychosocial occupational therapy.* Thorofare, NJ: SLACK Incorporated.

Bruce, M. & Borg, B. (1993). *Psychosocial occupational therapy: Frames of reference for intervention* (2nd ed.). Thorofare, NJ: SLACK Incorporated.

Bundy, A. (1991). The process of planning and implementing intervention. In A. Fisher, E. Murray, & A. Bundy (Eds.), *Sensory Integration Theory and Practice.* Philadelphia, PA: F.A. Davis Company.

Carlsen, P. (1975). Comparison of two occupational therapy approaches for treating the young cerebral palsied child. *American Journal of Occupational Therapy, 29,* 267-272.

Carter, L., Oliveira, D. O., Duponte, J. & Lynch, S. U. (1988). The relationship of cognitive skills performance to activities of daily living in stroke patients. *American Journal of Occupational Therapy, 42,* 449.

Catalano, J., & Kleiner, B. (1984). Distant transfer and practice variability. *Perceptual and Motor Skills, 58,* 851-856.

Christiansen, C., & Baum, C. (1997) *Occupational therapy: Enabling Function and Well-Being* (2nd ed.) Thorofare, NJ: SLACK Incorporated.

Clark, F., Mailloux, Z., & Parham, D. (1985). Sensory integration and children with learning disabilities. In P. Clark & A. Allen (Eds.), *Occupational therapy for children* (p. 384). St. Louis, MO: C.V. Mosby.

Clark, F., Mailloux, Z., & Parham, D. (1992). Sensory integration and children with learning disabilities. In P. Pratt & A. Allen (Eds.), *Occupational therapy for children* (2nd ed.) (pp. 457-507). St. Louis, MO: C.V. Mosby.

Colangelo, C. (1999). The biomechanical frame of reference. In P. Kramer & J. Hinojosa (Eds.), *Frames of reference for pediatric occupational therapy* (2nd ed.) (pp. 257-322). Baltimore, MD: Williams & Wilkins, Inc.

Compas, B. (1997). Coping with stress during childhood and adolescence. *Psychological Bulletin, 101,* 393-403.

Daniels, L., Sparling, J., Reilly, M., & Humphry, R. (1995). Use of assistive technology with young children with severe and profound disabilities. *Infant Toddler Intervention, 5*(1), 91-112.

d'Avignon, M. (1981). Early physiotherapy ad modum Vojta or Bobath in infants with suspected neuromotor disturbance. *Neuropediatrics, 12*(3), 232-241.

DiBuono, E. (1982). *A comparison of the self-concept and coping skills of learning disabled and non-handicapped pupils in self-contained classes, resource rooms and regular classes [Dissertation].* West Covina, CA: Walden University.

Dunn, W. (1991). Motivation. In C. Royeen (Ed.), *Neuroscience foundations of human performance.* Rockville, MD: AOTA.

Dunn, W., Brown, C., McClain, L., & Westman, K. (1994). Ecology of human performance: A framework for thought and action. In C. B. Royeen (Ed.), *ATOT self study series on occupation.* Bethesda, MD: American Occupational Therapy Association.

Dunn, W., Brown, C., & McGuigan, A. (1994). The ecology of human performance: a framework for thought and action. *American Journal of Occupational Therapy, 48*(7), 595-607.

Dunn, W. (1999). *Sensory profile manual.* San Antonio, TX: The Psychological Corporation.

Fisher, A., Murray, E., & Bundy, A. (1991). *Sensory integration theory and practice.* Philadelphia, PA: F.A. Davis Company.

Ford, A. (1975). *Teaching dressing skills to a severely retarded child.* American Journal of Occupational Therapy, 29(2), 87-92.

Forssberg, H., Grillner, S., & Rossignol, S. (1975). Phase dependent reflex reversal during walking in chronic spinal cats. *Brain Research, 85,* 103-107.

Gibson, J. (1966). *The senses considered as perceptual systems.* Boston, MA: Houghton Mifflin.

Goodgold-Edwards, S., & Cermak, S. (1990). Integrating motor control and motor learning concepts with neuropsychological perspectives on apraxia and developmental dyspraxia. *American Journal of Occupational Therapy, 44,* 431.

Greene, P. (1972). Problems of organization of motor systems. In R. Rosen & F. Snell (Eds.), *Progress in theoretical biology* (pp. 304-338). San Diego, CA: Academic Press.

Hainsworth, F., Harrison, M., Sheldon, T., & Roussounis, S. (1997). A preliminary evaluation of ankle orthoses in the management of children with cerebral palsy. *Developmental Medicine and Child Neurology, 39*(4), 243-247.

Held, J. (1987). Recovery of function after brain damage: theoretical implications for therapeutic intervention. In J. Carr, R. Shepherd, J. Gordon, et al. (Eds.), *Movement sciences: Foundations for physical therapy in rehabilitation* (pp. 155-177). Rockville, MD: Aspen Systems.

Horowitz, L., Oosterveld, W., & Adrichem, R. (1993). Effectiveness of sensory integration therapy on smooth pursuits and organization time in children. *Upadiatrie und Grenzgebiete, 31*(5), 331-344.

Humphries, T., Wright, M., Snider, L., & McDougall, B. (1992). A comparison of the effectiveness of sensory integrative therapy and perceptual-motor training in treating children with learning disabilities. *Journal of Developmental and Behavioral Pediatrics, 13*(1), 31-40.

Jodrell, R., & Sanson-Fisher, R. (1975). Basic concepts of behavior therapy: An experiment involving disturbed adolescent girls. *American Journal of Occupational Therapy, 29*(10), 620-624.

Jonsdottir, J., Fetter, L., & Kluzik, J. (1997). Effects of physical therapy on postural control in children with cerebral palsy. *Pediatric Physical Therapy 9*(2), 68-75.

Kandell, E., Schwartz, J., & Jessell, T. (1997). *Principles of neural science* (3rd ed.). New York, NY: Elsevier.

Kaplan, M., & Bedell, G. (1999). Motor skill acquisition frame of reference. In P. Kramer & J. Hinojosa (Eds.), *Frames of reference for pediatric occupational therapy* (2nd ed.) (pp. 401-430). Baltimore, MD: Williams & Wilkins, Inc.

Kemmis, B. & Dunn, W. (1996). Collaborative consultation: The efficacy of remedial and compensatory interventions in school context. *American Journal of Occupational Therapy, 50*(9), 709-717.

Kennedy, B. (1984). *The relationship of coping behaviors and attribution of success to effort and school achievement of elementary school children* [Dissertation]. Albany, NY: State University of New York.

Kielhofner, G. (1992). *Conceptual Foundations of Occupational Therapy.* Philadelphia, PA: F. A. Davis Company.

Kimball, J. (1999). Sensory integrative frame of reference. In P. Kramer & J. Hinojosa (Eds.), *Frames of reference for pediatric occupational therapy* (2nd ed.) (pp. 169-204). Baltimore, MD: Williams & Wilkins, Inc.

Kugler, P., & Turvey, M. (1987). *Information, natural law, and self-assembly of rhythmic movement.* Hillsdale, NJ : Erlbaum.

Law, M. (1991). The environment: A focus for occupational therapy. *Canadian Journal of Occupational Therapy, 58,* 171-179.

Law, M., Cadman, D., Rosenbaum, P., Walter, S., Russell, D., & Dematteo, C. (1991). Neurodevelopmental therapy and upper extremity inhibitive casing for children with cerebral palsy. *Developmental Medicine and Child Neurology, 33,* 379-387.

Law, M., Cooper, B., Stewart, D., Letts, L., Rigby, P., & Strong, S. (1994). Person-environment relations. *Work 1994,4,* 228-238.

Law, M., Cooper, B., Strong, S., Stewart, D., Rigby, P., & Letts, L. (1997). Theoretical contexts for the practice of occupational therapy. In C. Christiansen & C. Baum (Eds.), *Occupational therapy: Enabling function and well-being* (2nd ed.) (pp. 73-101). Thorofare, NJ: SLACK Incorporated.

Law, M., Cooper, B., Strong, S., Steward, D., Rigby, R., & Letts, L. (1996). The person-environment-occupational model: A transactive approach to occupational performance. *Canadian Journal of Occupational Therapy, 63*(1), 9-23.

Lazarus, R., & Folkman, S. (1984). *Stress, appraisal, and coping.* New York, NY: Springer Publishing.

Leibowitz, J., & Holcer, P. (1974). Building and maintaining self-feeding skills in a retarded child. *American Journal of Occupational Therapy, 28*(9), 545-548.

Lemke, H., & Mitchell, R. (1972). A self-feeding program: Controlling the behavior of a profoundly retarded child. *American Journal of Occupational Therapy, 26*(5), 261-264.

Lilly, A., & Powell, N. (1990). Measuring the effects of neurodevelopmental treatment on the daily living skills of two children with cerebral palsy. *American Journal of Occupational Therapy, 44*(2), 139-145.

Lockhart, J., & Law, M. (1994). The effectiveness of a multisensory writing program for improving cursive writing ability in children with sensorimotor difficulties. *Canadian Journal of Occupational Therapy, 61*(4), 206-214.

Lorch, N. (1981). *Coping behavior in preschool children with cerebral palsy* [Dissertation]. Hempstead, NY: Hofstra University.

Magnus, R. (1926). Some results of studies in the physiology of posture. *Lancet, 2,* 531-585.

Menken, C., Cermak, S., & Fisher, A. (1987). Evaluating the visual-perceptual skills of children with cerebral palsy. *American Journal of Occupational Therapy, 41,* 646.

Newell, K. (1991). Motorskill acquisition. *Annual Review of Psychology, 42,* 213-237.

O'Brien, V., Cermak, S., & Murray, E. (1988). The relationship between visual-perceptual motor abilities and clumsiness in children with and without learning disabilities. *American Journal of Occupational Therapy, 42,* 359.

Odom, S., & Karnes, M. (1988). *Early intervention for infants & children with handicap.* Baltimore, MD: Paul H. Brookes Publishing Co.

Ogburn, K., Fast, D., & Tiffany, D. (1972). The effects of reinforcing working behavior. *American Journal of Occupational Therapy, 26*(1), 32-35.

Ottenbacher, K. (1991). Research in sensory integration: Empirical perceptions and progress. In A. Fisher, E. Murray, & A. Bundy (Eds.), *Sensory integration: Theory and practice.* Philadelphia, PA: F. A. Davis.

Palmer, F., Shapiro, B., Wachtel, R., Allen, M., Hiller, J., Harryman, S., Mosher, B., Meinert, C., & Capute, A. (1988). The effects of physical therapy on cerebral palsy: A controlled trial in infants with spastic diplegia. *New England Journal of Medicine, 318,* 803-808.

Prout, S., & Prout, H. (1998). A meta-analysis of school-based studies of counseling and psychotherapy: An update. *Journal of School Psychology, 36*(2), 121-126.

Rawlings, E., Rawlings, I., Chen, C., & Yilk, M. (1972). The facilitating effects of mental rehearsal in the acquisition of rotary pursuit tracking. *Psychonomic Science, 26,* 71-73.

Riccio, C., Nelson, D., & Bush, M. (1990). Adding purpose to the repetitive exercise of elderly women. *American Journal of Occupational Therapy, 44,* 714.

Scherzer, A., Mike, V., & Olson, J. (1976). Physical therapy as a determinant of changes in the cerebral palsied infant. *Pediatrics, 58,* 47-51.

Schkade, J., & Schultz, S. (1992). Occupational adaptation: Toward a holistic approach for contemporary practice, part 1. *American Journal of Occupational Therapy, 46,* 829-837.

Schmidt, R. (1988). *Motor control and learning* (2nd ed.). Champaign, IL: Human Kinetics.

Schmidt, R., & Young, D. (1987). Augmented kinematic information feedback for skill learning a new research paradigm. *Journal of Motor Behavior, 24*(3), 261-273.

Schoen, S. & Anderson, J. (1993). Neurodevelopmental treatment frame of reference. In P. Kramer & J. Hinojosa (Eds.), *Frames of reference for pediatric occupational therapy* (2nd ed.) (pp. 83-118). Baltimore, MD: Williams & Wilkins, Inc.

Sharpe, K. (1992). Comparative effects of bilateral hand splints and an elbow orthosis on stereotypic hand movements and toy play in two children with Rett's syndrome. *American Journal of Occupational Therapy, 46*(2), 134-140.

Sherrington, C. (1947). *The integrative action of the nervous system* (2nd ed.). New Haven, CT: Yale University Press.

Shumway-Cook, A., & Woollacott, M. (1995). *Motor control: Theory and practical applications.* Baltimore MD: Williams & Wilkins.

Singer, R. (1980). *Motor learning and human performance* (3rd ed.). Macmillan, NY.

Spence, S. (1994). Practitioner review: Cognitive therapy with children and adolescents: From theory to practice. *Journal of Child Psychology and Psychiatry and Allied Disciplines, 35*(7), 1191-1228.

Soper, G., & Thorley, C. (1996). Effectiveness of an occupational therapy program based on sensory integration theory for adults with severe learning disabilities. *British Journal of Occupational Therapy, 59*(10), 475-482.

Stein, F. (1982). A current review of the behavioral frame of reference and its application to occupational therapy. *Occupational Therapy Mental Health, 2*(4) 35-62.

Thelen, E., Kelso, J., & Fogel, A. (1987). Self-organizing systems and infant motor development. *Developmental Review, 7,* 39-65.

Todd, V. (1993). Visual perceptual frame of reference: an information processing approach. In P. Kramer & J. Hinojosa (Eds.), *Frames of reference for pediatric occupational therapy* (pp. 177-232). Baltimore, MD: Williams & Wilkins.

Turnbull, A., & Turnbull, H. (1990). *Families, professionals, and exceptionality: A special partnership* (2nd ed.). Columbus, OH: Merrill Publishing.

Van Sant, A. (1987). Concepts of neural organization and movement. In B. Connolly & P. Montgomery (Eds.), *Therapeutic exercise in developmental disabilities* (pp.1-8). Chattanooga, TN: Chatanooga Corporation.

Weber, N. (1978). Chaining strategies for teaching sequenced motor tasks to mentally retarded adults. *American Journal of Occupational Therapy, 32*(6), 385-389.

Wehman, P., & Marchant, J. (1978). Improving free play skills of severely retarded children. *American Journal of Occupational Therapy, 32*(2), 100-104.

Weisz, S. (1938). Studies in equilibrium reaction. *Journal of Nervous Mental Disorders, 88*, 150-162.

Werner, E., & Smith, R. (1982). *Vulnerable but invincible: A study of resilient children.* New York, NY: McGraw-Hill.

Williamson, G., Zeitlin, S., & Szczepanski, M. (1989). Coping behavior: Implications for disabled infants and toddlers. *Infant Mental Health Journal, 10,* 3-13.

Williamson, G., Szczepanski, M., & Zeitlin, S. (1993). Coping frame of reference. In P. Kramer & J. Hinojosa (Eds.), *Frames of reference for pediatric occupational therapy* (pp. 395-436). Baltimore, MD: Williams & Wilkins.

Williamson, G., & Szczepanski, M. (1999). Coping frame of reference. In P. Kramer & J. Hinojosa (Eds.), *Frames of reference for pediatric occupational therapy* (2nd ed.) (pp. 431-468). Baltimore, MD: Williams & Wilkins.

Winstein, C. (1991). Knowledge of results and motor learning-implications for physical therapy. *Physical Therapy, 71,* 140-149.

Winstein, C., & Schmidt, R. (1990). Reduced frequency of knowledge of results enhances motor skill learning. *Journal of Experimental Psychology (Learning, Memory, and Cognition), 16,* 677-691.

Woollacott, M., & Shumway-Cook, A. (1990). Changes in posture control across the life span-a systems approach. *Physical Therapy, 70,* 799-807.

Wright, T., & Nicholson, J. (1973). Physiotherapy for the spastic child: An evaluation. *Developmental Medicine and Child Neurology, 15,* 146-163.

Yeargan, D. (1982). *A factor-analytic study of adaptive behavior and intellectual functioning in learning disabled children* [Dissertation]. Denton, TX: North Texas State University.

Zeitlin, S. (1985). *Coping Inventory.* Bensenville, IL: Scholastic Testing Service.

Zeitlin, S. & Williamson, G. (1990). Coping characteristics of disabled and nondisabled young children. *American Journal of Orthopsychiatry, 60,* 404-411.

Zeitlin, S., Williamson, G., & Rosenblatt, W. (1987). The coping with stress model: A counseling approach for families with a handicapped child. *Journal of Counseling and Development, 65,* 443-446.

5

The Screening, Referral, and Pre-Assessment Processes

Winnie Dunn, PhD, OTR, FAOTA

As occupational therapy becomes more integrated within community service systems, colleagues and team members solicit our participation in population-wide services. Population-wide services are those activities that professional staff engage in to survey the needs of cohort groups (i.e., groups that share features, such as their age and interests), provide direction for service exploration, and construct preventative strategies to support successful performance within natural contexts.

The purpose of population-wide services is to use professional knowledge and expertise to identify potential performance difficulties early so that a plan for supporting the child can be implemented before problems occur. The most frequent population-wide services are screening and pre-assessment; we will discuss both of these processes in this chapter. We will also discuss the referral process and other service supports that occur in relation to these identification activities.

SCREENING

Screening is a process of comparing a person's general performance to general standards of performance for the cohort group. For children, screening usually involves comparisons to developmental norms and expectations to see if the child is within, below, or above age expectations (Collier, 1991). There are three typical outcomes from screening: the child is performing within expectations and requires no further services, the child is definitely outside of expectations and needs to be referred for further assessment, and the child needs to be checked again periodically because some performance standards are questionable (Collier, 1991).

Principles for a Typical Screening Program

Screening programs have been around for a very long time in related disciplines, such as medicine and education. These established programs offer best practice guidance about the criteria for excellent screening programs (Collier, 1991; Frankenburg, 1975).

Screening Tools Must Meet the Standards for Valid and Reliable Measures

Many times screening is the first contact the family has with the service system. During this initial contact, it is very important that the family receives accurate and helpful information. When screening tools meet the same standard as other measures, we can feel safer that the decision we make based on screening results

Outcome of Screening Activity			
		Child is OK	**Child has a problem**
Actual Status of the Child	OK	TRUE NEGATIVE (A) The child is OK and the test says the child is OK.	FALSE POSITIVE (B)* The child is OK, but the test says the child has problem.
	Has a problem	FALSE NEGATIVE (C)* The child has problem, but the test says the child is OK.	TRUE POSITIVE (D) The child has a problem, and the test says the child has a problem.
*The status and conditions don't match; well-designed measures find very few children in these categories.			

Figure 5-1. Summary of possible findings from screening tools.

will be correct. Figure 5-1 illustrates the relationships between the possible decisions (i.e., screening outcome) and the actual status of the child (i.e., child outcome). As you can see, conditions A and D yield correct decisions for the family; in condition A the child is ok and the screening tool says the child is ok, while in condition D, the child has a problem and the screening tool says that the child has a problem. The errors occur in conditions B and C, in which the child's actual status and the screening tool finding do not match. Valid and reliable measures find very few children in conditions B and C.

Screening tools must also be simple to learn, administer, and interpret; many screening programs have some volunteer staff supporting them. There must be cost-effectiveness in the screening program as well, including costs of materials and supplies, personnel, and space to conduct the program. Table 5-1 summarizes the characteristics of some traditionally used screening tools.

When professionals conduct a screening, there must be evidence that providing intervention after the screening period results in better outcomes than intervention provided later. Literature strongly supports the premise that providing early intervention services is effective at improving outcomes for children (see Odom & Karnes, 1988). Community-based screening programs for children are typically directed at younger children in an effort to identify the potential difficulties early and provide supports for improved outcomes.

There must be additional services available after the screening, i.e., assessment procedures to evaluate the problem in more depth than the screening and intervention services to address the problem. Best practice dictates that communities have a cascade of services and professionals available to families. It is inappropriate to use community and family resources to conduct and participate in screening programs if there will be no follow-up activities for families whose children are at risk. The essential nature of screening is to identify potential needs and issues that can be minimized or resolved if dealt with efficiently; it is inappropriate to give parents feedback about difficulties without offering guidance about what to do next.

Screening is reserved for those performance features that are prevalent and/or have serious (negative) impact. Community screening programs are designed to locate those children for whom early intervention will improve their overall outcomes. Although theoretically we may think that we should screen all children for all possible issues, this is not a good use of community resources or family time and resources. For example, there are enough developmental issues that impact school performance to justify early school screening. We also want to screen everyone for problems that may be rare but which have a very negative impact; for example, all infants are screened for phenylketonuria (PKU) in the hospital. Very few children have this condition, but we have a very effective treatment and the early intervention prevents severe retardation. Therefore, the cost/benefit makes this type of screening worthwhile. On the other hand, it may not be cost-effective to conduct community screenings for the presence of warts or moles; these do not impact overall performance.

The Screening Process

There are two aspects to the screening process that safeguard errors in screening decisions. The first type of screening is "population screening", in which professionals see all individuals in a cohort group (e.g., all children of preschool age, all children entering kindergarten, all children born). When we find children who are at risk or demonstrate clear delays, we conduct follow-up activities to add to our database and confirm or deny our original conclusion. The second type of screening is screening for service eligibility. When children are referred for possible assessment it is appropriate to review records and other available data to determine whether assessment is warranted.

Population Screening

Population screening is a process of checking everyone in the cohort group on a variable of interest. Typical population screening programs for communities check children's developmental status during the toddler and preschool years. These programs are staffed by a combination of professional staff (which may or may not include occupational therapists) and volunteers from the community. Professional staff train the volunteers in procedures for all aspects of the screening program, including registering the families, administering portions of the screening, and recording findings for the files.

Every state has an early identification program (called "Child Find" in legislation), typically held in the spring prior to the coming school year. The local school districts sponsor these screening programs, advertise in the community so parents are aware of the services available, schedule appointments for a prescribed amount of time, and follow-up the phone calls with materials in the mail. Screening officials ask parents to bring completed forms with history information (e.g., shot records, developmental information) to facilitate moving them through the process efficiently. With toddlers and preschoolers, it is important to be time-efficient, since the children can lose attention or become fatigued and irritable at these ages.

In some population screening programs, each "testing" station worker provides the family with feedback about the child's performance (e.g., "his vision is fine", or "most of her gross motor skills are at age level; she needs to work on balance in the next few months"). In other programs, the findings are collected and one person counsels with the parents at the end of the screening process. Occupational therapists might be asked to serve in either of these roles, or to supervise others in carrying out these tasks.

When there are concerns, best practice dictates that the screening program offer parents alternatives for addressing the concerns. If the child's performance is "at risk" (i.e., we don't know whether a problem will develop or not), the professionals will set a reschedule time (usually 3 to 6 months) to check the child again. The program staff will also give these parents suggestions about what to watch for and what to work on in the interim period. If the child's screening finds that there is a definite problem, the screening staff will direct the family to additional resources. This may include referral to an assessment team, suggestions about specialized therapy, or ideas about early intervention or preschool programs. Many screening programs provide handout materials about community services, developmental milestones, and developmental play activities so the parents go home with resources.

At the end of this chapter there are a series of figures that illustrate typical materials for a district-wide population screening program in Kansas. This particular Child Find program is called Count Your Kid In (Figures 5-2 to 5-13).

Screening for Service Eligibility

We screen for service eligibility to determine whether further assessment is warranted and what assessment strategy might be appropriate. Children might be part of the pre-assessment process or someone might have submitted a referral as a result of population screening or due to a performance concern. This type of screening provides a safeguard against "over-assessment" of children. With this additional step, we conduct another check to see if comprehensive assessment is absolutely necessary.

Occupational therapists are frequently called upon to conduct this type of screening. In this capacity, we might conduct a records review (including history information), observe the child, and/or interview the current care providers. In some situations, it is appropriate to administer a screening measure to augment the information available. The outcome of these activities is to make a decision whether to go on to a comprehensive assessment or provide other guidance that is sufficient to address the concern. The most common time to screen for service eligibility is during the pre-assessment process described below.

Table 5-1.

Summary of Primary Characteristics of Screening Instruments Frequently Used by Occupational Therapists

	Short Sensory Profile	Miller Assessment for Pre-schoolers (MAP)	Developmental Profile II (Interview)	Denver Developmental ScreeningTest Revised (DDST-R)	Quick Neurological Screening Test	Therapist Generated Developmental Screening Checklists
AGE RANGE	3 to 10 years	2 years 4 months 5 years 8 months	0 to 9 1/2 years	0 to 6 years	5 to 18 years	typically 0 to 9 years
TESTING TIME (Minutes)	10minutes	20 to 30 minutes	20 to 40 minutes	5 to 7 minutes	20 minutes	15 to 20 minutes
SCORING TIME (Minutes)	5 minutes		10 to 20 minutes	5 minutes	5 to 10 minutes	
MAJOR AREAS TESTED: Personal/social			X	X		X
Communication			X	X		X
Cognition		X	X			
Self-help			X	X		X
Gross motor		X	X	X	X	X
Praxis		X			X	X
Reflexes						X
Fine motor		X		X	X	X
Visual-motor integration		X			X	X
Visual perception		X			X	X
Sensory Processing						
TYPE OF TEST: Norm referenced	X	X				
Criteria referenced				X		
Informal structured		X			X	X
Observation			interview		X	X
SCORES OBTAINED: Age level			X	X		X
Percentile		X		X		
Standard	X					
Quantified observations						

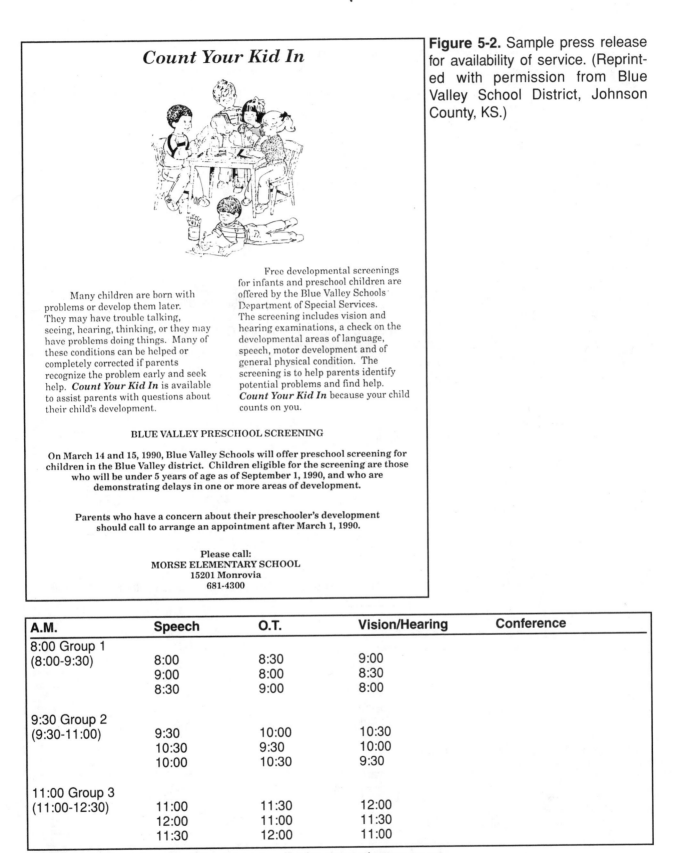

Count Your Kid In

Many children are born with problems or develop them later. They may have trouble talking, seeing, hearing, thinking, or they may have problems doing things. Many of these conditions can be helped or completely corrected if parents recognize the problem early and seek help. *Count Your Kid In* is available to assist parents with questions about their child's development.

Free developmental screenings for infants and preschool children are offered by the Blue Valley Schools Department of Special Services. The screening includes vision and hearing examinations, a check on the developmental areas of language, speech, motor development and of general physical condition. The screening is to help parents identify potential problems and find help. *Count Your Kid In* because your child counts on you.

BLUE VALLEY PRESCHOOL SCREENING

On March 14 and 15, 1990, Blue Valley Schools will offer preschool screening for children in the Blue Valley district. Children eligible for the screening are those who will be under 5 years of age as of September 1, 1990, and who are demonstrating delays in one or more areas of development.

Parents who have a concern about their preschooler's development should call to arrange an appointment after March 1, 1990.

Please call:
MORSE ELEMENTARY SCHOOL
15201 Monrovia
681-4300

Figure 5-2. Sample press release for availability of service. (Reprinted with permission from Blue Valley School District, Johnson County, KS.)

A.M.	Speech	O.T.	Vision/Hearing	Conference
8:00 Group 1 (8:00-9:30)	8:00	8:30	9:00	
	9:00	8:00	8:30	
	8:30	9:00	8:00	
9:30 Group 2 (9:30-11:00)	9:30	10:00	10:30	
	10:30	9:30	10:00	
	10:00	10:30	9:30	
11:00 Group 3 (11:00-12:30)	11:00	11:30	12:00	
	12:00	11:00	11:30	
	11:30	12:00	11:00	

Figure 5-3. Sample schedule sheet for district screening program.

STUDENT HISTORY FORM (CONFIDENTIAL)

General

NAME _____ SEX_____ AGE ____
            (Last)   (First)   (Middle)

ADDRESS _____ CITY/STATE_____ ZIP _____

PHONE _____ DATE OF BIRTH _____

AGE AT TIME OF HISTORY _____ PLACE OF BIRTH _____

FATHER OR GUARDIAN'S NAME _____ AGE _____

OCCUPATION _____ HEALTH _____

MOTHER'S NAME _____ AGE _____

OCCUPATION _____ HEALTH _____

CHILD'S PHYSICIAN _____ PHONE _____

RELATIONSHIP OF INFORMANT TO CHILD _____

HOME SCHOOL _____ SUBDIVISION _____

Family

A. Are parents separated? _____ Divorced? _____

B. Has either parent remarried? _____ Which one? _____

C. With whom does the child live? _____

D. Check one: ( ) Natural Child   ( ) Adopted Child   ( ) Foster Child

E. Name of children in family (eldest to youngest – giving age): _____

F. Other living in the home: _____

Developmental and Medical Background

1. Prenatal: Was there any illness, infection, or unusual condition of mother during pregnancy?_____

2. Birth: Length of pregnancy? _____ Weight at birth? _____

Difficult or forced labor? _____ Instrument delivery? _____

Was there a delay in starting the baby to breathe? _____

Other comments: _____

Child's Health History: _____

3. A. Has the child ever had: Convulsions? _____ Seizures? _____
      Give details: (Identify illness being discussed with exact dates or ages when it occurred, etc.) _____

   B. Unexplained high fever: _____ How high? _____ Duration? _____
      When? _____ Circumstances: _____

   C. Is your child on medication or has he/she been on any in the past? _____
      Type? _____ Reason? _____ Date? _____

D. Present physical condition: Good _____ Fair _____ Poor _____

E. Please list any preschools and/or special programs your child has attended including therapy for speech, motor, etc.: _____

Physical Factors

A. At what age was he/she potty trained? _____

B. Does your child now have or has he/she ever had any of the following conditions?
   Difficulty: Talking? _____ Seeing? _____ Hearing? _____
   Falls or accidental injuries? _____ Does your child have trouble running or walking? _____
   How well does your child use: Scissors? Good _____ Fair _____ Poor _____
                                 Pencils? Good _____ Fair _____ Poor _____
                                 Crayons? Good _____ Fair _____ Poor _____
                                 Right handed? _____ Left handed? _____

C. Has your child had any of the following?
   Serious accidents? _____ Date? _____
   Operations? _____ Date? _____
   Unusual illnesses? _____ Date? _____
   Unusual diseases? _____ Date? _____

D. To what things is the child allergic? _____

Figure 5-4. Legal Guardian's report of student's history form. (Reprinted with permission from Blue Valley School District, Johnson County, KS.)

E. Has the child had any special problems in visual function? (Prolonged wandering of the eyes in infancy, crossed eyes, eyes turned out, drooped lids, failure to follow light or motions, reverses numbers or letters, i.e., sees "b" for "d" or "p" for "g", sees a "6" as a "9") _____
Has vision been tested? _____ Date or age tested? _____ Results: _____
F. Has the child even had his ears examined by a physician? _____ At what age? _____
Results: _____
Has hearing been tested? _____ Was an audiometer used? _____ At what age? _____
Has your child even had earaches/otitis media? _____ How often? _____
Have these been recurring? _____
G. Medical treatment being given out; for what conditions and by whom? _____

Family and Home Situation
A. What types of discipline do you use most often in guiding your child? Give examples: _____
B. Are there any adults besides the parents who play an active part in guiding your child? If so, whom?___
C. Is he/she afraid of certain things, persons, animals, or situation? _____
Explain: _____
D. Has he ever had temper tantrums? _____ At what age? _____
Explain: _____
E. What particular talents does your child have? _____
F. Are your child's sleeping habits regular? _____
G. Are your child's eating habits regular? _____
Does your child have strong likes or dislikes toward food textures? _____
Likes? _____ Dislikes? _____
H. How does your child respond to other siblings? _____
I. How do other siblings respond to this child? _____
J. Did he seem to understand what was said to him before he learned to talk? _____
K. Were the child's wants anticipated before he attempted to speak? _____
L. Did your child use much gesture or sign language? _____
M. Did anyone "baby talk" to your child? _____
N. Is your child easily distracted or does he/she have trouble functioning if there is a lot of noise around? _____

Figure 5-4 continued. Legal Guardian's report of student's history form. (Reprinted with permission from Blue Valley School District, Johnson County, KS.)

Count Your Kid In
Preparation Procedures Checklist

Initial Preparation of Team

Meeting of the specialists to determine the date of C.Y.K.I.

A press release is then distributed to:
- Elementary buildings for their newsletters
- Private preschools
- Multipurpose Center
- Newspapers in the area
- Grocery Stores

Developmental Council

Meeting of the principal and the preschool specialists to determine:
- Rooms to be used
- Date for staffings for those who qualify for the Special Needs Preschool Program after the C.Y.K.I. evaluation is completed

Individual Preparation

Preschool Specialist.
1. Review call-in procedures with secretary and give them the "office folder" with the basic information form, cover letter for appointment time, press release, social history form and time schedule.

Figure 5-5. Count Your Kid In (C.Y.K.I.) preparation procedures. (Reprinted with permission from Blue Valley School District, Johnson County, KS.)

- Parents call in and C.Y.K.I. basic information form is filled out over the telephone.
- A time is then assigned.
- The secretary then sends the cover letter for appointment time and the social history form to be filled out and returned when they arrive.

2. Meet with other specialists assigned to evaluation during C.Y.K.I. to review procedures and give them a specialist's folder with:
   - date of evaluation
   - individual duties
   - place assigned for testing
   - list of children and times of each evaluation
   - copy of the press release form

3. Prepare each child's folder with information on Basic Information Form stapled inside the folder on the left side. Inside the folder are Consent for Evaluation form, Parent's Rights form, two Results forms (with carbon) and a Cover Letter for Results form.

4. Be sure enough extra Cover Letter for Results forms, Results forms, Social History forms, and Special Needs Preschool Information forms are available.

5. Have name tags for evaluators and children typed.

6. Have small prizes available for the children as they leave.

7. Be sure signs are made and put up directing parents to waiting area as they arrive.

8. Get camera and film.

Nurse (Vision)
1. Get eye chart and response forms and any other equipment ready.
2. Set up room for testing – measure for eye examination, etc.
3. Get handouts, if applicable.
4. Be sure table, chairs, etc., are set up inside and outside the room.

Audiologist (Hearing)
1. Get audiometer set up along with other equipment.
2. Get response forms.
3. Set-up room for testing.
4. Get handouts, if applicable.
5. Be sure table, chairs, etc., are set up inside and outside the room.

Speech Pathologist
1. Get tests, other materials, and test fonts.
2. Get speech-language evaluation forms.
3. Get handouts, if applicable.
4. Be sure table, chairs, etc., are set-up inside and outside the room.

Psychologist, Guidance Counselor, or Designated Person
1. Get extra forms, name tags, and pens from Preschool Specialist.
2. Have handouts on behavior, discipline, thumb sucking, toilet training, etc., if applicable.

Occupational Therapist
1. Select screening tools and gather screening materials needed to perform the test.
2. Get screening tools ordered or copied and ready for screening.
3. Get handouts ready for a variety of problem areas a child might have (e.g., fine motor difficulty, gross motor, self-help, visual perceptual, etc.).
4. On the day of the screening, set-up testing room for screening—table, chairs, testing instrument, and materials.

Community Volunteers
1. Get waiting area for family and children set-up (i.e., chairs for adults and children, table for children to color while they wait, refreshment table, etc.).
2. Escort parent and child to each screening section.
3. Take folder with each screening result to each screening station.
4. Escort children to restroom, if needed.
5. Record screening information on forms, if asked by professional performing screening.
6. Set up games, toys, and fine motor activities in waiting room to help the time pass for children who are waiting for screening.

Figure 5-5 continued. Count Your Kid In (C.Y.K.I.) preparation procedures. (Reprinted with permission from Blue Valley School District, Johnson County, KS.)

Count Your Kid In Day Procedures

Parents and children arrive and follow signs to waiting area.

Give out name tags and take picture of each child.

Psychologist, Guidance Counselor, or designated person checks for social history form, has consent signed, and gives out Parent's Rights form. Then that person is available to parents for questions or concerns about the child's social and cognitive development, kindergarten expectations, behavior discipline, thumb sucking, toilet training, etc.

Speech Pathologist, Occupational Therapist, and Nurse take the first child assigned to each of them for the first session.

Each professional finishes evaluating and writes results on the appropriate form and signs his or her name. If there is an area of concern and services may be warranted, a star is placed in the left margin.

Each professional briefly reviews their own results with the parent after the evaluation.

The child and his folder are then taken to the next evaluator with handout information, if applicable.

The last specialist reviews with parents. If an area of concern is noted, the parents are told that a call will be made to them after the specialists meet and determine what services or further recommendations would most benefit the child. Cover letter for results is attached to one copy of the results form for the parents to take with them.

The child chooses a small prize to take home.

The team meets at the end of the day to determine which children warrant services—either the Preschool Program or individual speech and/or occupational therapy. A representative from the school speech therapists attends to make any followup recommendations on children only needing speech services.

Parents are called with recommendations for areas of concern. If the Preschool Program is recommended, a time is set-up for them to visit the classroom and arrange a staffing time.

Figure 5-6. Count Your Kid In day procedures. (Reprinted with permission from Blue Valley School District, Johnson County, KS.)

Summary of District Screening Battery

Developmental Area Screened	Name of Screening Tool(s)	Length of time to administer	Who can perform this screening
Vision	*Vision Screening	5 minutes	Nurse
Hearing (Pure Tone Screening) (Tympanometry)	Report of Hearing Test	10 minutes	Nurse
Speech and Language	Goldman Fristoe (Articulation Screening)	10 minutes	Speech Pathologist
	The Communication Screen (language & articulation)	10 minutes	
	Bankson Language Screening Test (language)	10 minutes	
	Peabody Picture Vocabulary Test (PPVT)	10-15 minutes	
	Preschool Language Scale	10-15 minutes	
Motor (Fine and Gross Self-help)	Denver Developmental Screening Test (0-6 yrs)	5-10 minutes	Occupational Therapist Physical Therapist Physical Education Trained Volunteer

Figure 5-7. District screening battery. (Reprinted with permission from Blue Valley School District, Johnson County, KS.)

Motor (Fine and Gross Self-help)	Miller Assessment for Preschoolers (ages 2.9 years to 5.8 years)	20-30 minutes	Administered by professional or non-professional, interpreted by professionals who have attended MAP seminar.
	*St. Lukes Gross, Fine, Self-help Screening, Checklist (2-5 years)	20 minutes	Occupational Therapist Physical Therapist
	Developmental Profile II (requires parent report) 0-9 ½ years	20-40 minutes (all sections given) Areas that are screened are physical, self-help, social, academic & communication. (*Can do only sections of this screening)	Professionals or para-professionals
	*Blue Valley School District Gross Motor Screening	5-10 minutes	Occupational Therapist Physical Therapist
Behavior	*Informal observation of child during screening, observation of parent/child interaction		Psychologist School Counselor

Figure 5-7 continued. District screening battery. (Reprinted with permission from Blue Valley School District, Johnson County, KS.)

Vision Screening

Functional Assessment   Date: _____

		OK	?
1. Pupillary Response (shine penlight into eye from 12")	(right) constrict dilate		
	(left) constrict dilate		
2. Corneal Light Reflex (penlight to bridge of nose from 14-16")	similar position of reflection in each eye		
3. Blind Reflex (hand moves toward face)	blink		
4. Alternate Cover Test	right eye left eye		
5. Tracking (14-16")	right/left above/below		
6. Visual Acuity-Lighthouse (if appropriate)	lighthouse score		
7. Near point convergence	near point		

Comments:

Additional Observations
1. Eyes crossed–turning in or out–at any time, or eyes that do not appear straight, especially when child is tired.
2. Has reddened eyes or eyelids.
3. Turns the head to use one eye only. L R (eye used)
4. Tilts the head to one side: L R
5. Places an object close to the eyes to look at it.
6. Squints while looking at objects.
7. Blinks excessively.
8. Covers or closes one eye: L R
9. Rubs eyes: L R
10. Sits close to the TV.

Figure 5-8. Vision screening form. (Reprinted with permission from Blue Valley School District, Johnson County, KS.)

Developmental Skills Screening

Name: _____   Examiner: _____
Birthdate: _____   Date: _____

B = requires assistance of examiner   *A = accomplishes activity within normal time*

Age
3 years

Gross Motor
1. Gets up from floor with partial trunk rotation
2. No longer walks with arms outstretched and shows uniformity of heel-toe gait
3. Balances on one foot for 1 second
4. Crawls through objects
5. Walks backwards
6. Catches large ball with arms fully extended
7. Throws small ball with torso participation
8. Alternates feet going upstairs holding rail
9. Jumps from bottom step with feet together

Fine Motor
1. Inserts circle, square and triangle into formboard with rotations
2. Picks up cube without touching table
3. Builds 9-block tower
4. Imitates train of 3 or more blocks
5. Screws lid on jar
6. Demonstrates preferred hand using 3 fingers and thumb to grasp crayon
7. Copies circle
8. Copies horizontal line
9. Imitates cross
10. Uses scissors to snip at paper

Visual and/or Tactile
1. Hesitates at top of stairs when descending (depth perception)
2. Recognizes halves and fits together
3. Identifies familiar objects by touching and handling

Self-Help Skills
1. Undresses but needs help with fastenings
2. Puts on shoes and socks; may be incorrect
3. Unlaces shoes
4. Washes hands in appropriate sequence
5. Drinks from glass with one hand
6. Drinks through straw
7. No turning of spoon with minimum spilling
8. Pours from small container into glass with assistance
9. Uses fork to pierce food
10. Has BM and urinates in potty when reminders and assistance in wiping–boys may stand

Figure 5-9a. Type 1 screening program tool. (Reprinted with permission from Blue Valley School District, Johnson County, KS.)

Developmental Skills Screening

Name: _____   Examiner: _____
Birthdate: _____   Date: _____

B = requires assistance of examiner   *A = accomplishes activity within normal time*

Age

4 years

Gross Motor

1. Walks with long swinging steps
2. Gets up from floor with no trunk rotation
3. Hops on toes with both feet
4. Balances on one foot for 2-5 seconds
5. Can touch end of nose with finger
6. Gallops
7. Walks on 3 ½" walking board stepping off 3 times
8. Catches large ball with hands moving in accordance with ball
9. Throws ball with elbow movement and no torso involvement
10. Holds rail to walk downstairs alternating feet
11. No evidence of ATNR

Fine Motor

1. Adult grasp of pencil
2. Copies cross
3. Imitates square
4. Traces diamond
5. Cuts straight line
6. Draws man with 3 parts
7. Copies train of blocks
8. Copies bridge
9. Imitates gate

Visual and/or Tactile

1. Can identify closer of 2 objects
2. Matches identically shaped objects by size
3. Tactually matches objects by size with vision occluded

Self-Help Skills

1. Undresses and unbuttons buttons
2. Puts coat on
3. Laces shoes
4. Identifies front and back
5. Uses fork appropriately
6. Pours from container without spilling
7. Blows nose
8. Goes to toilet on own – may need reminder to wipe
9. May call for mother at night for toileting

Figure 5-9b. Type 1 screening program tool. (Reprinted with permission from Blue Valley School District, Johnson County, KS.)

Developmental Skills Screening

Name: _____ Examiner: _____

Birthdate: _____ Date: _____

B = requires assistance of examiner   *A = accomplishes activity within normal time*

Age

5 years

Gross Motor
1. Arms held near body with narrow stance in gait
2. Stands up without using hands for support
3. Can change from sitting, standing and squatting in serial manner
4. Makes 90 degrees pivot in standing
5. Distinguishes between own right and left
6. Walks full length of 3 ½" walking board
7. Sits up straight in chair
8. Skips on alternating feet
9. Bounces ball
10. May catch and kick ball simultaneously
11. Walks up and down stairs on alternating feet without rail

Fine Motor
1. Copies square
2. Copies triangle
3. Draws man with 6 parts
4. Reach and placement of blocks show good accuracy
5. Copies gate of blocks
6. Cuts gate
7. Cuts curved line
8. Alternates supination and pronation irradically
9. Serial opposition with overflow and poor rhythm

Visual and/or Tactile
1. Differentiates square from rectangle
2. Localizes tactile stimuli to specific body part (arm, leg, etc.)
3. Mean of nystagmus to left – 8.9 seconds to right – 8.7 seconds

Self-Help Skills
1. Fastens buttons that are within sight
2. Washes and dries hands
3. May dress without prodding, but needs help with back fasteners
4. Brushes hair
5. Brushes teeth
6. Slow but independent feeding
7. Uses knife to spread
8. Needs reminders to wipe
9. No longer needs night toileting

Figure 5-9c. Type 1 screening program tool. (Reprinted with permission from Blue Valley School District, Johnson County, KS.)

Developmental Skills Screening

Name: _____   Examiner: _____
Birthdate: _____   Date: _____

B = requires assistance of examiner   A = accomplishes activity within normal time

Age
6 years

Gross Motor
1. Bows with feet together, legs and knees straight
2. Balances on one foot with eyes open
3. Walks on 1 ½" walking board with 2-3 falls
4. Jumps over one foot obstacles
5. Reaches for objects beyond arm's length with ease
6. Kicks ball from running start
7. Catches small ball and throws using optimal use of upper extremity
8. Jumps from bottom step on toes
9. Balances well on toes
10. TLR prone and supine held for 20-30 seconds
11. Body righting diminished
12. Heel-toe walks forwards

Fine Motor
1. Shows good thumb and index finger flexion in writing
2. Draws square with sharp corners
3. Copies diamond

Visual and/or Tactile
1. Nystagmus mean to left – 10.5 seconds to right – 9.2 seconds

Self-Help Skills
1. Dresses self; may need minimal assistance
2. Ties shoe laces loosely
3. Bathes self except for head and neck
4. Uses fork to cut food to bite size
5. Toilets self completely

Figure 5-9d. Type 1 screening program tool. (Reprinted with permission from Blue Valley School District, Johnson County, KS.)

Pupil Observation and Parent Interview

Pupil's Name: _____
Age: _____
Date: _____

Interviewer: _____
(Psychologist or school counselor)

Brief 1 counselor:

Brief summary of developmental and medical history:

Discussion with parent pertaining to their concern for bringing their child to Count Your Kid In:

Interviewer's observation of child during screening: (The interviewer at this time looked at how the child interacted with the examiner either in speech or motor screening. The interviewer looked at the child's attending

Figure 5-10. Pupil observation and parent interview form. (Reprinted with permission from Blue Valley School District, Johnson County, KS.)

skills, compliance, ability to follow directions, or any other appropriate or inappropriate behaviors observed during the screening.)

Interviewer's observation of the child's interaction with parent:

Summary of Interviewer's observation of parent-child Interaction and child Interaction during the screening:

Recommendations by Interviewer:

Review of Psychological Testing: (This section will be completed by the psychologist either by review of reports the parents have brought to screening or by interviewing the parent concerning any intellectual functioning questions the parent might have about the child during the screening.)

Figure 5-10 continued. Pupil observation and parent interview form. (Reprinted with permission from Blue Valley School District, Johnson County, KS.)

Count Your Kid In Results for: _____
                                        (Child's Name)
                              Date: _____

SPEECH/LANGUAGE _____Speech/Language Pathologist
Articulation:
Language: receptive:
                 expressive

MOTOR _____Occupational Therapist
Gross motor:
Fine motor:
Self-help:

BEHAVIORAL _____Psychologist
Parent observations:
Interactions:
Interview data:

VISION _____Nurse
Functional assessment:
Additional observations:

HEARING _____Audiologist
Audiometric:
Tympanometric:

RECOMMENDATIONS:
1.
2.
3.
4.

REFERRAL DATES:
*Denotes area(s) of concern. Person screening a child will use (*) to denote a concern or delay in developmental area being screened.

Figure 5-11. Count Your Kid In results form. (Reprinted with permission from Blue Valley School District, Johnson County, KS.)

Fine motor activities involve the use of the small muscles of the hands. Many school tasks such as writing, drawing, and cutting require good fine motor skills, so it is helpful if these skills can be stressed at home.

1. Paper provides a medium that has a lot of fine motor possibilities. Tearing, cutting, folding, coloring, and pasting are all good activities. Making paper chains requires cutting, folding, and pasting; making paper airplanes can include folding and coloring.

2. Clay or play dough is fun to play with and requires strength and coordination. Have your child make shapes or structures; roll it out and cut shapes with cookie cutters.

3. Clothing fasteners such as buttons, shoe strings, snaps and zippers require hand control. Help your child practice fastening.

4. The use of simple tools may be motivating for some children, while developing fine motor control. Screw drivers, saws, manual egg beaters, or rolling pins can be used in play or to "help" mom and dad during activities.

5. Finger games like Teensie Weensie Spider, The Wheels on the Bus, Little Bunny Fu-fu, or any game that requires finger movements can be incorporated into travel time in the car.

6. Let your child sort small objects for you. Nails, screws, and bolts can be sorted at the tool bench; paper clips, safety pins, and rubber bands can be sorted from the desk.

7. Sewing cards require coordination of both hands and rely on the child being able to watch the hands as they move. Tube macaroni, cranberries, or popcorn can be strung as an alternative to purchasing sewing cards.

8. A number of commercially available toys require fine motor coordination; these make good gifts (e.g., Lite Brite, pot holder loom, pop beads, chalkboard, craft kits, simple model kits, blocks, puzzles).

9. Coloring books, dot-to-dot books, cut and paste books, and sticker books are useful; parents may need to guide these activities to ensure success.

10. Blow soap bubbles and pop them with different fingers or hand patterns.

11. Blow up a balloon or wad up a piece of paper and play games with it as if it were a ball; hit it into the air with a paddle, racquet, paper plate, or hands. These activities encourage development of eye and hand coordination.

12. Playing with marbles or jacks facilitates controlled hand movements.

13. Purchase a piece of Masonite with the holes in it and get some golf tees. Have your child put one golf tee into each hole to make patterns.

14. Purchase spring-type clothes pins. Let your child use them to clip things together or to secure notes around the house.

Figure 5-12. Activities which can aid in the development of fine motor skills. (Reprinted with permission from Dunn, W. (1991) *Pediatric Occupational Therapy: Facilitating Effective Service Provision.* Thorofare, NJ: SLACK Incorporated.)

Gross motor skills involve the coordinated and efficient use of the body in movement. Balance, control and patterns of movement are all part of gross motor development.

Controlled movements such as walking, jumping, hopping, and skipping are all good gross motor activities. Vary the activities so that your child remains challenged to master harder skills. For example, have your child:
- Jump over various sizes of objects, such as a book or a box.
- Jump off a step or box.
- Jump/hop with feet together around a box, table, the yard.
- Hop on one foot and then the other; change the speed; demonstrate a pattern and have your child repeat it.
- Hop into and out of objects such as hoops or a box.
- Walk on a 2" x 4" board, 8 – 10 feet long, positioned on the floor. Vary the method, such as walking sideways, backwards, or heel to toe.
- Gallop or skip around objects.
- Play hopscotch. Begin with simple hopscotch patterns; vary the pattern of boxes on the cement.

Construction toys with large pieces encourage the use of both hands, motor planning and imagination. Encourage your child to make anything; be creative; later guide him to make what is on the picture directions, by showing him the piece, then helping him find it, if necessary, and putting it together.

Ball or bean bag activities require gross motor coordination:
- Throw and catch a large ball. Adjust the distance, speed, and type of ball.
- Throw a ball or bean bag into a box or wastebasket.
- Bounce/dribble large ball with one hand and then the other hand; create patterns the child can copy.
- Kick balls of various sizes and weights; sometimes use stationary positions, other times roll or throw the ball.
- Set targets up, have your child throw bean bags toward the parts of the target.

Figure 5-13. Activities which can aid in the development of gross motor skills. (Reprinted with permission from Dunn, W. (1991) *Pediatric Occupational Therapy: Facilitating Effective Service Provision.* Thorofare, NJ: SLACK Incorporated.)

PRE-ASSESSMENT

The pre-assessment process is a proactive part of serving children in their natural contexts. When children have difficulties in their schoolwork, it is important for the team members to investigate all avenues of support prior to assuming the child will need a comprehensive assessment and special education programming. Pre-assessment enables the school personnel to explore options for supporting the child's learning as part of the natural course of instruction. Each service agency might name their pre-assessment process differently, such as Developmental Team, Teacher Support Team, or Troubleshooters. It is important to find out which team serves this function.

The Pre-Assessment Team

The pre-assessment team typically consists of professionals within a building. It is common for classroom teachers to form the core of the team with special education, administrative, and related service personnel serving as supports to the pre-assessment team.

The Pre-Assessment Process

When a teacher notices that a student is having difficulty in school, the teacher makes changes in directions, assignments, etc., in an attempt to find a successful strategy for the student. At some point if those changes are not working, the teacher brings this concern to the pre-assessment team. The team reviews the work the teacher has done (see Figure 5-14 for an example of a teacher documentation form for pre-assessment) and collaborates with the teacher to identify additional methods for supporting the student. The pre-assessment team also designs data collection strategies for monitoring the effectiveness of the new strategies. The teacher then implements the new strategies and collects data to see if they are working to support the student's successful performance.

Occupational therapy can be involved in pre-assessment in a number of ways. First, the occupational therapist can serve as a member of the pre-assessment team; this usually occurs after a therapist has been part of a system for a period of time and the teachers have come to trust the therapist's contributions. Second, the occupational therapist can be called in to assist the team on particular cases (the therapist serves on the team for that child's needs only). Third, the occupational therapist can serve as a resource to the pre-assessment team, providing them with checklists, materials, and suggestions to facilitate their overall work.

Figure 5-15 contains an example of suggestions an occupational therapist might formulate for the pre-assessment team's use in their problem-solving activities. You will see ideas on this form that are related to the most common concerns expressed by school personnel. The student does not have to go through comprehensive assessment and placement in special education services to profit from the occupational therapist's expertise. In fact, it is in children's best interest for occupational therapists to offer those suggestions that are safe for others to implement during the pre-assessment process. This supports the children to remain in their natural context, the overall goal of both education and therapy.

Outcomes of Pre-Assessment

The pre-assessment process can lead to two primary outcomes. First, the child can perform successfully with the supports provided and remain in regular education. Second, the team can determine that they will need a comprehensive assessment to investigate the child's needs further. In either case, the team has been vigilant in meeting the spirit of the "least restrictive environment" initiative (i.e., children must be served in the most natural setting for their interests and age, see Chapter 9).

Example of Pre-Assessment Teamwork

Let's consider an example (adapted from Collier, 1991). Barry is a second grade student. His teacher has begun to notice that Barry is slow to complete his seatwork, drops his pencil a lot, continues to reverse letters and produces messy papers. She had tried to support Barry by giving him more time, but this did not help his work product. She then completed the Teacher Intervention Checklist (Figure 5-14) and submitted it to the pre-assessment team at her school. She also tells the team that her concerns have increased as she has seen Barry act more self-conscious with his peers lately.

Student: _____   Teacher: _____   School: _____
Class/Subject:: _____   D.O.B.: _____   Date Completed: _____

Intervention Checklist
Classroom Teacher

What strategies have you tried to correct the problem? Please indicate those strategies you have applied to the problem and give an estimate of how long the strategy has been in effect in terms of days or weeks. Also comment on the success of these strategies in terms of "Yes" or "No":

	Specify:	(Days/Weeks) Duration	(Y-N) Success
Environmental Strategies			
1. Seating Change			
2. Isolation (how often?)		_____	_____
3. Change to a different hour/same teacher		_____	_____
4. Change to a different teacher		_____	_____
5. Other		_____	_____
		_____	_____
Organization Strategies			
1. Setting time limits for assignments/completion during class		_____	_____
2. Questioning at end of each sentence/paragraph to help focus on important information		_____	_____
3. Allowing additional time to complete task/take test		_____	_____
4. Highlighting main facts in the book		_____	_____
5. Organizing a notebook or providing folder to help organize work		_____	_____
6. Asking student to repeat directions given		_____	_____
7. Other		_____	_____
		_____	_____
Motivational Strategies			
1. Checking papers by showing "C's" for correct			
2. Sending home daily progress report		_____	_____
3. Immediate reinforcement of correct response		_____	_____
4. Keeping graphs and charts of student's progress		_____	_____
5. Conferencing with student's parents		_____	_____
6. Conferencing with student's other teachers		_____	_____
7. Student reading lesson to aide, peer tutor or teacher		_____	_____
8. Home/school communication system for assignments		_____	_____
9. Using tapes of materials the rest of the class is reading		_____	_____
10. Student using tapes of materials at home or school		_____	_____
11. Classmate to take notes with carbon		_____	_____
12. Other		_____	_____
		_____	_____
Presentation Strategies			
1. Giving assignments both orally and visually			
2. Taping lessons so student can listen again		_____	_____
3. Allowing student to have sample or practice test		_____	_____
4. Providing legible material		_____	_____
5. Immediate correction of errors		_____	_____
6. Providing advance organizers		_____	_____
7. Providing tests in smaller blocks of questions/wider spaced		_____	_____
8. Providing tests in small segments/student hands in at end of each segment and gets next		_____	_____
9. Providing modified tests, fewer questions, simpler material		_____	_____
10. Giving tests orally		_____	_____
11. Other		_____	_____
		_____	_____
Curriculum Strategies			
1. Providing opportunities for extra drill			
2. Providing study guide (outline, etc., to follow)		_____	_____
3. Reducing quantity of material		_____	_____
4. Providing instructional materials geared to lower level of basic skills		_____	_____
5. Vocabulary flash cards		_____	_____
6. Vocabulary words in context		_____	_____
7. Special materials		_____	_____
8. Other		_____	_____
		_____	_____

Are there any other strategies you have used that are not listed above? If "yes", please describe: (Duration and success):

Figure 5-14. Intervention checklist for the classroom teacher. (Reprinted with permission from Dunn, W. (1991) *Pediatric Occupational Therapy: Facilitating Effective Service Provision.* Thorofare, NJ: SLACK Incorporated.)

Classroom Adaptations to be Considered for Common Related Service Referral Complaints Prior to Comprehensive Assessment

Referral Complaint*	Possible Adaptations**
Poor lunch skills/behaviors	Provide a wheeled cart to carry lunch tray Provide large handled utensils Clamp lunch tray to table to avoid slipping Serve milk in sealed cup with straw
Poor toileting skills	Provide a smaller toilet Provide looser clothing Provide a step stool for toilet/sink
Can't stay in seat; fidgety	Allow student to lie on floor to work Allow student to stand to work Provide lateral support to hips or trunk (e.g., rolled towels) Adapt seat to correct height for work Be sure feet are flat on floor when seated Provide more variety in seatwork
Clumsy in classroom/halls; gets lost in building	Move classroom furniture to edges of room Send student to new locations when halls are less crowded Provide visual cues in hall to mark locations Match student with partner for transitions
Can't get on or off bus independently	Allow student to back down stairs Provide additional smaller steps
Can't get jacket/coat on/off	Place in front of student, in same orientation each time Provide larger size for easier handling
Drops materials; can't manipulate books, etc.	Place tabs on book pages for turning Provide small containers for items Place all items for one task on a lunch tray
Poor attention, hyperactive, distractible	Decrease availability of distracting stimuli (e.g., visual or auditory) Provide touch cues only when student is prepared for it Touch student with firm pressure Provide frequent breaks in seatwork
Poor pencil/crayon use	Use triangle grip on pencil/crayon Use fatter writing utensil Provide larger sheets of paper Provide paper without lines Provide paper with wider-spaced lines
Poor cutting skills	Provide adapted scissors Provide stabilized paper: e.g., tape it down, use large clips, C-clamps
Unable to complete seatwork successfully	Provide larger spaces for answers Give smaller amounts of work Put less items per page Give more time to complete task Change level of difficulty
Loses personal belongings; unorganized	Make a map showing where items belong Collect all belongings and hand them out at the beginning of each activity
Doesn't follow directions	Provide written or picture directions for reference Provide cassette tape of directions Allow student to watch a partner for cues

*More serious problems usually require immediate involvement of the occupational and/or physical therapist.
**If these strategies are unsuccessful, involvement of the occupational or physical therapist is appropriate.

Figure 5-15. Classroom adaptations that can be used in the preassessment process.

The occupational therapist at Barry's school serves on the pre-assessment team. They meet every other week to review Intervention Checklists and concerns filed by other classroom teachers. The team decides that for Barry, the occupational therapist is the best person to provide support in the classroom. They decide that an 8-week period of observation and intervention trials will provide enough time to review progress data and make further decisions. The teacher and the occupational therapist agree on a meeting schedule and times for the therapist to observe in the classroom during the pre-assessment period. The occupational therapist also gave the teacher a handout about adaptations that are appropriate for the classroom and asked her to review it before their meeting (with similar suggestions to those in Figure 5-15).

After two observations and one meeting with the teacher, they decide to try several strategies. The therapist gets a pencil grip for Barry's pencil to stabilize his grip and suggests using unlined paper for a while to see if the decreased "pressure to be inside the lines" will reduce Barry's frustration. The teacher and therapist also designed a data collection strategy for these interventions so they could monitor Barry's progress.

After three weeks the teacher reported that Barry was demonstrating less frustration (i.e., he had only been in one "altercation" with a peer) and had only thrown away three papers. He was not dropping his pencil, but was fidgeting with it a lot, so the therapist provided the teacher with three other types of grips to try. After six weeks, Barry seemed more comfortable with one of the grips and asked to keep that one. When they went back to the pre-assessment team, everyone agreed with the teacher that Barry did not require further assessment.

THE REFERRAL PROCESS

Referral is the process of either receiving a request from or making a request to others in a child's and family's interest. We use the referral process to provide the family or care provider with additional resources for problem solving, i.e., to broaden the perspectives in an attempt to understand the needs more clearly. Occupational therapists can receive referrals or make referrals, and therefore need to understand how to use this process effectively.

Receiving Referrals

The most common sources for referrals are team members from early intervention, preschool, and school-based programs. These individuals might make a referral to the occupational therapist as a result of population screening, pre-assessment processes, or as part of comprehensive assessment for special education services. We might also receive referrals from physicians who have particular medically-related concerns with daily life, or from parents who need guidance in supporting their children at home. Some states require particular documentation of referrals as part of the licensing or registration laws, be sure to check these regulations in your state.

It is common for occupational therapy personnel to design referral checklists to make it easy for others within their systems to express concerns. Referral forms also enable the therapist to guide others' thinking to be consistent with the domain of concern of occupational therapy. Some referral checklists are general in nature, sampling a wide range of skills and domains (Figure 5-16). Other referral forms have a more specific focus; these are appropriate when the therapist already has some idea of the referral concern and can ask for information that is more directed. Figure 5-17 is an example of a referral form related to sensory processing difficulties that might be used for a child with learning or behavior difficulties in school.

Novice therapists may be hesitant to make referrals, fearing that they are making poor judgements about a situation (either too leniently or too strictly). It is always good to use a more experienced professional to guide these early decisions about referrals because many times this brings up the availability of resources that the novice would not know about, and provides a mechanism for learning the system while providing services.

Making Referrals

It is also appropriate for occupational therapists to make referrals to others who may support the child and family. When we have medically-related concerns, we make referrals to physicians or nurse practitioners. We might see that a related discipline such as social work, physical therapy, speech pathology, or psy-

Occupational Therapy Referral Form

_____ has been referred for an occupational therapy evaluation. To help with the evaluation, your input is very important. Please complete this questionnaire and return to the occupational therapist. The evaluation will be completed on _____. Thank you very much for your help!

Date of Referral: _____ Teacher: _____

Why do you feel this child should be evaluated by the occupational therapist? _____

Formal Evaluations:
1. I.Q./Name of Test: _____
   Date Given: _____
   Full Score: _____
       Verbal: _____
       Performance: _____
2. Academic Levels:
   Reading: _____ Date of Assessment: _____
   Spelling: _____ Date of Assessment: _____
   Math: _____ Date of Assessment:: _____
3. Other Pertinent Evaluations:
   Speech Evaluation Results: _____
   Special Evaluations (Given by Counselor or Special Teacher of LD resource teacher): _____
   VMI: _____
   Peabody Picture Vocabulary Test: _____
4. Health Evaluation:
   Medical Problems: _____
   Health Screening Results: _____
   Medications: _____

Checklist for Occupational Therapy

Please check the statements that are pertinent to this child.

Gross Motor
_____ Seems weaker than other children his/her age
_____ Does not have the endurance other children his/her age have for an activity
_____ Difficulty with hopping, jumping, skipping, or running as compared with others his/her age
_____ Appears stiff and awkward in his/her movements
_____ Clumsy, does not appear to know how body works, bumps into others or objects, never quite sits in chair correctly
_____ Does not seem to understand concepts such as right, left, front, or back as it relates to his/her body
_____ Shies away from playground equipment. May only play on one particular item
_____ Poor posture (always seems to be leaning against something, shoulders slump forward)

Fine Motor
_____ Difficulty with drawing, coloring, tracing
_____ Performs these activities quickly and result is usually sloppy
_____ Avoids fine motor activities
_____ Problem holding pencil, grasp may be very loose or very tight
_____ Printing is too dark, too light, too large, too small
_____ Does not seem to have a dominant hand

Academic
_____ Distractible
_____ Restless
_____ Slow worker
_____ Disorganized, messy desk
_____ Short attention span
_____ Hyperactive

Figure 5-16. Occupational therapy referral form and behavior checklist. (Reprinted with permission from Dunn, W. (1991) _Pediatric Occupational Therapy: Facilitating Effective Service Provision._ Thorofare, NJ: SLACK Incorporated.)

_____ Can't follow directions
_____ Never completes assignments

Tactile Sensation
_____ Withdraws from touch
_____ Tends to wear only certain types of clothing
_____ Touches everything
_____ Avoids being close to others (doesn't like to be hugged)

Vestibular Sensation
_____ Fearful of being off the ground
_____ Doesn't like playground equipment like the merry-go-round, slide
_____ Can't seem to stop moving, craves swinging, rocking

Auditory
_____ Has difficulty pronouncing words
_____ Does not appear to understand other people
_____ Tends to repeat things to himself/herself

Visual Perception
_____ Trouble discriminating shapes, letters, or numbers
_____ Cannot complete puzzles appropriate for age
_____ Difficulty copying designs, letters or numbers
_____ Difficulty tracking (i.e., as in reading in a book or following teacher's arm movements)

Emotional
_____ Does not care to have routine changed
_____ Is easily frustrated
_____ Cannot get along with others
_____ Accident prone
_____ Deals better with a small group situation or one-to-one
_____ Frequently involves self in other people's activities

Additional information:
Please attach a sample of the child's seatwork. An example of this would be a drawing or a printing exercise.

Signature of person completing form: _____ Date: _____

Figure 5-16 continued. Occupational therapy referral form and behavior checklist. (Reprinted with permission from Dunn, W. (1991) *Pediatric Occupational Therapy: Facilitating Effective Service Provision.* Thorofare, NJ: SLACK Incorporated.)

Overreactive	**Underreactive**
Somatosensory (touch) system	
___ defensive about others touching body	___ slow to respond
___ reacts emotionally or aggressively to touch	___ doesn't notice others
___ avoids selected textures in clothing selection	___ uses poor judgment regarding personal space
___ narrow range of clothing choices	___ mouths objects frequently
___ rigid rituals in personal hygiene	___ chews on pencils
___ extremely negative about dental work	___ doesn't seem to notice when someone brushes
___ picky eater, especially regarding textures	or touches arm or back
___ avoids haircuts, hair washing	___ allows drool to remain on face
___ withdraws from splashing water	___ leaves clothing twisted on body
___ pushes washcloth/towel away	
___ cries when hair is washed and dried	
___ pulls at hats and accessories	
___ gags easily with food textures/utensils in mouth	
___ avoids tasks that are wet/messy	
___ complains about tape or glue on skin	

Figure 5-17. Common observations when sensory systems are poorly modulated. (Reprinted with permission from Dunn W. (1991) The sensorimotor systems: A framework for assessment and intervention. In F.P. Orelove & D. Sobsey (Eds.), *Educating children with multiple disabilities: A transdisciplinary approach* (2nd ed.) Baltimore, MD: Paul H. Brookes.)

Overreactive	Underreactive
Vestibular (movement) system	
___ insecure about movement experiences	___ clumsy, lethargic
___ avoids or fears movement	___ slow to respond to movement demands
___ holds head upright, even when bending/leaning	___ poor endurance, tires easily
___ avoids new positions, especially of head	___ rocks in desk/chair
___ holds onto walls or bannisters	___ craves movement
___ very clumsy on changeable surfaces, such as a field	
___ becomes disoriented after bending over sink, table	
___ becomes overly excited after a movement activity	
___ turns whole body to look at you (rather than just head)	
Proprioceptive (body position) system	
___ tense muscles	___ weak grasp
___ rigidity, diminished fluidity of	___ poor endurance for tasks
___ locks joints to stabilize movement	___ tires easily, collapses
	___ hangs on objects for support
	___ can't lift heavy objects
	___ props to support self
Visual system	
___ avoids bright lights, sunlight	___ doesn't notice when people come into the room
___ covers eyes in lighted room	___ difficulty finding objects in drawer, desk, on paper
___ watches everyone when they move around	___ trouble locating desired object on shelf, in drawer
___ covers part of the page when reading	
Auditory system	
___ overreacts to unexpected sounds	___ doesn't respond to name being called
___ easily distracted in classroom	___ seems oblivious within an active environment
___ holds hands over ears	___ makes sounds constantly
___ can't work with background noise	
___ cries about sounds in environment (e.g., hair dryer)	

Figure 5-17 continued. Common observations when sensory systems are poorly modulated. (Reprinted with permission from Dunn W. (1991) The sensorimotor systems: A framework for assessment and intervention. In F.P. Orelove & D. Sobsey (Eds.), *Educating children with multiple disabilities: A transdisciplinary approach* (2nd ed.) Baltimore, MD: Paul H. Brookes.)

chology needs to be involved in a case. It is also appropriate to make referrals to other occupational therapists with expertise that the family needs. For example, a school-based occupational therapist is not likely to be skilled at fabricating splints, even though he learned it in college. If a child needed a splint, this therapist would make a referral to another therapist with splinting expertise to ensure that the family receives the best possible services.

We also make referrals to other community agencies (see Chapter 2 on interagency collaboration) if their mission and resources will be supportive to the family. Community referrals can also include resources such as karate classes, swimming, scouts, and activity or support groups. In order to be effective as a community service provider, therapists must familiarize themselves with the options available.

REFERENCES

Collier, T. (1991). The screening process. In W. Dunn (Ed.), *Pediatric occupational therapy: Facilitating effective provision* (pp. 11-33). Thorofare, NJ: SLACK Incorporated.

Frankenburg, W.K. (1975). Criteria in screening test selection. In W. K. Frankenburg & B.W. Camp (Eds.), *Pediatric screening tests.* Springfield, IL: Thomas.

Odom, S., & Karnes, M. (1988). *Early intervention for infants & children with handicap.* Baltimore, MD: Paul H. Brookes Publishing Co.

6.

Best Practice Occupational Therapy Assessment

Winnie Dunn, PhD, OTR, FAOTA

Occupational therapists have a unique knowledge base and perspective to offer their teams; the assessment process provides a way to employ that perspective on behalf of children and families. Teams use assessment findings and interpretations to make a number of decisions about placement, programming, and service options, so skill and integrity are critical in this aspect of service provision. Tests and other assessment methods are powerful tools that must be used carefully in service to children and families (Cook, 1991); for example, certain evaluations require specific training for administration, while others require broad-based knowledge for proper interpretation. The AOTA has provided standards that outline the appropriate use of standardized tests and other evaluation techniques (Maurer, Barris, Bonder, & Gillette, 1984). Most recently, however, the AOTA endorsed the American Psychological Association's standards for test design and development (see APA, 1999).

DEFINING ASSESSMENT AND EVALUATION

Assessment is a comprehensive process through which professionals obtain information about a child and family. The term "assessment" refers to the entire process of gathering information for decision-making. The term "evaluation" refers to a specific strategy that a professional uses to gather data; we can use formal and informal evaluation methods as described below.

__Important Note:__ As this text is being written, the official AOTA position on assessment and evaluation is just the opposite of the one just described. In this single case, I will deviate from official AOTA positions in describing best practices to you. All other professionals who serve on teams serving children and families use the designation "assessment" for the overarching process, and "evaluation" for the specific activity. Therefore, in this text, we will use this more generally accepted reference so we are consistent with the interdisciplinary world of child and family practice.

All team members participate in assessment; the product of assessment may be a diagnosis, determination of eligibility, construction of an intervention plan, or a determination of whether or not comprehensive services are still required. Any activity that constitutes data-gathering can be considered part of the assessment, including records reviews, interviews, skilled observations (including by videotape), checklists, developmental, or criterion measures, and formal tests. The goal of assessment is to compile comprehensive information about a child's strengths and needs, thereby necessitating a team approach. The members of an assessment team serving a child and family can include such professionals as a special educator, psychologist, speech pathologist, classroom teacher, physician, audiologist, social worker, occupational therapist, and/or a physical therapist (along with the child, family, and/or other care providers). With each of these persons engaging in unique "perspective taking", the team can conceptualize the child's overall performance patterns and identify possible supports and barriers to performance.

Conducting evaluations as part of comprehensive assessment requires various skills. Each evaluation strategy or tool requires the professional to draw on particular abilities. Skilled observations and interviews require the professional to understand the possible reasons for performance difficulties (expressed in the referral or request), so that the professional can solicit (when interviewing) or notice (when observing) factors that will be informative to the decision-making process. Some formal assessments require special training because their administration is standardized or because advanced knowledge is necessary for proper interpretation.

PROFESSIONAL KNOWLEDGE AND SKILLS FOR BEST PRACTICE ASSESSMENT

Professionals set the tone for the assessment process, and so must be prepared to create the optimal situation. First, the professionals must be prepared with the background and competence to conduct the assessment properly; this ensures that the team can count on the data to provide a reliable picture of the child's performance and on the therapist to report and interpret the data accurately.

Professionals must focus on establishing rapport with the child and family. The characteristics of good rapport building are empathy, genuineness, warmth, respect for children, and a sense of humor (Sattler, 1988). It is the professionals' responsibility to make the child (and family and teachers) feel comfortable; professionals must display an openness to information and an acceptance of the child and family in order to put them at ease. For new professionals, it is helpful to solicit feedback regarding rapport building, including having peers watch a video of several interactions to see what patterns are present and how different individuals respond.

During assessment procedures, professionals must be so skilled at their own recording and manipulation tasks that they are "transparent" to the child (i.e., they can get the information they need without distracting or interrupting the child's performance). Any feedback or encouragement from the professional must be of a benign nature and must avoid revealing any indication of the success of the performance (i.e., "You are really working hard on this", not "that was correct").

MEASUREMENT OPTIONS IN BEST PRACTICE ASSESSMENT

There are several options for gathering data during assessment. Each option gives professionals a specific way to understand the factors that might be contributing to or interfering with performance. Occupational therapists focus attention on the referral concern to construct the overall assessment plan; knowing the characteristics of assessment options enables the therapist to select a combination of measures that reveal the child's performance strengths and needs.

Records Reviews

When we receive referrals, it is common that other team members have gathered information about the child. This can include history (including birth history, age, family structure, developmental milestones reached, achievement test history), referral concerns, or even some initial testing. When children are older, their files can contain previous testing and school records as well. It is prudent as part of assessment for the occupational therapist to review the available records. This review can provide a background for the child's needs, avoid duplication of questions for the family or teacher, and guide choices for further assessment procedures. If another professional has already given a particular measure recently, it is appropriate to use this data in your assessment interpretation rather than administering the evaluation again. Some therapists think they must administer each evaluation so they can observe the child themselves; this is not an effective use of the child or therapist's time. It is best practice to glean whatever we can from the records and then proceed with other assessment strategies.

Norm-Referenced Measurement

Norm-referenced measures (also called standardized measures) have been designed to evaluate particular behaviors; the developers collect data on typical individuals as a comparison group (i.e., the normative group). Because we are comparing the person we are testing to a comparison group, we must use the same directions and procedures for testing each time. We cannot compare performance of the person we are testing to the comparison group if we allow the person to perform in a different way.

Typically, there are very clear parameters for acceptable use of standardized measures, including an acceptable age range, type of disability and intelligence level. If a professional uses a standardized tool with an individual outside of the parameters, then the professional cannot calculate scores for this performance and must limit assessment remarks to observations.

Most norm-referenced measures yield specific score results that are translated into standard scores in order to easily compare performance against the comparison group. Figure 6.1 illustrates the relationship among the most common types of standard scores and the bell curve. The bell curve is the pictorial representation of a normal distribution of scores on any test (Sattler, 1988). The shaded area in the center represents the range of scores that are considered the "normal range". Scores above this area are better than the norm group and scores below this area are worse than the norm group.

It is important to note that percentile scores do not distribute evenly across the bell curve as other scores do. The percentile score reflects the ratio of people that scored at or above a certain level. If a person obtains a 70% score, this means that the person performed as well as or better than 70% of the people in the norm group. Because the bell curve does not evenly distribute the scores (see the middle of the bell contains 68% of the people, while the edges contain only 2%), the percentiles are more densely represented in some parts of the bell curve than others.

Teams frequently use norm-referenced measures to establish a child's performance status (e.g., level of intelligence, level of motor performance). Remember, a status measure only records the child's current capacity in an area, the nature of the standardized task does not lend itself to intervention planning. Norm-referenced measures establish a child's eligibility; you need other measures to gather data for program planning. Frequently used status measures are plotted on Figure 6-1 so you can see the comparison of a standard score on each of them. For example, an IQ score of 85 on intelligence tests is comparable to a score of 40 on the Bruininks-Oseretsky Test of Motor Proficiency. You can see what other scores would be comparable to any score by drawing a vertical line on the figure.

Criterion-Referenced Measurement

Criterion-referenced measures are designed to compare a person's performance to a previously established standard of performance (Cook, 1991). In norm-referenced testing, we are comparing the person to other individuals, while in criterion measures we are comparing him or her to a performance standard (Sattler, 1982). We use criterion measures to investigate mastery, readiness, and skill acquisition, so this information enables the team to plan programs. These are only suggested procedures for testing with criterion measures. Table 6-1 contains a summary of the features of criterion measures in comparison to norm-referenced measures.

Many developmental tests are criterion measures. Developmental tests include skills that we have come to believe represent particular age levels (e.g., when a child can stand on one foot for 10 seconds, how many one inch cubes the child can stack). When we determine that a child can do certain behaviors and not others on the criterion list, we hypothesize about the child's developmental level. There are more difficult items beyond the child's performance on criterion measures; these form the structure for designing the intervention process and ultimately provide the structure for charting progress.

Figure 6-1. Relationship of frequently used standard scores to the bell curve. Shaded area denotes normal range. (Reprinted with permission from Sattler, J. M. (1988). *Assessment of Children* (3rd Edition). San Diego, CA: Jerome M. Sattler, Publisher, Inc.)

Percent of cases within sections of bell curve	2%	13.5%	34%	34%	13.5%	2%	
Standard deviations	-3.0	-2.0	-1.0	0.0	+1.0	+2.0	+3.0
Cumulative Percentages	0.1%	2.0%	16%	50%	84%	98%	99.9%
Percentile Equivalents		1	5 10 20 30 40 50 60 70 80		90 95 99		
Z Scores	-3.0	-2.0	-1.0	0.0	+1.0	+2.0	+3.0
T Scores	20	30	40	50	60	70	80
Stanines	1	2	3 4 5 6 7		8 9		
Percent in Stanines	4%	7%	12% 17% 20% 17% 12%		7% 4%		
IQ Composite Score (SB)	52	68	84	100	116	132	148
IQ Subtest Scores (SB)	26	34	42	50	58	66	74
IQ Composite Scores (Wechsler, KABC)	55	70	85	100	115	130	145
IQ Subtest Scores (Wechsler, KABC)	1	4	7	10	13	16	19
Bruininks–Oseretsky Composite Scores	20	30	40	50	60	70	80
Bruininks–Oseretsky Subtest Scores	0	5	10	15	20	25	30
Motor Free Visual Perception Test (Perceptual Quotient)	55	70	85	100	115	130	145
Test of Visual Perceptual Skills (Composite Scores)	55	70	85	100	115	130	145
TVPS Subtest Scores	1	4	7	10	13	16	19

Table 6-1.

Comparison of Norm-Referenced and Criterion-Referenced Tests

Norm-Referenced Tests

1. Purposes: to examine individual performance in relation to a representative group; can be used to establish age levels; used for diagnosis and placement.

2. Test construction: items developed from activities hypothesized to top specified skill or performance; test items usually not related to the objective of instruction (intervention).

3. Administration: must be administered in a standard manner as specified in test manual.

4. Scoring: based on standards relative to a group; normal distribution, variability of scores (bell curve with means and standard deviations) is desired.

5. Psychometric properties: test should demonstrate reliability and validity.

6. Standards, or reference points, are the average, relative points derived from the performance of a group.

7. Evaluates individual performance in comparison to a group of persons; student competing against others.

8. May or may not have a relationship to the specific instructional content.

9. Tests may have a low degree of overlap with actual objectives of instruction.

10. Does not indicate when individuals have mastered a segment of the spectrum of instructional objective.

11. Designed to maximize variability and produce scores that are normally distributed.

12. Designed to maximize differences among individuals.

13. Requires very good diagnostic and interpretive skills, otherwise a poor aid in planning instruction.

14. Tests not sensitive to the effects of instruction.

15. Is generally not concerned with task analysis.

16. Is more formative (used at various points during instruction) than summative though it can be used both ways.

17. Interpret test scores in relation to established norms.

18. Broadly sample the domain of a particular achievement area.

19. Provide a concise summary of overall outcomes of components of achievement and ability.

20. Encourage and reward individual excellence in achievement. Emphasize performance in relation to the reference group (e.g., age, group, males).

21. Treat learning as consisting of building a structure of numerous relations among concepts.

Criterion-Referenced Tests

1. Purposes: to examine individual performance in relation to a criterion or external standards; used for program planning and evaluation because items are sensitive to effects of instruction (intervention).

2. Test construction: items developed from task analysis; test items are related to the objective of instruction (intervention).

3. Administration: may or may not be administered in a standard manner.

4. Scoring: based on absolute standards; variability of scores is not obtained because mastery of skills is desired.

5. Psychometric properties: test should demonstrate reliability and validity.

6. Reference points are fixed at specific cut-offs, which are predetermined by consensus of experts.

7. Evaluates individual performance in relation to a fixed standard; student competing against self.

8. Is content specific.

9. Tests are directly referenced to the objectives of instruction.

10. Identifies those segments of the spectrum of objectives the individual has mastered.

11. Variability of scores is not desired; mastery is expected.

12. Designed to discriminate between successive performances of one individual.

13. Geared to provide direct information for use in planning instruction.

14. Tests are very sensitive to the effects of instruction.

15. Depends on task analysis.

16. Is more summative (used at the end of instruction) than formative or is strictly diagnostic.

17. Report which, or how many, of a set of specific achievement goals the individual has reached.

18. Sample a limited number of specifically defined goals.

19., Report specific and detailed information on pupil achievement.

20. Emphasize mastery of specific subject matter by all pupils.

21. Treat learning as if it were acquired by adding separate, discrete units to the collection of things learned.

Adapted from Gilfoyle, E. M. (Ed.) (1981). Training: Occupational therapy education management in schools. Rockville, MD: AOTA.

Some criterion measures report age or grade equivalent scores. They are calculated by finding the average score for children of the specified age (i.e., in years and months) or grade (i.e., in grade and tenth of a grade level). **The American Psychological Association (1999) strongly urges that we discontinue using age equivalent scores because they are misleading.** The units of measure are not equivalent as they are in standard scores, and yet people can view them in the same way that they view standard scores. For example, a preschooler's development of fine motor skills is much more rapid than a third grader's, therefore a 3 month change at 4 years will represent much more skill development than that same amount of change (i.e., 3 months) when the child is 8-years-old.

Informal Measures

An informal measure is a tool constructed by the professional to gather data about a particular situation or performance. We can construct a plan for observation, completing a questionnaire, or engaging the child in a set of movements or other actions. When therapists select informal measures they rely on their scientific reasoning knowledge to guide their data-recording and interpretations. We might design a list of questions for the teacher to respond to regarding the child's behaviors in the classroom or ask the teacher's aide to collect data on a particular behavior for a period of time to get a record of the patterns of performance. Sometimes there are informal tools that have been designed in a particular work setting, and all the therapists in that setting use the forms as part of their agency's assessment process.

When the referral concern is about a particular performance, the therapist might work with the child on that activity, changing aspects of it as they go to see how the child responds. For example, if a teacher states that the child is having trouble with math worksheets, the therapist might first observe the child in the classroom and then take the math worksheets and the student into a separate space (to watch the performance carefully to hypothesize about what might be interfering with the task performance). During this type of informal assessment, the therapist is formulating ideas for intervention while conducting the assessment.

Commonly used techniques for informal assessment are skilled observations, interviewing, ecological assessment, and activity analysis.

Skilled Observations

Skilled observation is the most critical assessment tool available to occupational therapists. Because occupational therapists are trained to notice and interpret behaviors in a particular manner (based on our knowledge and skills), we call this process *skilled* observation. Skilled observation enables us to capture the nature of the behavior in its natural context, and therefore reveals what might be supporting or interfering with the desired performance. Skilled observation is also the most difficult assessment method because it requires the therapists to bring all of their knowledge to bear (e.g., all their practice model knowledge, their clinical reasoning skills) on the moment-by-moment interaction between the person and the environment.

Through skilled observation, we can determine a child's use of cognition, sensory processing, motor, and psychosocial skills during daily life. We can identify what environmental stimuli enable a child to focus or what is distracting. We can see the process the child uses to solve problems, and how the child selects to engage when not being directed by others. All of these aspects of performance can be tested in isolation, but we do not know whether they are interfering with performance until we conduct a skilled observation in the natural context. For example, perhaps the therapist observed that the child took a longer time to gather materials for the reading group than the other children, perhaps the mother complained about the child's frustration when trying to find his favorite toy. Both the mother and the therapist provide skilled observation data. The therapist hypothesizes that there may be a visual perception problem and so decides to administer the Test of Visual Perceptual skills to test this hypothesis. The score profile indicates that the child has visual figure ground perception difficulties (when compared to the norm group), thus verifying the hypothesis and linking poor visual figure ground perception to difficulty with performance at home and school. This formal test score merely verifies the nature of the problem that occurs in this child's daily life.

There are several particular competencies required to conduct a skilled observation, including monitoring engagement, attending to environmental features, and defining behaviors in observable and neutral terms (Cook, 1991).

Monitoring Engagement

When conducting a skilled observation, the therapist must be careful not to interfere with the natural course of events being observed. This means that we must remain in the background of the activity and not become the person directing the activity or creating reinforcement by responding to the child directly. When a therapist becomes overly engaged, he or she becomes part of the activity and loses the vantage point that facilitates good data recording. For example, the therapist who gets too involved in a conversation with a child during the skilled observation may miss the directions from the teacher to the class or may not notice the other children's responses to the target child. We must make sure that we are available for all possible opportunities to notice what might be supporting or interfering with performance.

Attending to Environmental Features

Occupational therapists are interested in the child's performance in daily life. Skilled observation provides an excellent window for noticing what the environmental features are and to begin hypothesizing how these features are contributing to or interfering with performance. Initially, the therapist records objective statements about the environment and then later can consider the impact of these environmental features on the child's performance. The therapist must record information about all aspects of context as outlined in the AOTA Uniform Terminology document (see Appendix A), i.e., physical, social, cultural, and temporal features. Some aspects of context remain stable during a skilled observation (e.g., physical room layout) and form the backdrop, while other aspects of context are fluid and interact with the child's performance (e.g., the teacher giving directions and the children following along) and must be recorded along with the child's responses. By recording in this manner, the therapist can review and interpret the information later, remaining open and available to observe during the session.

Defining Behaviors in Observable and Neutral Terms

Skilled observation requires therapists to record the actual behaviors that have occurred, without interpreting the meaning of the behavior or generating hypotheses. This is an important skill when working on an interdisciplinary or transdisciplinary team because colleagues from other disciplines might interpret a behavior differently than we do from an occupational therapy perspective. If we only record our interpretations, it is difficult to get others' perspectives about the meaning of the core behavior.

For example, an infant squirms, cries, and pushes away from the care provider when she tries to pick the child up from the bassinet. A sensory processing interpretation would be that the child is having difficulty organizing the vestibular input provided when moving from supine to upright. A psychoanalytic interpretation would focus on the child's difficulty attaching to a person other than the mother. A behavioral interpretation would address the child's association of this care provider and activities that are undesirable (the developmental "work" to come). If the occupational therapist records "the child is hypersensitive to movement" (i.e., the interpretation of the behavior, not the behavior itself), then the other possibilities offered by the other perspectives become unavailable to the team for consideration. In order to have the best possible chance for accurate interpretations of our assessment data, we must stay open to possibilities. The quality of our intervention plans is dependent on the accuracy of our observations and interpretations of them.

Interviews

Interviewing is an artful task in which the professional is seeking information from an informant (e.g., the teacher, the parent, a sibling or friend, and/or the child being evaluated). Although this is a data-gathering tool, interviewing is also a time for establishing rapport. The comfort (or discomfort) a person feels will influence the amount of information they feel comfortable providing.

There are a number of ways to conduct an interview, and each needs to be selected based on the information needed and the comfort level of the interviewee. Parents may feel more comfortable in their homes, or may wish to get away for a little while and be interviewed at a coffee shop. Some teachers will select the teacher's lounge at school, while others will find this environment less private than they like and will choose another location. Most of the time a face to face interview is better, but there may be situations in which the person will suggest a phone interview (usually related to time or distance restraints). There are also occasions when the therapist will send a questionnaire along ahead of time so the person has time to formulate their thoughts before the interview; as with other techniques, it is important to invite the person to help you decide what is best. You can say, "would it be helpful for you to receive some questions ahead of time, or would you prefer to just chat with me when we meet?" This gives the person an opportunity to participate in the process in the most comfortable way.

Interviewing requires the therapist to be very focused on both the information needed and what the person is relaying in the conversation. Some interviews require very explicit information (e.g., developmental milestones), while others need to be more open-ended to elicit descriptive information (e.g., "tell me about mealtime"). When we begin with specific questions and work toward more general ones, it is called a "reversed funnel" sequence interview; when we begin with very general questions and work toward specific information, this is called a "funnel" interview (Cook, 1991). For example, if we ask a parent to discuss their specific referral concern, and then branch to other issues as the parent talks, it would be a reversed funnel sequence. But if we ask the parent to describe their home life, and work toward their specific concerns, it would be a funnel-sequenced interview.

When formulating interview questions, it is important to ask mostly open-ended questions that do not indicate a right or wrong response. We use words like "describe" to encourage the person to elaborate on the issue (Cook, 1991). Questions that encourage a "yes" or "no" response do not encourage elaboration. It is helpful to reflect back to the person what they have just said to make sure that you clearly understand their perspective, and to indicate that you are listening actively to what they are saying. Additionally, it is important to use positive nonverbal communication, such as eye contact, open postures, leaning forward, and facial expressions, to indicate involvement in the conversation. Therapists can also take notes during the interview to indicate their interest in the person's comments. All of these strategies increase the likelihood that the informant will share their perspectives and concerns candidly and therefore increase the possible insights into the performance situation.

Ecological Measures

Ecological assessment includes measurement of the environmental variables themselves and measurement of the interaction among the child, the environment, and the task. Ecological assessment is critical to best practice occupational therapy; it provides the backdrop for the child's performance and can either interfere with or support performance. Children's skills and liabilities in performance are only relevant in their natural contexts; without ecological assessment data, we cannot know the relationship between the children's skills and the environmental features. Sometimes the environment is helpful to the child (e.g., the toothbrush and toothpaste on the sink cues the child to brush his or her teeth). Other times the environment is interfering (e.g., when there is too much clutter on the sink to see the toothbrush). Ecological assessment is dynamic so that the professional can capture the salient features of the environmental supports and barriers to performance.

There are a number of strategies for conducting ecological assessment, and we frequently conduct these assessments with other discipline colleagues. Figure 6-2 illustrates an ecological assessment method for adapting environments and activities to support children in their natural context. In this strategy, we consider both what the typical child in the situation does and what the target child does; this comparison helps the team to figure out possible adaptations to support the child. Table 6-2 contains a list of additional measures available; they are reviewed in Law, Baum, & Dunn (2000) if you require additional information.

Activity Analyses

Activity analysis is a hallmark of occupational therapy practice. The purpose of activity analysis is to identify the features of the task so that we can change some aspects when needed to support more efficient and satisfying task performance. For example, when analyzing the task of completing seatwork, the therapist con-

Ecologically-Based Individualized Adaptation Inventory

Environment: Classroom snack time area
Activity: Eating snack, drinking juice
Plan

A Nonhandicapped Toddler Inventory	An Inventory of Beth	Skills Beth Can Probably Acquire	Skills Beth May Not Acquire	Adaptation Possibilities	Observation Assessment	Daily Plan
Moves to snack area	Cannot get to table by self	Can learn to walk		Adult can assist by using facilitation	Beth walked well when facilitation at hips was used	Teacher will fade assistance as demonstrated by therapist. Aim for walking well with 1 hand held w/in 1month
Position self at table	Cannot get chair out to sit down	Can learn to get chair out; rotate to sit		Adult can assist with pulling chair out & facilitating rotation to sit	She pulled out chair with hand over hand; rotated & sat with facilitation from trunk	Fade assistance in hand over hand for pulling chair; aim for pulling w/o increased tone in arms; teacher will fade facilitation for rotating to sit as demonstrated by therapist.
Take utensils when passed out	Can grasp large items					Beth will take utensils by self
Take food when passed out	Can grasp large items (cookies) but not small pieces		May not learn to grasp very small items	Try smaller fork for small pieces or only give large finger foods	Fork worked with "stabbable" foods	Use toddler fork
Hold cup for liquid to be poured into	Cup is held sideways	Can learn to hold cup straight		Use cup with two handles	Beth held cup sides with hands through handles	Use two-handled cup
Eat food	Can finger feed					Beth will finger feed by self
Drink liquid	Can drink but not hold cup to mouth	Can learn to hold cup		Adult assistance to facilitate cup to mouth pattern	Minimal help needed to raise cup to mouth	Fade assistance to verbal cues "pick up cup" to no cues
Request more if desired	Vocalizes for more		May not learn to talk	Use picture communication board during snack	A picture board with cup & correct food was used when prompted "Do you want more?" She vocalized at same time	Teacher will make picture board daily with cup and correct food. Place board before Beth and watch for her to use alone. If she does not indicate that she wants more, verbally prompt. Use magnetic stove board & magnet pictures. Reinforce all joint points and vocalizations.

Figure 6-2. Sample ecological assessment for a preschooler at snack time. (Reprinted with permission from *The Journal of the Association for the Severely Handicapped.*)

Table 6-2.

Measures of Person-Environment-Occupation Variables

Aspect Measured	Title of Measure	Source Information
Person/ Environment	The Parenting Stress Index	Psychological Assesment Resources (P.O. BOX 998, Odessa, FL 33556, (800) 331-TEST)
	Coping Inventory	By Shirley Zeitlin (1985). Scholastic Testing Service Inc., Bensenville, IL 60106-1617
	Early Coping Inventory	By Shirley Zeitlin, Gordon Williamson, and Margery Szczepanski (1988). Scholastic Testing Service Inc., Bensenville, IL 60106-1617
	Play History	Bryze, K. (1997). Narrative contributions to the Play History. In Parham, L. D., & Fazio, L. S. (Eds.). *Play in occupational therapy for children*, (pp. 23-34). St. Louis, MO: C.V. Mosby.
		Behnke, C., & Fetkovich, M. M. (1984). Examining the reliability and validity of the Play History, *American Journal of Occupational Therapy*, 38, 94-100.
		Takata, N. (1974). Play as a prescription. In M. Reilly (Ed.). *Play as exploratory learning* (pp. 209-246). Beverly Hills, CA: Sage.
	Pediatric Evaluation of Disability Inventory	PEDI Research Group, Dept. of Rehabilitation Medicine, New England Medical Center Hospital, #75 K/R, 750 Washington Street, Boston, MA, 02111-1901
	Assessment of Ludic Behavior	Ferland, F. (1997). *Play, children with physical disabilities and occupational therapy.* Ottawa, Ontario, Canada: University of Ottawa.
	Sensory Profile	By Winnie Dunn (1999). The Psychological Corporation, 555 Academic Court, San Antonio, TX 78204-2498, (800) 211-8378, www.tpcweb.com
	Infant Toddler Sensory Profile	By Winnie Dunn (in press). The Psychological Corporation, 555 Academic Court, San Antonio, TX 78204-2498, (800) 211-8378, www.tpcweb.com
Person/ Occupation	Test of Playfulness	Currently available primarily for research purposes by contacting the author: Anita Bundy, ScD, OTR, Department of Occupational Therapy, OT Building, Colorado State University, Ft. Collins, CO 80523. fax: (970) 491-6290. Bundy@cahs.colostate.edu
	Revised Knox Preschool Play Scale	Knox, S. (1997). Development and current use of the Knox Preschool Play Scale. In L. D. Parham & L. S. Fazio (Eds.), *Play in occupational therapy for children*, (pp. 35-51). St. Louis, MO: C.V. Mosby.
	AAMD Adaptive Behavior Scales	American Association on Mental Deficiency, 5101 Wisconsin A Avenue NW, Washington DC 20016
	Woodcock Johnson Scales of Independent Behavior	By R.Bruininks, R. Woodcock, R. Weatherman & B.Hill, DLM Teaching Resources, Allen, TX 75002
	Vineland Adaptive Behavior Scale	By S. Sparrow, D. Balla, & D. Cicchetti, American Guidance Service Inc., Circle Pines, MN 55014-796
	Child Behavior Inventory of Playfulness	Rogers, C. S., Impara, J. C., Frary, R. B., Harris, T., Meeks, A., Semanic-Lauth, S., & Reynolds, M. R. (1998). Measuring playfulness: Development of the Child Behaviors Inventory of Playfulness. In S. Reifel (Ed.). *Play & Culture Studies* (Vol. 1), (pp. 121-136). Greenwich, CT: Ablex.

Table 6-2 continued.

Person/ Environment/ Occupation	School Function Assessment	Psychological Foundation, Skill Builders Division (555 Academic Court, San Antonio, TX 78204, (800) 228-0752).
	Canadian Occupational Performance Measure	Law, M., Baptiste, S., Carswell, A., McColl, M. A., Polatajko, H., & Pollock, N. (1998). *The Canadian Occupational performance measure* (3rd Edition). Toronto, Canada: CAOT.
	Transdisciplinary Play Based Assessment	Linder, T. W. (1993). *Transdisciplinary Play-Based Assessment: A functional approach to working with young children* (Rev. edition). Baltimore, MD: Paul H. Brookes.
Environment	Test of Environmental Support-iveness	Currently available primarily for research purposes by contacting the author: Anita Bundy, ScD, OTR, Department of Occupational Therapy, OT Building, Colorado State University, Ft. Collins, CO 80523. fax: (970) 491-6290. Bundy@cahs.colostate.edu
	Home Observation for Measure-ment of the Environment	Infant Toddler, Early Childhood and Middle Childhood versions are available from Home Inventory LLC, c/o Lorraine Coulson, 13 Saxony Circle, Little Rock, AR 72209. Phone and fax: (501) 565-7627; e-mail lrcoulson@ualr.edu. Cost for the manual, containing all three scales is $15.00 plus $6.00 shipping and handling. Protocol sheets for the Infant Toddler Scale are $7.50/50. Others are $.35 each. Information about the Adolescent version is available from Dr. Robert Bradley (rhbradley@ualr.edu).
	Early Childhood Environment Rating Scale	National Network for Child Care (NNCC). Parris, P.L. S. & DeBord, K. (1997). *Early Childhood Environment Rating Scale*. Raleigh, NC: North Carolina State University Cooperative Extension Service.
	School-Age Care Environment Rating Scale	National Network for Child Care (NNCC). Parris, P.L. S. & DeBord, K. (1997). *School-Age Care Environment Rating Scale*. Raleigh, NC: North Carolina State University Cooperative Extension Service.

Information from Law, M., Baum, C., & Dunn, W. (2000). Measuring Occupational Performance: A guide to best practice. Thorofare, NJ: SLACK Incorporated.

siders the child's sitting posture and position, the grip on the pencil, the type of materials (e.g., paper, workbook, textbook), the cognitive demands of the task, and the length of time required for a typical child to complete the task. The therapist would assess the contribution or barrier created by each feature as part of the activity analysis. This information leads directly into intervention planning (e.g., if the child is writing too randomly on the page, the therapist might suggest lined paper, or might even enhance the lines with a marker to make them more obvious to the child). If the task is too hard for the child, the therapist might suggest smaller amounts to complete at a time or the use of a peer tutor.

Activity analysis is a strong tool that occupational therapists bring to their teams; it is part of our core knowledge for the discipline. We understand the nature of task performance (i.e., what it takes to be successful and satisfied when doing things). We also have scientific reasoning information regarding the individual's capacity to perform, the characteristics of objects and materials, and the cognitive and psychosocial features of the actual task performance. We therefore recognize how to make things harder or easier, simpler or more complex by changing some aspect of the situation. Other team members may recognize the nature of the problem, but have not been trained in the art of "adjusting" task features to support performance.

PARAMETERS FOR BEST PRACTICE ASSESSMENT

Occupational therapists are concerned with performance in daily life. This focus needs to be evident throughout the occupational therapy process, but is particularly important during assessment because assessment sets the stage for all subsequent intervention and follow-up activities. The first and primary focus of best practice occupational therapy assessment is finding out *what the person wants and needs to do*. The second issue in best practice assessment is determining *where the person needs to perform*. After these two issues are addressed, the occupational therapist *identifies the person, task, and environmental variables that are supporting and creating barriers to performance*; this is the data from which we build intervention recommendations.

In standard practice, there is a greater focus on assessing the child's skills and liabilities and speculating how these person variables are having an impact on performance. In best practice assessment, we maintain our focus on the performance issues in their natural contexts.

STRUCTURE OF BEST PRACTICE OCCUPATIONAL THERAPY ASSESSMENT

When designing best practice occupational therapy assessment, the occupational therapist organizes the work by beginning with the performance in context and ending with assessment of *only those person variables* that need further attention to understand the performance issue more clearly.

We might characterize the evaluations available for assessment in accordance with the Person Environment Occupation conceptual framework (Law, Baum, & Dunn, 2000). Table 6-2 provides a summary of assessment tools in these categories (i.e., P=person variable measure; E= environmental variable measure; O= occupation variable measure; PE= person/ environment measure; EO= environment/ occupation measure; PO= person/ occupation measure; PEO= person/ environment/ occupation measure).

Occupationally-Focused Assessment: What the Child/Providers Want and Need for the Child to Do

The referral concern provides the best starting place for guidance about the performance focus for assessment. A parent may be concerned about how to play with the child, a teacher might be concerned that a student with severe disabilities needs to develop eating skills, or a school-to-work coordinator may want assistance in selecting a well matched job for an adolescent. These statements about needs for performance indicate where the occupational therapy assessment begins.

The most common strategies for assessing occupation are skilled observation and interviewing. These two techniques provide a means for understanding why this performance is a priority, the factors that may be supporting and creating barriers to performance, and what would constitute satisfying performance. Therapists also need to characterize the child's current approach to the task of interest; sometimes children approach performance in an unusual, but successful manner (i.e., they are satisfied with how they do it), but others may wish for the child to conduct themselves differently or believe that a different approach would solve the performance problem.

For example, it is common for teachers to want children to have a mature tripod grasp of writing utensils for classroom work; since this is how most children write the best, they believe this grasp is related to completing schoolwork efficiently. However some children will hold the writing utensil a different, but functional way while working. In addressing performance, the occupational therapist can determine the need, utility, and feasibility of changing the grasping pattern. The therapist will use clinical reasoning to determine whether the current grasping pattern is efficient for the child in completing schoolwork, and whether the grasping pattern presents any risks for malformations, skin breakdowns, or joint deformities (which would ultimately interfere with schoolwork performance). The therapist can also consider whether it is possible for the child to use a different grasping pattern and, if possible, the length of time it would take for the child to change and regain efficiency. The therapist will also be thinking about adaptations to using the writing utensil in consideration of all possibilities for functional written communication in schoolwork.

There are several evaluation tools available to characterize overall occupational performance. *The Canadian Occupational Performance Measure* (COPM) is a tool that solicits the child (if appropriate), family, and/or teacher to identify performance issues in activities of daily living, productive activity, and leisure. The COPM also asks the person to characterize the level of competence; and rate satisfaction of that performance competence (Law, Polatajko, Pollock, McColl, Carswell, & Baptiste, 1994). One of the most interesting things about the COPM is that it supports the idea that less than perfect performance is still satisfying and therefore acceptable. Intervention planning and goal setting emerges from the COPM in relation to those performance areas that are not satisfying to the person and family. In the case study of Tammy, the therapists used the COPM as part of their assessment plan (see Chapter 10).

The *School Function Assessment* (SFA) is also a performance in context measure. Teachers complete the form, rating the child's level of function in 14 performance areas at school; they report whether the child needs accommodations or assistance to complete the school tasks of interest. In the case study of Peter, we illustrate the SFA in use (see Chapter 10).

Several authors have also created adaptive behavior scales, or measures of the child's ability to engage in purposeful interaction with persons, objects, and situations (Cook, 1991). Typically, the rater characterizes the child's ability to perform the functional life tasks, including personal care skills, functional communication, money handling, social interactions, self direction and coping skills. The Vineland Adaptive Behavior Scales and the Woodcock Johnson Scales of Independent Behavior are most commonly used by interdisciplinary team members. The Coping Inventory (Williamson & Szczepanski, 1999) characterizes the person's responses to internal and external forces; we illustrate the Coping Inventory with Peter (see Chapter 10).

Occupational therapists have addressed the issue of play as a critical role for children (Knox, 2000; Bundy, 1997). As Table 6-2 indicates, there are several measures available to evaluate aspects of play in children. Linder (1993) developed the Transdisciplinary Play-Based Assessment strategy, which enables the team to work collaboratively to identify children's performance issues while observing the child playing. This is a great team strategy because everyone learns about the others' perspectives while conducting the assessment; additionally, the child is frequently more comfortable in this assessment setting because the activities can be familiar.

Contextually-Based Assessment

Although many of the occupational performance assessment strategies include performance in context, it is also important to consider assessment of the environment itself. This information is helpful for placement decisions (i.e., is this or that setting a better match for the child) and for resource acquisition (i.e., what will it take to make this environment user-friendly, or accessible to the child). For example, the Home Observation for Measurement of the Environment (HOME) measures the content, quality, and responsiveness of home environments (Caldwell & Bradley, 1978). Other scales measure the service setting environment (e.g., the Early Childhood Environment Rating Scale and the School Age Care Environment Rating Scale, see Table 6-2).

Other contextual measures consider the relationship between the person and the environment. The Coping Inventory and the Early Coping Inventory provide a structure for characterizing the child's responses to internal and external stressors, with the recognition that there is a level of stress that is motivating to act and a level that interferes with performance. The Pediatric Evaluation of Disability Inventory (PEDI) provides a method for recording the impact of the child's disability on function within their living environments. The Sensory Profile and the Infant Toddler Sensory Profile solicit the caregivers perspective on how their children respond to sensory events in the daily living environment. By reviewing these tools, therapists can determine which would provide useful environmental function information for the occupational therapy assessment process. Table 6-2 contains a list of measures that evaluate the environment and the person/environment variables.

Person Variable Assessment

The final area for best practice occupational therapy assessment is the evaluation of the child's skills and difficulties in relation to the occupational performance need. When using a best practice assessment strategy, the occupational therapist already has quite a bit of information about the child's skills and difficulties from the records reviews, skilled observations, and interviews related to the occupational performance of interest. We must not discount or ignore this vital information about the child's abilities, because use of one's abilities during performance is more important than any assessment of skills in isolation. We use formal evaluations to verify a child's skills (or difficulties) or to obtain more specific information to support more refined program planning. In this section we will discuss both skilled observation during performance (thereby embellishing information from the section on occupationally-focused assessment) and the use of formal tests to verify and specify performance component skills and difficulties. For occupational therapy, "person variables" fall into three categories: sensorimotor, cognitive, and psychosocial aspects of performance (see Appendix A).

Skilled Observation During Performance to Reveal Performance Component Skills and Difficulties

The most artful part of best practice occupational therapy assessment is recognizing the performance component skills and difficulties as they present themselves during performance in daily life. With appropriate training and practice, anyone can administer a formal test of skills. However, it takes clinical reasoning skills to glean this information from day-to-day activities. In this section we will consider some ways to recognize the sensorimotor, cognitive, and psychosocial performance components in children's daily performance.

The best way to develop these skills is to practice. Watch others perform and identify the sensorimotor, cognitive, and psychosocial aspects of the performance. View videotapes with your peers and talk about the performance components that are characterized in the people's behaviors. Make this aspect of your clinical reasoning part of the fabric of your everyday thinking.

Sensory Processing

Sensory information forms the basis for our brain's ability to recognize and derive meaning from the world. Children can have difficulty receiving sensory information due to a structural defect in the sensory organ itself (e.g., with visual and hearing impairments), or they can have difficulty deriving meaning from the sensory information they receive (Kandel, Schwartz, & Jessell, 2000; Dunn, 1997). To discriminate these functions, we look for any signs of noticing stimuli. For example, even premature infants will have autonomic nervous system (ANS) responses to stimuli when they notice them (e.g., eyes dilating). Children with non-functioning sensory organs will not have ANS reactions because their nervous systems have not taken in any information.

Processing Touch Input. The tactile system is one of the basic sensory systems whose job is to tell the child where the child ends and the world begins (i.e., the "boundary" of the child's body) (Dunn, 1997). As with all sensory systems, the tactile system is modulated between arousing and calming, organized touch; modulation is frequently disrupted in children who have disabilities affecting the CNS. Children with too little arousal to touch may have a lot of cuts, bruises, or burns that indicate the child's lack of awareness of the stimuli causing the injuries. Children who are overly attentive to touch may be very active during observations in daily life because they are trying to "get away" from the uncomfortable stimuli. These children may also get into fights a lot at school, thinking others are "shoving" them when they are merely bumping into them in the normal course of moving about the room. Parents may report narrow clothing or food choices, suggesting some intolerance for textures.

Processing Proprioceptive Input. The brain receives information from the muscles, tendons, and joints to provide a map of our body positions (i.e., proprioception). Therefore, we can take note of behaviors that indicate joint, muscle, and postural integrity to evaluate proprioception. When children tire easily, seem lethargic, prop their heads in their hands, or hang on others, we can suspect poor proprioceptive feedback. Children can also demonstrate too much proprioceptive activity when they have heightened muscle tone; this suggests poor inhibitory control from higher brain centers onto the neurons and muscles at the limbs. In Figure 6-3, Nicholas is playing cards. He needs to use his proprioceptors to hold his wrist, hand, and forearm in a stable position. If Nicholas had poor proprioception, he might drop the cards, prop his forearms on the table, or display a more imprecise finger pattern to hold the cards.

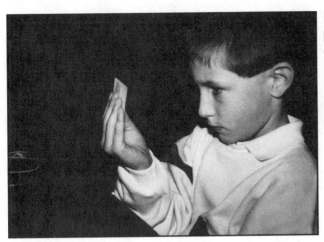

Figure 6-3. Nicholas demonstrates a modified pincer grasping pattern to hold the card and examine it. Proprioceptive feedback supports this hand position. (Reprinted with permission from Dunn W. (1991). *Pediatric Occupational Therapy: Facilitating Effective Service Provision.* Thorofare, NJ: SLACK Incorporated.)

Processing Vestibular Input. The vestibular system tells the brain about the movements we make in relation to gravity. Children tell us with strong behavioral messages about their responsiveness to movement. Some children will seek out movements, even those that appear dangerous; other children will demonstrate fear or avoid activities that have vestibular challenges, such as climbing or riding roller coasters. But this system can affect simple daily life activities as well. A child who is overly sensitive to vestibular input might become disoriented after turning to reach the soap in the shower a few times or from bending over to tie shoes.

Processing Visual Input. The visual system maps the environment. During skilled observations we look for children to attend to tasks with their eyes; skilled hand use is thwarted if the child is not watching the hands during tasks. When children's movement accuracy is poor (e.g., can't stay between lines when writing or cutting, misses the glass when reaching), we can suspect poor visual processing (see the following Perceptual Skills section for more information).

Processing Auditory Input. Although the auditory system is not the primary domain for occupational therapists, we can contribute to the team's understanding of this system from a functional perspective through our skilled observations. We observe whether the child is distracted by particular sounds or whether the child makes sounds during activities. Making sounds can provide an even auditory background for activity or it can interfere with performance, so we have to be careful to record and interpret our observations correctly.

Processing Olfactory and Gustatory Input. These are the chemical senses; they have obvious impact on eating, but they can also affect the child's level of arousal for tasks. If an examiner is wearing strong cologne or has used scented soaps, this can affect the child's level of arousal. For some people, sweet smells are irritating, while for others it may be calming because it reminds them of a comforting time.

Recognizing the sensory processing features of a child's performance is a unique gift that occupational therapists give their teams and families. No other discipline studies sensory processing in their entry preparation; this perspective enriches the discussion of performance needs and it is the occupational therapists' responsibility to provide guidance and leadership regarding this perspective.

Perceptual Skills

Perception is a cognitive ability to interpret the sensory information the brain receives. There are many types of perception, based on the many ways that the brain receives and makes sense out of the information available. Perceptual difficulties can interfere with many aspects of daily life; as occupational therapists we are concerned about perceptual difficulties as they impact living. Although there are formal tests of perceptual skills, these scores are irrelevant if the child is functioning successfully at school and at home. Table 6-3 contains a list of perceptual terms, their definitions, and an example of when this perceptual ability is used in daily life. Figures 6-4 and 6-5 illustrate the difference in the impact of perceptual abilities of Jake, a 2-year-old, and Jamie, a six-year old, as they try to use scissors. Jake is watching his hands and can open and close the scissors,

Table 6-3.

Functional Application of Common Perceptual Terms

Word	Definition	Example
Discrimination	The ability to identify the similarities and differences among stimuli.	Recognizing a pencil from a pen. Hearing the differences between similar words (e.g., bat and pat).
Sequencing	The ability to place stimuli in their proper order.	Completing a task in specified order. Writing letters of one's name in correct order.
Memory	The ability to recall stimuli.	Remembering phone number. Remembering what someone has asked you to do.
Closure	The ability to recognize existence of the whole form with only a portion of the stimulus available.	Knowing that it is a shoe and the rest of it is under the bed.
Figure-Ground	The ability to focus on the important stimuli and screen out unimportant background.	Finding an item in the junk drawer. Finding something in a busy picture. Focusing on boarding call and screening out the other airport noises.
Matching	The ability to identify the critical features of stimuli and categorize them by these characteristics.	Coordinating an outfit to wear. Picking out all the black jelly beans.
Visual-Motor/Auditory-Motor	The ability to coordinate the stimulus with the corresponding motor actions.	Tracing a picture. Following an oral direction. Stringing popcorn for the tree.
Spatial Relationships	The ability to recognize the proper relationships among stimuli.	Placing picture puzzle pieces in their proper orientation. Putting appliances in their proper place on the shelf.
Form Constancy	The ability to recognize the critical features of stimuli.	Sorting the laundry. Collecting all the cups from around the house after a party.

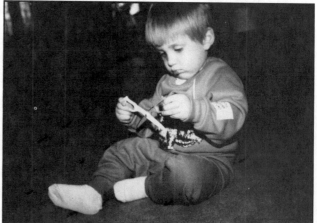

Figure 6-4. Jake (2-year-old) understands the use of scissors but cannot orient them properly for use. (Reprinted with permission from Dunn W. (1991). *Pediatric Occupational Therapy: Facilitating Effective Service Provision.* Thorofare, NJ: SLACK Incorporated.)

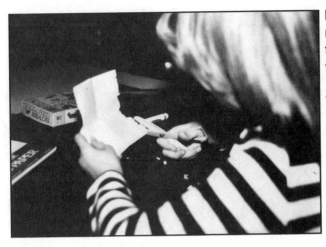

Figure 6-5. Jamie (6-year-old) has mastered both motor and perceptual performance components to use the scissors. (Reprinted with permission from Dunn W. (1991). *Pediatric Occupational Therapy: Facilitating Effective Service Provision.* Thorofare, NJ: SLACK Incorporated.)

but cannot orient them properly for cutting. Jamie can integrate her hand use and eye hand coordination to cut precisely. (Incidentally, they both demonstrate good postural control.)

Neuromuscular Performance

The neuromuscular system provides the background for our movements (i.e., the stability and postural control to maintain our relationship to gravity while we do other things). Because of this essential function, occupational therapists must document neuromuscular integrity as part of every skilled observation.

Influence of Reflexes. Particularly with very young children, therapists attend to the influence of primitive reflexes on performance. During early development the reflexes introduce the child to movement possibilities. For example, the asymmetrical tonic neck reflex places the child's head and eyes in position with an extended arm, a preliminary introduction to reaching out for objects in the environment. Other reflexes introduce the possibility of rolling or stepping. For most children, these early patterns become integrated with more volitional movements as they explore the environment and their own bodies.

When conducting skilled observations, occupational therapists look for the residual influence of primitive reflexes, that is, they consider whether any reflex patterns are interfering with the child's performance. For example, if a child had difficulty keeping legs bent for crawling during play, we may hypothesize that the tonic labyrinthine reflex is interfering with play (i.e., because when the child raises the head to look, there would be a tendency for the legs to straighten).

Range of Motion, Muscle Tone, and Soft Tissue Integrity. When serving children, it is best practice to evaluate range of motion, muscle tone, and soft tissue integrity during daily life. Are there movement restrictions that appear to be due to structural limitations; does the child compensate for typical use of joints with other movement patterns? Do some muscle groups appear more predominant in functional tasks than others? For example, if a child moves the entire trunk to reach, we might want to check on the range of motion and soft tissue integrity in the shoulder because this movement adaptation could be due to restrictions in the shoulder region. We might also hypothesize that increased muscle tone is "locking" the joint in place. The therapist can follow up by palpating the muscles during movement to determine the nature of the restriction in movement.

Strength and Endurance. To evaluate strength during functional tasks, we consider the amount of resistance the child faces during performance. For example, pedaling a bicycle requires the child to move against the resistance of the bicycle, body weight, and the surface tension on the ground. Walking up stairs requires moving against the resistance of gravity and the weight of the leg when lifting it to step. We consider endurance in relation to time (i.e., how long the child can participate before fatigue interferes with performance). We must be sure to discriminate the child's interest or tolerance for the task from endurance (Cook, 1991). A child may be able get dressed in the morning (task tolerance) but it may take an hour to finish (endurance), which is likely to interfere with the family's morning routine.

Figure 6-6. Jake demonstrates adequate posture control to interact with objects. (Reprinted with permission from Dunn W. (1991). *Pediatric Occupational Therapy: Facilitating Effective Service Provision.* Thorofare, NJ: SLACK Incorporated.)

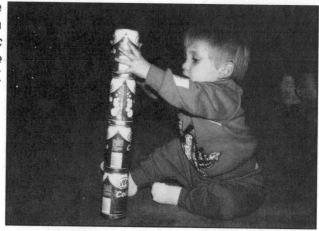

Postural Control. Postural control provides the infrastructure for performance. When conducting skilled observation, we note the child's ability to use postural control to support task engagement. For example, Jake displays trunk postural control to support his intention to explore the possibilities of manipulating the scissors in Figure 6-4. We also note the child's fluidity of moving into and out of different postural suppot positions. In Figure 6-6, Jake is using lower trunk postural control while shifting his weight to reach during this stacking activity. When children have difficulty with postural control they either collapse (indicating low stability and lack of control) or they tip over (usually related to rigidity of postural control) during tasks.

Motor Performance

The motor systems enable us to interact with the environment and learn about our bodies at the same time. The motor systems rely on the sensory and neuromuscular mechanisms to provide information and background support respectively, so it is important to discriminate these functions from motor performance during skilled observation. This requires careful consideration because what we observe on the surface is the motor performance. Skillful therapists observe to determine whether a particular difficulty with motor performance is due to poor sensory input and processing, poor postural control to support the movement, or is indeed related to poor motor performance.

We can discriminate these features in several ways. First, we can consider performance across activities, determining what features are consistent when there are different demands on the child. For example, if the child falls every time a reaching movement is required, we might hypothesize that the postural control system is unable to provide adequate support for the movement. Second, we can manipulate environmental variables and see how this changes, or does not change, the child's performance. For example, if we provide additional support for the reaching task (e.g., a chair with higher sides, or simply holding the pelvis in place ourselves) and the child can then reach efficiently, we would conclude that it is a postural control issue and not a motor performance problem. If we suspect poor sensory processing support we can test it in the same way. Let's say the child is seated and needs to tie his shoes. He or she bends down to do so, then begins, but does not finish, the task. We can ask the child to put his foot up on the chair to tie the shoe; this eliminates the vestibular stimulation from bending over. We can then see whether the child is able to complete the motor task when we reduce this sensory arousal during the task.

Large Motor Movements. Large motor movements enable a person to engage in the environment. We want to observe the child's ability to move the two body sides, cross the midline effectively, and move fluidly throughout space. Some bilateral integration tasks require a balance of stability in one body area to support movement in another body area. In Figure 6-6, Jake demonstrates the stability/mobility pattern by stabilizing the lower trunk to move bilaterally with his arms. Dani demonstrates a reciprocal pattern in Figure 6-7 as she holds the peg in her left hand and moves the hammer with her right hand. We can also see these gross motor patterns in kicking or throwing a ball, pushing a grocery cart, and wiping off the counter top.

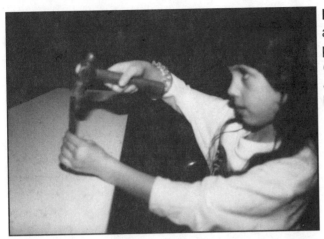

Figure 6-7. Dani demonstrates reciprocal bilateral integration as she hammers. (Reprinted with permission from Dunn W. (1991). *Pediatric Occupational Therapy: Facilitating Effective Service Provision.* Thorofare, NJ: SLACK Incorporated.)

Small Motor Movements. Small motor movements enable a person to manipulate objects. We want to observe the child's ability to move objects around in the hand, hold things, and use utensils (including writing, eating, and building tools). We also want to see if the child watches while using the hands to determine the synchrony of visual perception and fine motor performance.

Michael (Figure 6-8) is displaying a palmar grasping pattern with the cracker; this immature pattern limits Michael's ability to bite the cracker. If he used a more mature pincer grasp, the cracker would be more exposed and would enable him to eat more easily. Jake is using visual perception to watch his hands while he colors (Figure 6-9), but he is using a gross grasp, which affords less control on the pen for writing. We might also note in this picture that Jake is demonstrating postural flexibility by spreading his legs out for a wider base of support and propping on his left hand to support himself while coloring. So even though we might have been most interested in the fine motor tool use, we can collect other data at the same time. Jamie uses a pincer grasp (Figure 6-10) that gives her more control over the pen for drawing. She is using her left arm to stabilize as she draws, and her postural control is automatically supporting her body so she can concentrate on drawing.

Oral Motor Movements. The two performance areas that are most affected by oral motor development are eating and communication (Cook, 1991). Mealtime is the best time to evaluate the child's ability to use the oral motor structure for eating; we look at lip and tongue control, biting, chewing and swallowing patterns. Efficient sucking requires the child's ability to create a seal around the spout or straw (which means lip and tongue control). We can detect poor tongue control and weak swallowing patterns when food pouches in the cheeks and around the gums. We also consider the sensory aspects of eating, i.e., the temperature and texture of foods; children who have negative reactions to particular textures or who limit their food options are indicating their inability to process the sensory aspects of eating. We collaborate with the speech language pathologists to consider the integrity of the oral motor structures for vocalizing and functional communication.

Praxis. Praxis is the cognitive process of conceiving and planning new motor acts. When motor sequences become familiar they no longer require praxis (Ayres, 1979). For example, if a person gets on a bike and has not ridden one for years, the person will be a bit rusty at first, but the motor schemas to support this activity are still available and will support bike riding in a short time. This is very different from a person who has never ridden a bike before. Although this second person may have the balance, bilateral integration, and postural control needed, the person has never before put them together into a schema for bike riding. Therefore, to develop the new schema called "bike riding" would require praxis.

There are two primary areas of difficulty in praxis. First, children can have difficulty with "ideation", or coming up with the ideas needed to explore the environment and engage in discovery (Ayres, 1979). These children appear very dull and uninterested in play, and may just sit quietly or engage in a repetitive movement (e.g., opening and closing a door). They lack the ability to retain or develop play patterns that they can build on for increasingly complex play.

Figure 6-8. Michael demonstrates a palmar grasp, which is an ineffective strategy for eating a cracker. (Reprinted with permission from Dunn W. (1991). *Pediatric Occupational Therapy: Facilitating Effective Service Provision.* Thorofare, NJ: SLACK Incorporated.)

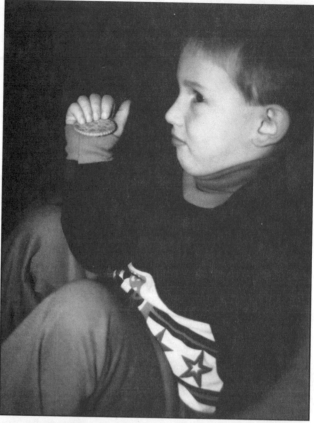

Figure 6-9. Jake demonstrates a gross grasp and emerging visual motor integration for coloring. (Reprinted with permission from Dunn W. (1991). *Pediatric Occupational Therapy: Facilitating Effective Service Provision.* Thorofare, NJ: SLACK Incorporated.)

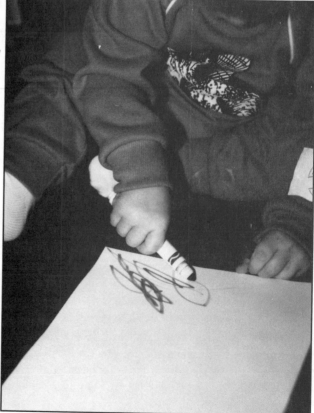

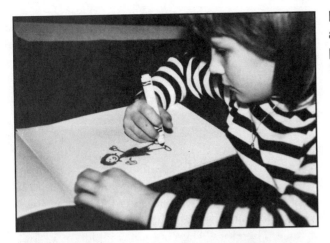

Figure 6-10. Jamie demonstrates age-appropriate visual motor skills for drawing. (Reprinted with permission from Dunn W. (1991). *Pediatric Occupational Therapy: Facilitating Effective Service Provision.* Thorofare, NJ: SLACK Incorporated.)

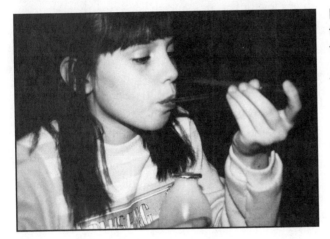

Figure 6-11. Jessica demonstrates the complexities of praxis ability. (Reprinted with permission from Dunn W. (1991). *Pediatric Occupational Therapy: Facilitating Effective Service Provision.* Thorofare, NJ: SLACK Incorporated.)

Second, children can have difficulty with "planning", or constructing the way to move to act out one's ideas (Ayres, 1979). These children are active and engaging, but their movements are ineffective and clumsy. They understand what they want to do, but have difficulty making their bodies do the correct patterns (enacting the idea). These children display signs of frustration due to awareness of the plan and their inability to "do it right", may refuse to try new things (or may direct others to do things for them to avoid the failure from trying it themselves), and may be labeled as "destructive" (their incoordination can lead to breaking toys). We must be careful to consider difficulty with praxis when we see these behaviors and not assume they reflect psychosocial difficulties.

If children have motor performance difficulties without dyspraxia, they will profit from feedback and practice. Children with dyspraxia need more carefully constructed interventions to improve performance. When practice and feedback help quickly, then the child does not have a praxis problem.

Jessica combines several skills to demonstrate her praxis as she plays with her drink (Figure 6-11). She is watching the liquid in the straw (visual perception), creating a seal around the straw with her mouth (oral motor), combining stability and mobility with her left hand to both hold the straw and manipulate the air in the end (fine motor dexterity), stabilizing the head and neck to support the task (postural control), and solving the problem of obtaining the liquid, holding it in the straw, releasing it, and swallowing the liquid in a well timed sequence (praxis and cognitive ability). Children create complex activities for themselves all the time, thereby challenging their systems to integrate more and more possibilities. During skilled observation, the occupational therapist watches the child in an attempt to sort out the aspects of complex performance and make hypotheses about what is interfering; this forms the basis for intervention planning.

Cognitive Performance

The use of cognitive abilities to perform in daily life is within the domain of concern for occupational therapists and other team members. Colleagues from other disciplines are more likely to use formal tests to measure cognition (i.e., intelligence and achievement tests). The occupational therapy contribution is in relation to the child's use of cognitive skills in daily life, or the application of cognition within performance. We must infer a child's cognitive ability from the behaviors we observe; there is no direct way to watch cognition as it is an internal process that supports performance.

Indications of Arousal and Attention. All persons have varying arousal states throughout the day; for functional performance, there must be a match between the person's arousal state and task requirements. Some environments are more familiar, and therefore require less generalized arousal; unfamiliar environments typically require more arousal to remain vigilant about unknown variables. As with all nervous system operations, people need to be able to modulate arousal states; too much arousal leads to distractibility, while too little arousal leads to inertia. Both of these states interfere with performance. Therefore, when observing children, we look for three factors. First, we look for a match between the child's level of arousal and the activity, then we identify what internal (i.e., body sensations) or external (i.e., environmental stimuli) factors alter the arousal state, and finally, we determine whether the child is able to regulate arousal within a reasonable range.

Attention requires directed cognitive effort. Appropriate attention is related to the task and the child's age. Some tasks require sustained attention, while for other tasks, intermittent attention is sufficient. For example, when the teacher gives directions orally to the class, the students must sustain attention during this time or they will miss what the teacher said. However, written directions provide the latitude to "drift away" because they will still be available when the student comes back to the task. When observing attentional skills, we must relate the child's attention to the task requirements and to age-appropriate attention.

Memory, Sequencing Skills, and Concept Formation. Most daily life tasks require memory, sequencing, and/or concept formation skills. Memory and concept formation are key factors in determining a child's ability to learn. Sometimes adults have ideas about what they want children to remember, and therefore judge the child's memory and learning on these criteria. When conducting skilled observations, we must recognize all signs of memory, not just those that we deem important. For example, if a child interrupts the care provider to tell about what happened on the weekend, the care provider might be bothered by the interruption, but the child's behavior indicates memory across time.

We must look at concept formation in the same manner. Children's abilities to organize objects and ideas into groups may be present, but not in the mature groupings adults consider with their mature schemas. For example, a young child may understand the concept of "four-legged animals", but name all such objects "doggies" even when they are cats. The error is in a finer distinction between four-legged animals, but the child is still demonstrating the basic skill of concept formation.

Only some daily life activities require sequencing, which is placing things in the correct order. It is important to get the steps of making a grilled cheese sandwich in the right order, but to place the items at a table setting, the spatial arrangement matters but not the order of placement. As with other cognitive observations, we must consider the demands of the task and the child's ability to operate within these demands.

Indications of Problem-Solving and Generalization of Learning. Problem-solving and generalization of learning are more complex cognitive functions, and indicate higher order thinking. When conducting skilled observations, it is important to record the child's approach to tasks that are difficult, not just whether the child succeeded in the task or not. The approach a child takes reveals the child's problem-solving abilities; successful performance may only mean that the child practiced and learned that particular skill. For example if you are watching an adolescent baking brownies, you can observe following directions and organizational strategies and may have naturally occurring opportunities to observe problem-solving (e.g., if there are no knives to cut the brownies, can the child come up with an alternate tool to "'cut" with; if the available pans are the wrong size, can the child select two pans that will hold the batter properly). In a follow-up interview with the parent, you can determine generalization of learning by finding out about the child's cooking participation at home. Sometimes children will say "oh, this is just like if I ....", this phrase also indicates generalization of learning because they are applying a strategy from one situation to another one.

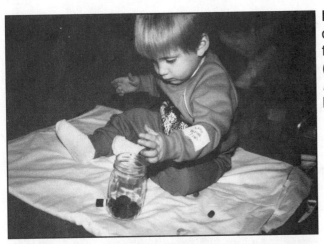

Figure 6-12. Jake demonstrates cognitive abilities during the motor task of placing objects in a container. (Reprinted with permission from Dunn W. (1991). *Pediatric Occupational Therapy: Facilitating Effective Service Provision.* Thorofare, NJ: SLACK Incorporated.)

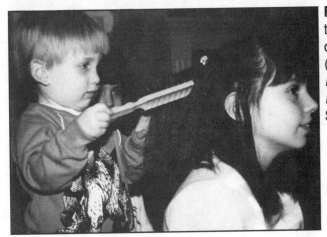

Figure 6-13. Jake understands how to perform the daily life task of combing, but demonstrates difficulty with certain performance components. (Reprinted with permission from Dunn W. (1991). *Pediatric Occupational Therapy: Facilitating Effective Service Provision.* Thorofare, NJ: SLACK Incorporated.)

Jake (Figure 6-12) illustrates the integration of cognitive, sensorimotor, and neuromuscular performance as he plays. He has figured out how to pick up the beads (pincer grasp) and release them into the jar. We see his visual attention to his hands as he plays. We hypothesize that this is a newly developing skill since his right hand is tense while his left hand is working to release the bead. He is providing himself with postural support by creating a wide base of support and weight-shifting to balance with his extended arms. With this information, we would not need to formally evaluate his postural mechanisms and would have a pretty good hypothesis about his fine motor and visual motor skill development and cognitive skill development. In Figure 6-13, Jake understands the task, but has not mastered the component skills yet.

Psychosocial Performance

Occupational therapists also collaborate with other disciplines to assess psychosocial performance components. As with each area in our domain of concern, our focus is on the supports or barriers created by the child's psychosocial skills. It is common for teams to gather this information across time so that there are multiple opportunities to see flexibility of responding and patterns that might be informative for intervention planning. Everyone on the team observes the child's behavior from different points of view so it is most likely for the group to discuss their observations before making conclusions and hypotheses.

During skilled observation, we look for those environmental or task features that influence the child's responses and the range of responsivity the child exhibits (i.e., does the child use the same strategy no matter what). We also examine the child's approach strategies (i.e., how the child engages others for help, to play, to talk, etc). For example, some children with poor self-concepts will shrink in group situations, refusing to try or to participate without a lot of coaxing; while other children will respond aggressively toward others to avoid engagement. Any extremes in responses are suspect and are brought to the team for consideration in interpretation and hypothesis generation.

Formal Assessment of Person Variables to Verify and Specify Performance Components

Best practice directs us to limit formal assessment of performance components to those aspects of performance that remain unclear after other assessment procedures have been completed. For example, it is inappropriate to formally evaluate a child's visual perceptual skills just to have "data" to present to the team or for the files. In best practice, we rely first on skilled observation in the natural context to determine whether there are possible visual perception concerns. If we can identify visual perceptual difficulties clearly through skilled observations, interviews, and/or records reviews (e.g., test scores already available), then this is all that we need to make conclusions and recommendations. In those cases that the nature of the visual perceptual skills and difficulties are still unclear after all other procedures, it would be appropriate to conduct a formal evaluation.

There are a number of measures available to evaluate the components of a child's performance. Table 6-4 provides a list of some of the more frequently used performance component tools. Occupational therapists and professionals from other disciplines use many of the tools on this list. It is common in settings that serve children and families for the team to decide who will administer particular tests that the team uses frequently; with the data collected, everyone can use it to gain insights for their interpretations.

FUNCTIONS OF ASSESSMENT IN CHILD AND FAMILY PRACTICE

There are five functions of assessment in child and family practice: determining eligibility for services, planning programs and interventions, monitoring progress, conducting comprehensive assessment and reassessment, and terminating services. We will discuss each separately.

Determining Eligibility

When serving children and families, professionals must support families to gain access to appropriate services. The first purpose of assessment, then, is to determine the child and/or family's eligibility for services. This is a process that must occur regardless of the community agency; each agency has parameters for their scope of service, and an initial assessment goal is to identify whether a child or family will be able (i.e., are "eligible") to receive services through that system. To determine eligibility, occupational therapists must identify a performance need and determine whether the child and/or family qualify for services in the system of interest.

Identifying the Performance Need

We identify performance needs through the referral process. Occupational therapists can receive referrals from parents, teachers, physicians, other therapists, and other care providers. Chapter 5 contains further details regarding this activity. In some states, therapists must obtain authorization from a physician to act on the referral, so it will be important to know the regulations for your state.

Determining Whether the Child and/or Family Qualify for Particular Services

Each service system has criteria that specifies who qualifies for services within that system. Some social service agencies have income requirements (e.g., Aid to Dependent Children), other agencies only serve a particular population (e.g., United Cerebral Palsy). The intake coordinators at the agencies typically determine these qualification levels.

In early intervention and public schools, there must be some difference between the child's capacity and current performance abilities in order for the child to be eligible for services. Each LEA must create criteria for these decisions; the criteria must be *at least* as inclusive as the federal mandates, but can be more inclusive. The professionals' roles in determining whether the child qualifies is to provide information that will facilitate the "yes" or "no" decision. For occupational therapists, this frequently means administering evaluations that con-

Table 6-4.

Assessment Tools Commonly Used by Occupational Therapists in Pediatric Practice

	Bayley Scales of Infant Development Mental and Motor Scales	Beery Developmental Test of VMI	Brigance Diagnostic Inventory of Early Development	Bruininks-Oseretsky Test of Motor Proficiency	Degangi-Berk Test of Sensory Integration	Test of Visual Perceptual Skills (Non-motor) (TVPS)	Hawaii Early Learning Profile (HELP)
Age Range	2 months to 2 1/2 years	2 to 15 years	0 to 7 years	4 1/2 to 14 years	3 to 5 years	4 to 12 years	0 to 36 months
Testing Time (minutes)	45 to 50	10 to 15	30 to 60	45 to 60	30	10 to 20	30 to 36
Scoring Time (minutes)	15 to 25	10	10 to 15	10	5 to 10	10	10 to 15
MAJOR AREAS TESTED: Personal/Social	X						X
Communication	X		X				X
Cognition	X		X				X
Self-help			X				X
Gross Motor	X		X	X	X		X
Praxis				X	X		
Reflexes	X				X		
Fine Motor	X		X	X	X		X
Visual Motor Integration (VMI)		X		X			X
Visual Perception						X	
Tactile							
Vestibular					X		
TYPE OF TEST: Norm-referenced	X	X		X		X	
Criteria-referenced			X		X		X
Informal Structured Observation							
SCORES OBTAINED: Age Level	X	X		X		X	X
Percentile		X		X		X	
Standard	X	X		X		X	
Quantified Observations					X		

Adapted from Cook, D. G. (1991). The assessment process. In Dunn, W. (Ed.), Pediatric Occupational Therapy: Facilitating Effective Service Provision (pp. 40-41). Thorofare, NJ: SLACK Incorporated.

Table 6-4 continued.

Assessment Tools Commonly Used by Occupational Therapists in Pediatric Practice

	Learning Accomplishment Profile-Diagnostic Ed	Learning Accomplishment Profile-Revised Ed (LAP-R)	Motor-Free Visual Perceptual Test (MVPT)	Movement Assessment of Infants	Peabody-Developmental Motor Scales	Sensory Integration and Praxis Test (SIPT)	Test of Visual Motor Skills (TVMS)
Age Range	12 to 72 months	36 to 72 months	4 to 8 years	0 to 12 months	7 years	4 years to 8 years 11 months	0 to 36
Testing Time (minutes)	1.5 to 2 hrs	2 to 2.5 hrs	10 to 20	15	40 to 60	75 to 100	10 to 15
Scoring Time (minutes)	15	15	10	10	15	45 to 60	5 to 10
MAJOR AREAS TESTED: Personal/Social		X					
Communication	X	X					
Cognition	X	X					
Self-help	X	X					
Gross Motor	X	X		X	X	X	
Praxis					X	X	
Reflexes					X		
Fine Motor	X	X			X	X	
Visual Motor Integration (VMI)		X			X	X	X
Visual Perception			X			X	
Tactile						X	
Vestibular						X	
TYPE OF TEST: Norm-referenced			X		X	X	X
Criteria-referenced	X	X			X		
Informal Structured Observation				X			
SCORES OBTAINED: Age Level	X		X		X	X	X
Percentile					X	X	X
Standard					X	X	X
Quantified Observations		X		X			

Adapted from Cook, D. G. (1991). The assessment process. In Dunn, W. (Ed.), Pediatric Occupational Therapy: Facilitating Effective Service Provision *(pp. 40-41). Thorofare, NJ: SLACK Incorporated.*

tain developmental or performance standards; we compare the child to an external standard to see if there is a discrepancy between this child's performance and the standard. When the discrepancy is large enough (based on the criteria set by the LEA), then the child will qualify for services.

When participating in qualification decisions, it is typical for occupational therapists to use norm-referenced measures because the normative information provides the external standard of performance. We also call them "status" measures because they record the child's current performance. Status measures do NOT provide information needed for designing interventions. Table 6-1 provides a summary of the characteristics of some norm-referenced measures.

Planning Interventions and Programs

In order to plan interventions and service programs for children and families, occupational therapists need information about performance. The criterion measures described above, along with skilled observations, interviews, and activity analyses are the best tools for intervention planning. These methods provide the texture and detail needed to tailor intervention options to be user-friendly for that child, family, and teacher team. Chapter 7 provides great detail about how to use assessment data to design best practice interventions.

Monitoring Progress

Best practice dictates that we incorporate ways to monitor the child's progress and the effectiveness of intervention strategies into the daily routines. In Chapter 8, Linder & Clark outline methods for collecting data to monitor progress in programs. The best monitoring methods are those that are part of the daily routine, rather than a measurement method that must be added onto the day.

Conducting Comprehensive Assessments and Reassessments

Initially (and periodically), it is important to conduct comprehensive assessments with children to be sure that all appropriate considerations are being made on the child's behalf. Some service systems require comprehensive assessments on a schedule (e.g., every 3 years), while in other systems the professionals make this determination. A comprehensive assessment is a set of activities to explore all possible areas of development, ability, and performance, and typically includes a variety of types of measures. Occupational therapists serve on these assessment teams, and in this role have the responsibility to report on the child's performance across the domain of concern (i.e., ADL, work and productive activity, play/leisure). Best practice comprehensive assessment includes assessment of performance in natural settings, along with a determination of the child/family/educator's satisfaction with current levels of performance. Additionally the therapist would have the responsibility to report to the team on the child's application and use of sensorimotor, cognitive, and psychosocial performance skills in daily life.

Terminating Services

Professionals conclude their services when the child and/or family they are serving has the skills and/or supports they need to live a satisfying life. This does not mean that we have "cured" the disability, but that we have provided all the strategies that enable the child and care providers to support functional performance. For school-aged children, this means that they have the supports and strategies to be a successful student. For young adults transitioning to community living and work, it might mean that we have supported a job search, placement, and the probationary period and have set natural supports in place (e.g., a supervisor or peer to help).

There are a number of strategies for conducting assessment to terminate services. The most efficient method is to have designed the intervention program with functional and measurable goals related to the child's performance so that when the child reaches the goals it is clear to everyone that services are no longer needed. The COPM is an excellent tool for concluding services because it is a reflection of the child and family's priorities and expectations about performance.

Sometimes families and teachers have come to rely on the occupational therapist and feel uncomfortable without this professional support themselves (on behalf of the child). Communication is critical to the process so the families and teachers feel supported; with good rapport, the therapist can also anticipate the source and features of the anxiety and can incorporate supports into the transition planning process. Therapists must also keep in mind that it is important to provide support without making boundaries unclear. Therapists provide a professional service, and need to avoid codependence that will hamper the child, family, or teacher's progress and competence to handle future situations.

We design probe assessment strategies to ensure that our "departure" was not premature and continue to address the other care providers' concerns. For example, a parent might be worried that her third grade daughter will "slide" back into poor social engagement patterns when the therapist is no longer supporting her. In this case, we would find out exactly what the parent fears will happen, and we set a transition goal related to the concern, e.g., "Karen will talk with a peer at lunch at least three times a week", or "Karen will play with a group of 2 to 4 children at least three times a week during recess". The team then agrees that if there ever is a week in the next quarter that Karen does not meet this criterion, the occupational therapist would immediately reenter Karen's educational program and collaborate with the teacher regarding this event. At the end of the quarter, the team and the parent can celebrate Karen's success. We have demonstrated Karen's ability to sustain performance and have been respectful of the parent's concerns all in one strategy.

There may also be times that we terminate services at one point in a child's life and will need to reenter the child's life a little later when task demands change. Many times if children have received consistent services in preschool and elementary school, they will not need services in the preadolescent period. This same child may need occupational therapy support in the transition to high school, or in career and life planning. It is completely appropriate to move in and out of children's lives.

TEMPLATE FOR BEST PRACTICE OCCUPATIONAL THERAPY ASSESSMENT

Sometimes the assessment process can seem overwhelming to a novice who wants to be sure to conduct a complete assessment in the most efficient manner. Figure 6-14 contains a template for planning a best practice assessment strategy. As you see, the rows contain the types of assessments available, and the columns indicate the areas for assessment. A complete assessment does not need to fill up all the boxes, but there should be some boxes completed in each column. The last column is shaded to remind you that we only conduct formal assessment of person variables when we need to clarify or verify the nature of the performance problem.

In Figure 6-15, you will see a completed assessment planning guide for a third grader named Rhegan. Rhegan did fine in school in the first and second grades, but is now struggling in third grade. His teacher reports in her referral that she is concerned about his performance in forming letters to write, particularly during seatwork, and his frustration during art class. He is tearing up his papers and kicking his desk when his work is unsatisfactory.

The therapist plans to conduct several assessment strategies to learn about Rhegan's difficulties and needs. You see that there are some measures listed in more than one box; these measures address the interaction between the variables, and so cover more than one area. For example, the *Coping Inventory* is a measure of the child in the environment, thus providing data on both variables. Measures such as these make the overall assessment process efficient and still complete. This plan will provide the occupational therapist and the team with the information they need to create a successful and satisfying seatwork time for Rhegan.

Summary

Best practice assessment is a complex process that draws on all of one's professional expertise. We must be able to construct a set of experiences that reveal the child's strengths and barriers to performance and form hypotheses about how to change the situation to support more successful performance. In this chapter we reviewed all the features of comprehensive assessment and offered methods for constructing a best practice assessment program.

Data collection strategy	Occupational performance: What they want and need to do	Context variable assessment	Person variables: Data during performance	Person variables: Formal assessment*
Records reviews				
Norm-referenced measurement				
Criterion-referenced measurement				
Informal measurement				
Skilled observation				
Interviews				
Ecological measures				

*Only included when necessary to verify or clarify; see text.

Figure 6-14. Best practice assessment planning guide.

REFERENCES

American Psychological Association (1999). Standards for Educational and Psychological Testing. Washington, DC: APA.

Ayres, A. J. (1979). *Sensory integration and learning disorders.* Los Angeles, CA: Western Psychological.

Bundy, A. (1997). Play and playfulness: What to look for. In L. D. Parham & L. S. Fazio (Eds.), *Play in occupational therapy for children* (pp. 52-66). St. Louis, MO: Mosby.

Caldwell, B. M. & Bradley, R. H. (1978). *Home Observation Measurement of the Environment.* Little Rock, AR: University of Arkansas Center for Child Development & Education.

Cook, D. G. (1991). The assessment process. In W. Dunn (Ed.), *Pediatric occupational therapy: Facilitating effective service provision* (pp. 35-74). Thorofare, NJ: SLACK Incorporated.

Dunn, W. (1997). Implementing neuroscience principles to support rehabilitation and recovery. In C. Christiansen and C. Baum. (Eds.), *Occupational Therapy: Enabling Function and well-being* (2nd Edition). Thorofare, NJ: SLACK Incorporated.

Kandel, E., Schwartz, J., & Jessell, T. (2000). *Principles of neural science.* New York, NY: McGraw-Hill Companies.

Knox, S. Measuring play practice (Knox preschool play scale). In M. Law, C. Baum, & W. Dunn (Eds.), *Measuring occupational performance: A guide to best practice.* Thorofare, NJ: SLACK Incorporated.

Law, M., Polatajko, H., Pollock, N., McColl, M. A., Carswell, A., & Baptiste, D. (Oct. 1994). Pilot testing of the Canadian Occupational Performance Measure: Clinical and measurement issues. *Canadian Journal of Occupational Therapy, 61*(4): 191-7 (7 ref).

Law, M., Baum, C., & Dunn, W. (2000). *Measuring occupational performance: A guide to best practice.* Thorofare, NJ: SLACK Incorporated.

Data collection strategy	Occupational performance: What they want and need to do	Context variable assessment	Person variables: Data during performance	Person variables: Formal assessment*
Records reviews	Seatwork and homework papers in file			Scores from intelligence and psycho-educational testing
Norm-referenced measurement	School Function Assessment	School Function Assessment		School Function Assessment
Criterion-referenced measurement		Coping inventory	Coping inventory	
Informal measurement				
Skilled observation	Seatwork period Lunch period (as contrast) Art class	Classroom setup Art room setup	Rhegan's sensori-motor, cognitive, and psychosocial features during seatwork, lunch, and at art	
Interviews	Teacher Rhegan			
Ecological measures		Ecological assessment of seatwork		
*Only included when necessary to verify or clarify; see text.				

Figure 6-15. Best practice assessment planning guide for Rhegan, a boy who needs to complete seatwork successfully and with satisfaction.

Linder, T. (1993). *Transdisciplinary play-based assessment: A functional approach to working with young children.* Baltimore, MD: Paul H. Brookes.

Maurer, P., Barris, R., Bonder, B., & Gillette, N. (1984). Hierarchy of competencies relating to the use of standardized instruments and evaluation techniques by occupational therapists. *American Journal of Occupational Therapy, 38*(12), 803-804.

Sattler, J. M. (1988). *Assessment of Children* (3rd ed.). San Diego, CA: Jerome M. Sattler, Publisher, Inc.

Sattler, J. M. (1982). *Assessment of Children's Intelligence and Special Abilities* (2nd ed.). San Diego, CA: Jerome M. Sattler, Publisher, Inc.

Williamson, G., & Szczepanski, M. (1999). Coping frame of reference. In P. Kramer & J. Hinojosa (Eds.), *Frames of reference for pediatric occupational therapy* (2nd ed.) (pp. 431-468). Baltimore, MD: Williams & Wilkins.

7

Designing Best Practice Services for Children and Families

Winnie Dunn, PhD, OTR, FAOTA

"A willingness to learn new patterns for providing services to students will be required by specialists as they apply their expertise in new organizational models. " McDonnell & Hardman, 1989

INTRODUCTION

Best practice service provision is a fluid and complex activity for the artful professional because it requires ongoing decision-making. In this chapter we will study ways to organize the service provision process that incorporates forward thinking philosophy (from Chapter 1), systematic attention to the range of salient variables (from Chapter 3), and an occupational therapy focus (from Chapter 4). Table 7-1 summarizes the core concepts from these chapters for your reference.

Services for children and families begin with an individualized plan that outlines the desired outcomes; within a family-centered care model, this means that we listen and respond to the family's and child's interests and desires about what they want and need the child to do. Depending on the service system and the child's age, the team might design an Individualized Family Service Plan (IFSP), an IEP, an Individualized Habilitation Plan (IHP), or another similar service plan. Therapists design service provision based on referral, pre-assessment, and assessment data (see Chapters 5 and 6), and in collaboration with other team members, family, and the child, if possible. The process we describe in this chapter provides a way to link assessment with intervention planning towards the desired outcomes.

Occupational therapists use their unique perspectives to create the links between families' needs and priorities for performance and the supports that other disciplines offer; this provides the infrastructure for performance. Additionally, the systematic model explained here provides methods for documenting and evaluating effectiveness as part of comprehensive services. Chapters 8 and 10 provide examples of documentation and effectiveness evaluations.

Many children receive services through more than one agency and provider. We also must take responsibility for integrating and coordinating these services for efficient use of resources so that the family can manage the complexity of supporting their child. Sometimes there is a professional who provides case management with the family, while at other times the family takes primary responsibility for coordinating their family's services. In service coordination situations, therapists and other professionals must be vigilant in making sure that the desired outcomes are clear and linked to various agency services.

Table 7-1.

Summary of Core Concepts to Recall for Intervention Planning

Clinical Reasoning	Practice Models	EHP Interventions	Philosophy Statement	Assessment Procedures

Scientific Reasoning
 	
Narrative Reasoning
 	
Pragmatic Reasoning
 	
Ethical Reasoning
	Developmental
	
	Sensory Integrative
	
	Neurodevelopmental
	
	Biomechanical
	
	Motor Control and Motor Learning
	
	Cognitive
	
	Coping
		Establish/Restore
		
		Adapt/Modify
		
		Alter
		
		Prevent
		
		Create
			Professionals have a particular knowledge base that represents their profession and enables them to derive particular meaning from situations; individuals expect professionals to provide services that **reflect the expertise of their discipline**
			
			Individuals have the **right to participate** in daily life activities of their choosing; communities have the resposibility to provide reasonable access to these activities
			
			Professionals who serve children and families have the responsibility to provide **family-centered care,** i.e., to honor the family's priorities and style in designing and implementing intervention plans.
			
			Professionals and families have the mutual and reciprocal right and responsibility to involve each other in the organization and structure of services within community-based systems.
			
			Individuals have the right to consider options and choose interventions; professionals have the responsibility to provide information regarding the effectiveness of the options we offer as potential solutions.
				Options:
				Records Review
				Norm-referenced
				Criteria-referenced
				Informal Measures
				Skilled Observation
				   Monitor Engagement
				   Environ. Features
				Beh./Obs. and Neutral Interview
				Economic Measures
				
				Structure:
				Occupationally-focused
				Contextual Base
				Person Variable
				   Skilled Observations
				   Formal Tests
				
				Functions:
				Eligibility
				Planning Interventions
				Monitoring Progress
				Comprehensive Assess.
				Termination

THE NEED TO PROVIDE INTEGRATED SERVICES

During the late 1970's and early 1980's, professionals debated over how to reconstruct services to transition from more traditional clinic-based services to public school and early intervention services (see Campbell, 1987a; Campbell, 1987b; Dunn, 1989a; Dunn, 1989b; Lyon, S. & Lyon, G., 1980; Sternat, Messina, Nietupski, Lyon, & Brown, 1977). A major issue in the transition to new settings for services has been the thrust to provide services that are integrated within the child's life rather than isolated from daily routines. Along with this emphasis is the need for occupational therapists to understand their role and functions within various structures of interdisciplinary teams (see Chapter 1).

The term "integrated therapy" evolved due to the prevalence of isolated therapy models (i.e., serving a child separate from the life environment, sometimes called pull-out services), which were developed in more clinical service settings. The criticisms of isolated therapy models for community settings involved what authors felt were erroneous assumptions about this type of service, i.e., that children would generalize from the isolated therapy to other life situations and that intermittent practice in the isolated therapy (i.e., once or twice a week) would be adequate to make performance changes (Sternat, Messina, Nietupski, Lyon, & Brown, 1977). When programs for children with special needs are separate from programs for children without disabilities, it is easier to perpetuate the "clinical" models of service, which have traditionally taken a more remedial or restorative approach to skill development.

Taylor (1988) reminds us that the concepts that have been our guideposts in the past can lead us astray tomorrow; to move closer to a society that represents more enduring human values, we must be prepared to implement new ideas when we have achieved certain goals. As community-based services have evolved, there has been an increasing emphasis on including children with disabilities in settings with their peers who do not have disabilities. Shifting to inclusion philosophies challenges our standard practices and requires different professional activities to support the success of this philosophical evolution.

Occupational therapists need to construct their service provision to ensure that services continue to be relevant to the children's lives, that the children and families continue to have access to occupational therapy philosophy (with its unique focus on living a satisfying life), and that children can continue to remain connected to those activities and environments that will sustain their satisfying life after the therapist is not actively involved. Because the shifts described above are occurring in the culture, occupational therapy must reconstruct the models and approaches for providing services as well.

MODELS OF SERVICE PROVISION

Models of service provision outline *the ways we use our time* in the intervention process. The AOTA (1989) outlined a continuum for services that enables therapists to be responsive to all children's and families' needs in a variety of service settings. The continuum includes direct service, integrated or supervised therapy, and consultation.

Direct Services

Therapists are providing direct therapy when they design individualized interventions and carry them out with the child individually or in small groups. We reserve a direct therapy model for those times when a child needs support from very specialized therapeutic techniques that cannot easily or safely be carried out by others. When therapists identify interventions that can be safely implemented by others (e.g., the family, siblings, teachers, friends), it is more desirable to imbed the intervention routines and activities into the child's daily life because there will be more naturally occurring opportunities for practice.

Best practice dictates that we never provide direct therapy without also providing one of the other service models; this ensures that the therapist is taking responsibility for generalization of skills to natural settings for performance. If a therapist provides direct therapy without other models, he or she cannot be sure that any changes that occur in the isolated setting are having any impact on the child's performance.

Since occupational therapy is concerned with participation in daily life, therapy is incomplete without goals and outcomes anchored in daily life. For example, although you might be addressing the child's need to establish equilibrium responses in a direct therapy situation, the only reason this matters to the child and family is so the child is safer to move about independently for playing, socializing, etc. It is best practice to establish goals related to playing and socializing, not equilibrium (because better equilibrium, as you would measure it in a direct therapy setting without better playing or socializing, is irrelevant to the child's life). The child must be able to use better equilibrium when challenged to do so in the course of daily routines for better equilibrium to matter.

In the case study of James (see Chapter 10), we see that he is clumsy when moving about. The therapist constructed one of his goals to be "James will transition among learning centers within 2 minutes 75% of the time so he can participate with peers in classroom activities". You see that the goal is focused on efficient movement so he has more time with peers. We could also write a goal about the nature and quality of James' participation with peers.

Neurobiologically-based intervention paradigms (e.g., sensory integration) contain the most common types of interventions that we apply in a direct service model. Practice models that require a strong background in neuroscience and biomechanics have aspects of their application that require constant and ongoing monitoring of the ANS, the sensory processing mechanisms, and the postural and motor output systems (Dunn & Campbell, 1991). Since occupational therapists have extensive background in the neurobiological systems and their application to the human experience, therapists can monitor changes that occur within these systems during an intervention activity and make changes to support positive nervous system actions (i.e., increasingly more complex adaptive responses) and diminish potentially negative responses (e.g., "fight or flight" reactions of the ANS). It would be difficult to train another care provider in some of the more subtle aspects of responsiveness in a short time.

For example, if a child is extremely hypersensitive to movement, the high level of activity and randomness of a preschool room may be overwhelming for the child. The occupational therapist might select direct service for several weeks to provide interventions to reduce the child's hypersensitivity so that the child can participate with peers more successfully during play. During that same time, the therapist would collaborate with the teacher to make adaptations to reduce the impact of the hypersensitivity on the child's school day (e.g., move his seat to a less active corner so there is less bumping, send him ahead of others to the bathroom). The therapist and teacher would also collaborate to collect data on the child's integration into more active play as the hypersensitivity is reduced. The case study of Peter (see Chapter 10) describes a situation similar to this one.

It is always most desirable to provide direct therapy in the child's natural setting. When a teacher sees that a particular child needs individualized instruction, the teacher pulls the child aside for a brief time, conducts problem-solving and feedback for the child's correct responses, and then immediately moves away from the child to see if the child can use the skill with less support and more naturally occurring events (e.g., returning to the reading group where other children are working). Therapists can do the same thing in direct therapy.

For example, a child is having difficulty with postural control that interferes with being able to stay in the desk during work time (i.e., the child falls out of his chair). The therapist can use a seatwork period to provide therapeutic interventions while enabling the child to work on seatwork. The therapist might support weight shift challenges by placing the work items on the counter next to the child's desk, requiring a little longer reach. This also provides the therapist the opportunity to see exactly where the control diminishes, enabling the therapist to develop more precise intervention opportunities. Conducting therapy within the setting also allows the teachers and aides to see what the therapist does to support the child, encouraging carry over throughout the week.

Integrated or Supervised Therapy

Integrated or supervised therapy is the second service provision category. Supervised therapy provides a mechanism for occupational therapy expertise to support children's performance within the natural environment. Because supervised therapy requires that we work with care providers that are with the child every day, it can provide the means for consistency and repeated practice, thereby increasing the chances for skill acquisition with contextual supports.

When using supervised therapy for service provision, the therapist conducts an assessment to identify the strengths and needs of the individual child. The therapist designs an intervention plan to meet individual needs and remains responsible for the outcome of the plan. The therapist trains another person within the child's natural environment to carry out the plan with accompanying progress monitoring (see Chapter 8), so that procedures will be implemented on a consistent basis and therefore have greater chance for generalization. The therapist remains in regular contact (i.e., at least biweekly) with the person who carries out the monitored program, so that necessary alterations in the program can be implemented in a timely manner (Dunn & Campbell, 1991).

Therapists must select an integrated service provision model carefully (AOTA, 1987, 1989). The overriding concern is to protect the health and safety of the child when we implement interventions; therefore, we must decide whether the person we train can conduct the intervention safely. Therapists must make sure the implementer can demonstrate the procedures without error and without cues. The therapist must be sure that the implementer can name the precautions, or the signs of risk or failure within the procedure as well. Therapists must never implement an integrated program if they cannot ensure that these criteria are met. Failure to meet these criteria would put the child at risk and the therapist in a position of defending a program that is not being carried out in the designed manner. Additionally, ongoing contact between the therapist and the implementer is essential to integrated therapy; the therapist must meet with the implementer at least biweekly to ensure high quality program implementation and to determine whether adjustments are needed and make adaptations in a timely manner.

Supervised therapy is a viable service provision alternative in many situations; it provides a method for making daily life "more therapeutic". Parents can incorporate programs within daily life routines such as bathing, diaper changing, eating, and dressing. Teachers and teacher's aides provide these programs within the daily school routine in areas such as positioning and handling, eating, functional mobility, and functional communication. Supervisors in a work environment provide programs that adapt tasks to facilitate the worker's timely task completion. Supervised therapy programs provide a means for occupational therapists to address the best fit between the individual's skills and needs and demands of the environment, by providing more opportunities for generalization and practice than would be possible through a direct service model.

Consultation

Consultation is the third model of service provision; consultation differs from direct therapy and supervised therapy in one significant way: the therapist is using expertise to address another person's issues (Dunn & Campbell, 1991; Dunn, 1991a). The therapist is not directly responsible for the outcome of the individual in the consultation model. Rather, the consultee is responsible for the outcome of the individual child; the therapist is responsible for the collaborative efforts with the adult who is carrying out the program.

Three types of consultation are important in pediatric therapy. The first is *case consultation,* in which the therapist collaborates with another care provider to address the needs of individuals. In case consultation, the therapist and teacher might meet to discuss the ways the teacher might facilitate greater participation of a student in the reading group. The second is *colleague consultation,* in which the therapist targets the needs of professional peers within a service environment. A therapist would use colleague consultation to collaborate with the teacher to design methods for the teacher to calm the children down after recess. The third is *system consultation.* This focuses on improvements of the system within which services are provided. Another name for this type of work is "population-based services" (see NBCOT, 1997; AOTA, 1999). Participation in a system-wide curriculum committee, or serving as a speaker in a pre-school Parents' Information Night, are examples of system consultation—where the objective is to improve how the system works so that all children will benefit. Case #10, "Service to the Westwood School" in Chapter 10 provides an example of population-based service to a Charter School. In each case, the therapist is using occupational therapy expertise to improve a situation of concern to others.

Best practice prescribes that we use a collaborative style of consultation, which acknowledges the specialized expertise of both the consultant and the consultee (Idol, Paolucci-Whitcomb, & Nevin, 1987). Dunn (1991b) found that a collaborative consultation approach with preschoolers yielded an equivalent number of achieved IEP goals (approximately 70%) when compared to a direct service condition. Additionally, teachers who participated in a collaborative consultation reported that the therapists contributed to goal attainment in 24% more instances than teachers whose children received isolated direct services.

When professionals collaborate, they share responsibility for identifying the problem, creating possible solutions, trying the solutions, and then altering them as necessary for greater effectiveness. The unique knowledge and skills of the occupational therapist lend themselves nicely to a collaborative style of consultation. Occupational therapists have backgrounds in behavior across the life span and understand the context of performance. These skills are easily translated into collaborative consultation. Other professionals have different expertise that contribute to the collaborative relationship in different ways. Classroom teachers focus on the products of learning, such as written work, verbal responses, staying on task to complete assignments, and attaining outcome competencies in subject areas. The combined perspectives of teachers and occupational therapists provide fertile ground for solving complex problems. There are several great sources for more detailed information about providing consultative services; use them to guide your practice (Dunn, 1991b; Jaffe & Epstein, 1993).

The person receiving consultation (i.e., the consultee) must be a willing participant in the consultative relationship. Dunn (1991b) provides strategies for determining a consultee's readiness for consultation and how to approach each type of readiness successfully. The therapist and consultee negotiate what the relationship will yield and what expectations need to be met. Without this negotiating process, a consultee that is not a willing participant can sabotage the outcomes for themselves and the child. As the consultant, the therapist must be careful to assess what would meet the consultee's needs and build this into the child's plan to ensure success. For example, if a therapist is working with a paraprofessional on the diapering routine, the paraprofessional may see all the therapist's suggestions as interference that will lengthen the time to get diapering completed. If the therapist can show how positioning and handling strategies can make it easier to get the diapers off and on (e.g., due to spasticity), then the paraprofessional will be more likely to implement the therapeutic intervention on the child's behalf because it also meets the paraprofessional's need to get finished quickly.

Factors in Selecting a Service Model

There are several factors that affect the choices therapists make about how to spend their time (i.e., the service model). Some performance challenges children face are more likely to require particular service models; for example, a child who is choking on foods may need some initial intense direct service so that the therapists (typically the occupational therapist and/or speech pathologist) can identify what is putting the child at risk. This situation would not be safe to turn over to an aide without additional information about precautions.

For other performance needs, supervised therapy or consultation are the best options. For example, an adolescent who needs to practice social engagement skills needs cues and supports throughout the school day; if the occupational therapist only worked on these skills using a direct service model, there would be little likelihood that the skills would generalize to the needed settings for performance. By using supervised therapy and consultation the therapist can design a rich context for supporting the child's skill development. We illustrate the occupational therapist collaborating in this way in the cases of Derek and Cameron in Chapter 10.

Since we do not provide services in isolation, contextual variables have a lot to do with the selection process as well. Therapists determine the amount and type of supports available to the target child when selecting a service provision model. For example, when working with a first-year classroom teacher, the therapist might decide on a short and intense period of direct service to identify the best strategies, following up with supervised therapy to support the teacher to learn the best ways to facilitate the child's performance. With a very experienced special education teacher, the therapist may select consultation immediately, knowing that this teacher will understand what the interventions look like and their purpose in the classroom environment.

Similarly with families, there will be some members that enjoy experimenting, and so the therapist will use consultation more readily and ask the family member to try several things and give feedback about the best strategy. Other family members will want the strategy that "works", thus dictating that the therapist will need to be more involved in the discovery process (i.e., using direct and supervised therapy models).

Therapists with less experience are frequently less comfortable with consultation because it requires an ability to conceptualize the problem in a more abstract way and size up situations efficiently. This is a great area to seek out mentoring, because consultation is a critical service model and skill set for a community-based therapist.

APPROACHES TO SERVICE PROVISION

Approaches to service provision *illustrate the focus of our interventions.* The Ecology of Human Performance conceptual framework (see Chapter 4) provides a comprehensive view of service approaches (Dunn, Brown, & McGuigan, 1994) by describing the focus in relation to the person-task-context interaction. When therapists consider several approaches to intervention planning, it is much easier to identify the best matched interventions for the child, the family, other service providers, and the life environments. The EHP outlines five approaches to intervention: establish/restore, adapt/modify, alter, prevent and create interventions.

Establish/Restore Interventions

The "establish/restore" intervention addresses a person's skills and barriers to performance; interventions are directed toward improving the person's repertoire of sensorimotor, cognitive, and psychosocial skills. For example, if a child has low endurance that is interfering with playing with friends on the playground and in intramural sports, the occupational therapist might consult with family and the school team to construct some endurance building activities into the child's weekly routines. The parents might sign the child up for gymnastics, karate, or swimming. The physical educator might work with the child to design a "personal fitness" program. The classroom teacher might include this child in cleaning the chalkboards and transporting books to the library. These activities address the "person variable" of low endurance that is interfering with play and socialization. When using this approach, the therapist is using occupational therapy knowledge and expertise to find ways to improve the child's skills to support performance.

Adapt/Modify Interventions

The "adapt/modify" intervention addresses the context and task characteristics that might be creating barriers to performance; the therapist changes aspects of the context or the task demands to make performance more possible. For example, if a child is having difficulty copying from the board the therapist might provide the child with slant board (i.e., a writing surface which changes the angle of work) to make the perceptual task of copying easier for the child. This change in the way the child performs the task does not make the child's perceptual skills better, but rather supports the child to complete the task in spite of perceptual challenges. For Cameron (see Chapter 10), the team designed adaptations to make the school more accessible.

Alter Interventions

The "alter" intervention takes advantage of the natural features of contexts; therapists select the best natural environment for the person without requiring the person to develop new skills and without requiring the context to be changed. For example, if a child has difficulty completing seatwork in the busy classroom, the occupational therapist might suggest that the child go to the library for work periods. The library has qualities that make it better for the child to work; the therapist hasn't improved the child's skills or asked the librarian to change the library. The therapist is taking advantage of the characteristics that are more suited to this child's current performance to advance his educational endeavors.

Prevent Interventions

The "prevent" intervention acknowledges the performance difficulties that *may* occur in the future, and sets a course to keep negative performance outcomes from occurring. For example, if a child has poor mobility, the therapist might anticipate that this child is at risk for developing pressure sores which would interfere with health and participation in the preschool program. The therapist would not wait for a pressure sore to develop, but would act on this knowledge about the risk. The therapist might develop a positioning program with the staff so that the child gets moved around throughout the day to prevent skin breakdowns. When we can anticipate a negative outcome, prevention enables us to use our expertise to redesign daily life to support a more positive outcome. It is not a prevention intervention if the problem already exists for the child; prevention is reserved for addressing potential problems, and by doing so, keeping them from happening in the first place (see Figure 7-7 later in this chapter).

Create Interventions

Finally, the "create" intervention uses the expertise and knowledge of occupational therapy in a way that promotes the availability of enriched contexts for everyone, without a specific focus on a disability or a person with a performance problem. Occupational therapy expertise is useful in designing universally accessible environments, such as community playgrounds. Making recommendations that are in everyone's best interest and not focused on a particular problem taps our discipline's expertise toward long-term community support outcomes. Occupational therapists serving children and families can serve on curriculum committees, community development boards, and charter school boards to infuse occupational therapy expertise into the daily routines of our communities. Case #10 in Chapter 10 illustrates an occupational therapist's involvement in the Westwood Charter School.

Factors in Selecting a Service Approach

We select service approaches in collaboration with families, team members, and when possible, the child. Best practice prescribes that occupational therapists design interventions using several different approaches and present them to the families, teachers, etc., so they can decide what might be the best match for them. This requires negotiation and a shared understanding of what the service will look like and how it will fit into the daily routine. This strategy of intervention planning requires therapists to have very creative and flexible thinking about performance problems, so that a variety of ideas emerge from planning. By only designing one approach, you limit the possibilities for the child and take the risk that the intervention won't be used, thereby diminishing any possible therapeutic benefit that might have been possible. In Chapter 10 we provide examples of how to design a multifaceted intervention approach with several children; in the next section, we present methods for organizing your thinking.

ORGANIZATIONAL TEMPLATES FOR BEST PRACTICE INTERVENTION PLANNING

There are many ways to organize your data, impressions, and recommendations for intervention planning; particular settings also have procedures for data-recording and documentation. It is important for you to learn the methods for each setting, while keeping in mind how to demonstrate the occupational therapy influence in any type of intervention planning forms and procedures. The methods we will introduce here provide templates for ensuring that the perspective of occupational therapy is clearly articulated in the intervention planning records. They can be adapted to be compatible with any system's documentation requirements.

Remember as you begin your career that you may want to be more structured in using templates such as these for your planning. Template structures provide you with a means to practice conceptually sound decision making; the worksheets contain cues to make sure you address all aspects of the situation and that you present the "domain of concern" and your expertise clearly to your teams and families. These early efforts will establish good intervention planning habits that will serve you well as you evolve professionally.

There are six templates for this intervention planning process. Figures 7-1 through 7-6 illustrate blank templates for you (see Dunn, Brown, McClain, & Westman, 1994 for completed examples across the life span).

Figure 7-1 illustrates a template for summarizing data related to person variables down the left side (i.e., sensorimotor, cognitive, psychosocial) and task variables across the top (i.e., activities of daily living, work/productive activity, play/leisure performance). Therapists complete this template using data collected from assessments of the child's performance in the area of interest. For example, if an adolescent wishes to plan a meal as part of job preparation, the therapist would record findings from interviews, observations, and evaluation relat-

Person Variables	Activities of Daily Living	Work/Productive Activity	Play/Leisure Performance
Sensorimotor			
Cognitive			
Psychosocial			

Figure 7-1. Data summary worksheet. (Adapted from Dunn, W., Brown, C., McClain, L., & Westman, K. (1994). The ecology of human performance: A contextual perspective on human occupation. In C. Royeen (Ed.), *The practice of the future: Putting occupation back into therapy.* Washington, DC: AOTA.)

ed to meal planning in the "work/productive activity" column. In the sensorimotor box, the therapist might write "good scanning skills in recipe books" and "maintains attention to cookbooks with others making noise around him". In the cognitive box, the therapist records "identifies protein and dessert, but misses fruits, vegetables, and grains", "persists in reviewing cookbooks to find alternatives". In the psychosocial box, the therapist might write "expresses fondness for particular foods that Grandma makes" and "avoids options that seem 'babyish' to him".

This template does not provide the details about the child's scores on particular assessments. What this template invites the therapist to do ahead of time (e.g., before the IEP meeting) is consider the relationship between the person variable data (e.g., visual perception skills, auditory figure ground perception, cognitive gaps, attention, and vigilance) and the performance of interest (in this example, meal planning). Keeping these factors linked makes the role and perspective of occupational therapy clear for others (i.e., performance).

Figure 7-2 illustrates a template for task analysis. On the left side of the template, record the typical performance features of the task of interest; on the right side of the template record this child's actual performance features. For example, using the previous story, typically a person would have ideas about the meal prior to beginning meal planning (e.g., I want something light and fruity, or I want something substantial). The adolescent in the story seemed to have no prior ideas about the meal; this might interfere with performance in that the school period will be over before the student can complete the task. Another aspect of the task analysis is to record the alternative strategies (when there are some) as they occur, without judging their effectiveness; people with disabilities may have effective and unusual ways to tackle a performance need.

There are many more complicated ways to conduct a task analysis (see Rainforth & York-Barr, 1997). This template is a worksheet for recording impressions and comparing typical and current performance.

Figure 7-3 illustrates a template for summarizing context data. There is a row for each aspect of context, and a column on the right hand side to code the contextual features as "supporting factors" to performance, or "barriers to performance"; there is also a code for features that have an unknown impact on performance. Using our example above, we might record that there are many cookbooks available as a physical feature with unknown impact (i.e., it could be helpful to some students and difficult for others to have lots of choices). In this school setting, there are many peers around (social), and they are very interested in the meal options this adolescent is considering (cultural). Sometimes therapists cannot code the context features until they have had multiple opportunities to consider the meaning of the student's performance.

Typical Performance Features of a Task	_____ 's Performance

Figure 7-2. Summary of task analysis worksheet. (Adapted from Dunn, W., Brown, C., McClain, L., & Westman, K. (1994). The ecology of human performance: A contextual perspective on human occupation. In C. Royeen (Ed.), *The practice of the future: Putting occupation back into therapy.* Washington, DC: AOTA.)

	Code
Physical	
Social	
Cultural	
Temporal	
Code: s=supporting factor; b=barrier to performance; ?= could be either a support or barrier	

Figure 7-3. Context Data Worksheet. (Adapted from Dunn, W., Brown, C., McClain, L., & Westman, K. (1994). The ecology of human performance: A contextual perspective on human occupation. In C. Royeen (Ed.), *The practice of the future: Putting occupation back into therapy.* Washington, DC: AOTA.)

Scientific Reasoning	Narrative Reasoning	Pragmatic Reasoning	Ethical Reasoning

Figure 7-4. Worksheet to outline clinical reasoning data. (Adapted from Dunn, W., Brown, C., McClain, L., & Westman, K. (1994). The ecology of human performance: A contextual perspective on human occupation. In C. Royeen (Ed.), *The practice of the future: Putting occupation back into therapy.* Washington, DC: AOTA.)

Figure 7-4 illustrates a template for summarizing one's clinical reasoning (see Chapter 3). This template enables a young therapist to systematically consider all the factors that might influence intervention options. In our example, scientific reasoning might include information about the class requirements and the student's particular disability (e.g., expected cognitive levels). Narrative reasoning might include the reason why this student is interested in this particular meal plan (e.g., he will get to invite 10 friends to the meal). Pragmatic reasoning might include information about the time restraints due to the school schedule. Using this template offers a means for organizing one's thinking before making recommendations.

Figure 7-5 illustrates a template for describing a range of interventions for each target performance. Record the target performance in the left column and then generate as many different intervention options as possible, taking into consideration all the information from the previous templates. This page represents your creative thinking about the ways to support better performance. For our example with meal planning, the therapist might record an establish/restore option of having the student assist the cafeteria staff with their planning, or have the student interview people about what they would want to eat. The therapist might also suggest a coding system for the cookbooks as an adaptation to deal with the pragmatic problem of time. To prevent a sense of failure, the therapist and teacher could design organized meal options for the student to select.

Figure 7-6 illustrates a more advanced version of the intervention planning template (see Figure 7-5). For this template, the intervention approaches are still across the top of the form; the left column contains the intervention models (i.e., direct, supervised therapy, consultation). The therapist and team members generate 15 possible interventions for each of the student's performance problems. This worksheet provides a tool for "brain aerobics". It is hard to think of 15 ways (i.e., the number of intersection boxes) to address the same problem, particularly when each way has to have unique qualities.

For example, the first box on the upper left is for "direct" and "establish/restore"; this is an easy box for experienced therapists and teachers because this has been the focus of our training in the past (i.e., fix the problem yourself). However, we can also provide direct service and use an adaptive approach (top box in third column). In this case, we might work with a child ourselves to design an adaptation for grasping and then move to consultation model (bottom box at left) to show the teachers and parents how to support the child to use it properly during performance. Figure 7-7 contains a completed form with options to support a student who has

Performance	Establish/Restore	Alter/Modify	Adapt	Prevent	Create

Figure 7-5. Worksheet for outlining therapeutic interventions. (Adapted from Dunn, W., Brown, C., McClain, L., & Westman, K. (1994). The ecology of human performance: A contextual perspective on human occupation. In C. Royeen (Ed.), *The practice of the future: Putting occupation back into therapy.* Washington, DC: AOTA.)

Models of Service	Establish/Restore	Alter/Modify	Adapt	Prevent	Create
Direct					
Supervised Therapy					
Consult					

Figure 7-6. Advanced worksheet for outlining therapeutic interventions. (Adapted from Dunn, W., Brown, C., McClain, L., & Westman, K. (1994). The ecology of human performance: A contextual perspective on human occupation. In C. Royeen (Ed.), *The practice of the future: Putting occupation back into therapy.* Washington, DC: AOTA.)

Models of Service	Establish/ Restore	Alter/Modify	Adapt	Prevent	Create
Direct	Therapist challenges the child's postural control using ball for a chair (moving it slowly) during a simpler, review part of the reading group (motor control and motor learning)	Therapist conducts an ecological assessment and identifies a better location for the reading group (e.g., in the "reading corner" of class, with pillows and other supports for posture)	Therapist constructs a chair with arms and sides for the child to use during reading group to reduce demand on postural control (biomechanical model)	Therapist teaches *only* the child (so others must use him as resource) new computer programs for reading follow-up to prevent social isolation from struggling in reading	N/A
Supervised Therapy	Therapist supervises the aide to support and challenge the child on the ball as a chair during reading		Therapist supervises the teacher to try devices/ strategies for turning the pages, which accommodate the child's clumsiness with the book (e.g., rubber fingers, bookmarks)	Therapist supervises a small group play activity with the reading group to prevent the child from experiencing social isolation within the group	N/A
Consult	Therapist and physical education teacher collaborate to design a posture and motor control intervention during an extra time during the week	Therapist and teacher identify the library "reading pit" as a better place for the reading group because there are no chairs and the children can lie down during the lesson	Therapist and teacher discuss other work postures, e.g., sitting backwards on the chair so back can support chest, placing a foam pillow in front of the child for support during reading	Therapist and teacher find an older child to record stories for this child's review to prevent reading skills from deteriorating	N/A

Figure 7-7. Advanced worksheet for outlining therapeutic interventions. **Intervention options for a student with too poor postural and motor control to participate in the reading group successfully.** (Adapted from Dunn, W., Brown, C., McClain, L., & Westman, K. (1994). The ecology of human performance: A contextual perspective on human occupation. In C. Royeen (Ed.), *The practice of the future: Putting occupation back into therapy.* Washington, DC: AOTA.)

poor postural and motor control, and cannot participate in the reading group. You will see that the "create" column is blank; this is because the example is about a specific child with a disability, and not about the community at large.

A final step in learning how to design best practice is to add a method for measuring effectiveness of the intervention option to each box as you generate ideas. This gets you into the habit of thinking about how to monitor and document progress as a natural part of the intervention. Chapter 8 provides details on how to monitor progress efficiently in practice settings.

USING PRACTICE MODELS IN BEST PRACTICE INTERVENTION PLANNING

The final aspect of intervention planning involves including practice model perspectives in your thinking. In Chapter 4, we discussed the most frequent practice models therapists use when serving children and families. Therapists use the worksheet (see Figure 7-6) in concert with specific practice models to generate intervention options. When learning to do this, therapists can use a separate worksheet for each practice model (i.e., make 4 copies and generate ideas using the biomechanical model on one, sensory integration on another, etc.), or can code each idea on the worksheet in relation to which practice model that idea is generated from (i.e., box 1 on Figure 7-7 employs a motor control and motor learning model, box 3 employs a biomechanical model). It is very important to be explicit with yourself in your thinking about which practice model is guiding idea generation; sometimes new ideas come from another practice model, rather than from using another approach to intervention. Figure 7-8 illustrates intervention options using biomechanical and sensory integration practice models on the worksheet.

Applying Practice Model Concepts in Community-Based Programs

It is important to understand how to translate concepts from occupational therapy practice models to community-based programs and concerns. In order for other discipline team members and families to feel committed to implementing occupational therapy ideas, we must be able to make the information accessible to them (i.e., use regular language to make the connections between our conceptual thinking and the daily life challenges they face).

In this section, I will introduce you to materials I developed to introduce the concepts of sensory processing to some preschool and school-based programs. I was interested in making sure that the sensory integration perspective was available to all the team members for our problem-solving. I wanted the team members and paraprofessionals to understand *why* I was asking them to conduct routines a certain way, so that they would feel a stronger commitment to carrying out some of the ideas that were based on sensory processing principles. Remember, this section only provides one example of how to make occupational therapy knowledge accessible to others. There are many ways to do this, and I look forward to your contributions in this area.

The first step was to translate some of the terminology into regular language. Table 7-2 contains a list of terms used to describe aspects of sensory input. The first column contains the names of the primary sensory systems, and then there are two more columns. The **"arousal/alerting"** column contains features of each sensory system that alert the nervous system. These features typically stimulate the reticular activating system, which sends generalized arousal messages to the brain. The **"discrimination/mapping"** column contains features of each sensory system that send specific, organized input to the brain to create maps of the body (i.e., the homunculi in the sensorimotor cortex) and the environment. The features in this column do not send messages through the reticular formation.

This table provides the team members with simple definitions of each sensory feature, along with a simple daily life example of when a person might receive this type of input. For example, the first entry for the somatosensory system is light touch, with the definition: gentle tapping on skin; tickling. After the definition, in parentheses, is the example: "loose clothing making contact with skin". The team members could read this definition and example and quickly understand the nature of "light touch". The information on this table provides common ground for initial discussions about the sensory processing perspective.

The team needs further information to be able to incorporate a sensory perspective into their planning. Table 7-3 is organized in exactly the same format as the previous table, but the purpose of this table is to provide the team members with the reasons they would select each sensory feature for a therapeutic benefit. This does not substitute for the therapist's thinking and contributions, but rather provides basic information so the team members can understand why the therapist might suggest a particular activity, or why something they are doing is not working.

Models of Service	Establish/Restore	Alter	Adapt	Prevent	Create
Direct	Guide exploration of movement on suspended and moving playground equipment during recess to facilitate responses to vestibular input *Improve postural alignment and head control for looking by stabilizing pelvis during circle time*	Select an isolated spot in the library with no traffic patterns nearby for the child's work time so that there are no opportunities for tactile arousal and "fight or flight" responses *Attend a showing at the IMAX theatre, which has chairs that support posture in relation to gravity*	Develop a verbal cueing system with a child who has motor planning problems so the child can complete self-care rituals *Design and fabricate a seating design to support a child with low muscle tone to enable access to socialization with peers*	Include peers in other intervention activities to prevent social isolation *Work in classroom to select proper seating to prevent asymmetry*	Encourage children to use a straw for all drinking to promote oral sensorimotor development *Place favorite toys in locations at the day care center to promote reaching and postural shift*
Supervised therapy	Supervise a sensorimotor exploration group run by the physical education teacher *Supervise all adults to provide physical guidance for a child who is working on reaching*	Supervise the team to review and select work site which has the quiet environment the student needs to minimize sensory overload *Supervise the job coach to select a job placement that contains supports on chairs for the desks to reduce the interference of postural instability at work*	Supervise the physical education teacher to modify the obstacle course to accommodate children with poor motor planning *Supervise development of a transporting routine that provides stability to minimize effects of a child's athetoid movements for efficient transport*	Supervise the teacher group as they design an art program that provides multisensory input to prevent fine motor delays *Supervise paraprofessional in jaw stabilization during meal time to prevent difficulties with lip closure*	Supervise the development of a pretend play area in the preschool classroom that provides enriched sensory exploration opportunities *Supervise the home toilet hygiene program so that parents promote alignment for sitting*
Consult	Identify heavy objects that can be incorporated into classroom tasks to increase proprioceptive input *Teach the classroom staff how to use several positioning strategies throughout the day to facilitate head realignment during copying tasks at the desk*	Collaborate with day care providers to select the group that supports the child's sensation-seeking behaviors as part of their rituals *Collaborate with educational team to select furniture for the cafeteria that supports children's sitting and moving postures*	Collaborate with the teacher to set up all work materials at waist level or higher to reduce vestibular stimuli in a child who is overly aroused by movement *Collaborate with team to design a schedule for positioning throughout the day that compensates for poor head control*	Collaborate with the teacher to control the amount and type of arousing stimuli in the classroom to prevent attentional and behavioral problems from erupting *Collaborate with teachers to design a "warm up" sequence of stretching to prevent stiffness for the day*	Work with administrative team to design a playground that provides sensory experiences and motor planning opportunities for everyone *Collaborate with third grade teacher team to match desk and chairs with students to facilitate postural alignment*

Figure 7-8. Advanced worksheet for outlining therapeutic interventions. Sensory integration framework is not italicized, biomechanical framework is italicized. (Adapted from Dunn, W., Brown, C., McClain, L., & Westman, K. (1994). *The ecology of human performance: A contextual perspective on human occupation.* In C. Royeen (Ed.), *The practice of the future: Putting occupation back into therapy.* Washington, DC: AOTA.)

Table 7-2.

Arousal/Alerting and Discrimination/Mapping Descriptors of the Sensory System

Sensory System	Arousal/Alerting Descriptors*	Discrimination/Mapping Descriptors**
For all systems	Unpredictable: The task is unfamiliar; the child cannot anticipate the sensory experiences that will occur in the task.	Predictable: Sensory pattern in the task is routine for the child, such as diaper changing—the child knows what is occurring and what will come next.
Somatosensory	Light touch: Gentle tapping on skin; tickling (e.g., loose clothing making contact with skin). Pain: Brisk pinching; contact with sharp objects; skin pressed in small surface (e.g., when skin is caught in between chair arm and seat). Temperature: Hot or cold stimuli (e.g., iced drinks, hot foods, cold hands, cold metal chairs). Variable: Changing characteristics during the task (e.g., putting clothing on requires a combination of tactile experiences). Short duration stimuli: Tapping, touching briefly (e.g., splashing water). Small body surface contact: Small body surfaces, as when using only fingertips to touch something.	Touch pressure: Firm contact on skin (e.g., hugging, patting, grasping). Occurs both when touching objects or persons, or when they touch you. Long duration stimuli: Holding, grasping (e.g., carrying a child in your arms). Large body surface contact: Large body surfaces, include holding, hugging; also includes holding a cup with the entire palmar surface of hand.
Vestibular	Head position change: The child's head orientation is altered (e.g., pulling the child up from lying on the back to sitting). Speed change: Movements change velocity (e.g., the teacher stops to talk to another teacher when pushing the child to the bathroom in his wheelchair). Direction change: Movements change planes, such as bending down to pick something up while carrying the child down the hall. Rotary head movement: head moving in an arc (e.g., spinning, turning head side to side).	Linear head movement: Head moving in a straight line (e.g., bouncing up and down, going down the hall in a wheelchair). Repetitive head movement: Movements that repeat in a simple sequence (e.g., rocking in a rocker).
Proprioception	Quick stretch: Movements that pull on the muscles (e.g., briskly tapping).	Sustained tension: Steady, constant action on the muscles pressing or holding on the muscle (e.g., using heavy objects during play). Shifting muscle tension: Activities that demand constant change in the muscles (e.g., walking, lifting, moving objects).
Visual	High Intensity: Visual stimulus is bright (e.g., looking out a window on a bright day). High contrast: A difference between the visual stimulus and surrounding environment (e.g., cranberry juice in a white cup). Variable: Changing characteristics during a task (e.g., a TV program is a variable visual stimulus).	Low Intensity: Visual stimulus is subdued (e.g., finding objects in the dark closet). High similarity: Small differences between visual stimulus and its surrounding environment (e.g., oatmeal in a beige bowl). Competitive: The background is interesting or busy (e.g., the junk drawer, a bulletin board).
Auditory	Variable: Changing characteristics during the task (e.g., a person's voice with intonation). High Intensity: The auditory stimulus is loud (e.g., siren, high volume radio).	Rhythmic: Sounds repeat in a simple sequence/beat (e.g., humming, singing nursery songs). Constant: The stimulus is always present (e.g., a fan noise). Competitive: The environment has a variety of recurring sounds (e.g., the classroom, a party). Noncompetitive: The environment is quiet (e.g., the bedroom when all is ready for bedtime). Low intensity: The auditory stimulus is subdued (e.g., whispering).
Olfactory/gustatory	Strong Intensity: The taste/smell has distinct qualities (e.g., spinach).	Mild intensity: The taste/smell has nondistinct or familiar qualities (e.g., cream of wheat).

*Arousal/alerting stimuli tend to generate "noticing" behaviors. The individual's attention is at least momentarily drawn toward the stimulus (commonly disrupting ongoing behavior). These stimuli enable the nervous system to orient to stimuli that may require a protective response. In some situations, an arousing stimulus can become part of a functional behavior pattern (e.g., when the arousing somatosensory input from putting on the shirt becomes predictable, a discriminating/mapping characteristic).

**Discriminatory/mapping stimuli are those that enable the individual to gather information that can be used to support and generate functional behaviors. The information yields spatial and temporal qualities of body and environment (the content of the maps), which can be used to create purposeful movement. These stimuli are more organizing for the nervous system.

From Dunn, W. (1991). The sensorimotor systems: A framework for assessment and intervention. In F. P. Orelove & D. Sobsey (Eds.), *Educating children with multiple disabilities: A transdisciplinary approach* (2nd ed.). Baltimore: Paul H. Brookes. Reprinted with permission.

Table 7-3.

Reasons for Incorporating Various Sensory Qualities into Integrated Intervention Programs*

Sensory System	Arousal/Alerting Descriptors	Discrimination/Mapping Descriptors
For all systems	Unpredictable: To develop an increasing level of attention to keep the child interested in the task/activity (e.g., change the position of the objects on the child's lap tray during the task).	Predictable: To establish the child's ability to anticipate a programming sequence or a salient cue; to decrease possibility to be distracted from a functional task sequence (e.g., use the same routine for diaper changing every time).
Somatosensory	Light touch: To increase alertness in a child who is lethargic (e.g., pull cloth from child's face during peek-a-boo). Pain: To raise from unconsciousness; to determine ability to respond to noxious stimuli when unconscious (e.g., flick palm of hand or sole of foot briskly). Temperature: To establish awareness of stimuli; to maintain attentiveness to task (e.g., use hot foods for spoon eating and cold drink for sucking through a straw). Variable: To maintain attention to or interest in the task (e.g., place new texture on cup surface each day so child notices the cup). Short duration: To increase arousal for task performance (e.g., tap child on chest before giving directions). Small body surface contact: To generate and focus attention on a particular body part (e.g., tap around lips with fingertips before eating task).	Touch pressure: To establish and maintain awareness of body parts and body position; to calm a child who has been overstimulated (e.g., provide a firm bear hug). Long duration: To enable the child to become familiar, comfortable with the stimulus; to incorporate stimulus into functional skill (e.g., grasping the container to pick it up and pour out contents). Large body surface contact: To establish and maintain awareness of body parts and body position; to calm a child who has been overstimulated (e.g., wrap child tightly in a blanket).
Vestibular	Head position change: To increase arousal for an activity (e.g., position child prone over a wedge). Speed change: To keep adequate alertness for functional task (e.g., vary pace while carrying the child to new task). Direction change: To elevate level of alertness for a functional task (e.g., swing child back and forth in arms prior to positioning him or her at the table for a task). Rotary head movement: To increase arousal prior to functional task (e.g., pick child up from prone [on stomach] facing away to upright facing toward you to position for a new task).	Linear head movement: To support establishment of body awareness in space (e.g., carry child around the room in fixed position to explore its features). Repetitive head movement: To provide predictable and organizing information; to calm a child who has been overstimulated (e.g., rock the child).
Proprioception	Quick stretch: To generate additional muscle tension to support functional tasks (e.g., tap muscle bell of hypotonic muscle while providing physical guidance to grasp).	Sustained tension: To enable the muscle to relax, elongate, so body part can be in more optimal position for function (e.g., press firmly across muscle belly while guiding a reaching pattern; add weight to objects being manipulated). Shift muscle tension: To establish functional movements that contain stability and mobility (e.g., prop and reach for a top; reach, fill, and lift spoon to mouth).

*Adapted from Dunn, W. (1991). The sensorimotor systems: A framework for assessment and intervention. In F.P. Orelove & D. Sobsey (Eds.), Educating children with multiple disabilities: A transdisciplinary approach (2nd ed.). Baltimore. Paul H. Brookes.

Table 7-3 continued.

Sensory System	Arousal/Alerting Descriptors	Discrimination/Mapping Descriptors
Visual	High intensity: To increase opportunity to notice object; to generate arousal for task (e.g., cover blocks with foil for manipulation task). High contrast: To enhance possibility of locating object and maintaining attention to it (e.g., place raisins on a piece of typing paper for prehension activity). Variable: To maintain attention to or interest in the task (e.g., play rolling catch with a clear ball that has moveable pieces inside).	Low intensity: To allow visual stimulus to blend with other salient features; to generate searching behaviors, since characteristics are less obvious (e.g., find own cubby hole in back of room). High similarity: To establish more discerning abilities; to develop skills for naturally occurring tasks (e.g., scoop applesauce from beige plate). Competitive: To facilitate searching; to increase tolerance for natural life circumstances (e.g., obtain correct tools from equipment bin).
Auditory	Variable: To maintain attention to or interest in the task (e.g., play radio station after activating a switch). High intensity: To stimulate noticing the person or object, to create proper alerting for task performance (e.g., ring a bell to encourage the child to locate the stimulus).	Rhythmic: To provide predictable/organizing information for environmental orientation (e.g., sing a nursery rhyme while physically guiding motions). Constant: To provide a foundational stimulus for environmental orientation; especially important when other sensory systems (e.g., vision, vestibular) do not provide orientation (e.g., child recognizes own classroom by fan noise and calms down). Competitive: To facilitate differentiation of salient stimuli; to increase tolerance for natural life circumstances (e.g., after child learns to look when his or her name is called, conduct activity within busy classroom).
Olfactory/gustatory	Strong intensity: To stimulate arousal for task (e.g., child smells spaghetti sauce at lunch).	Noncompetitive: To facilitate focused attention for acquiring a new and difficult skill; to calm a child who has been overstimulated (e.g., move child to quiet room to establish vocalizations). Low intensity: To allow the auditory stimulus to blend with other salient features; to generate searching behaviors since stimulus is less obvious (e.g., give child a direction in a normal volume). Mild intensity: To facilitate exploratory behaviors; to stimulate naturally occurring activities (e.g., smell of lunch food is less distinct, so child is encouraged to notice texture, color).

*Adapted from Dunn, W. (1991). The sensorimotor systems: A framework for assessment and intervention. In F. P. Orelove & D. Sobsey (Eds.), Educating children with multiple disabilities: A transdisciplinary approach (2nd ed.). Baltimore. Paul H. Brookes.

Let's look at light touch again. This time, the phrase tells the reader why to select light touch for a therapeutic purpose: "to increase alertness in a child who is lethargic". This simple definition points out that an arousing stimulus like light touch *is* a good choice to increase attention potential in a child with a flat affect; it is probably *not* a good choice for a hyperactive, distractible child. As with the previous table, the parentheses contain an example in daily life: "pull cloth from child's face during peek-a-boo". Examples such as these help the team member to associate the abstract concept with familiar life experiences.

With this background information, the team can practice taking a sensory processing perspective in their problem-solving. Figure 7-9 provides a Sensory Task Analysis worksheet that enables the team to consider a task from a sensory point of view. *Remember, we would never actually ask the team to take just one point of view for task performance, but rather use this process to practice a less familiar one for them.*

On this form, the team selects a task that the child is struggling with, and considers all the sensory features of that task. Figure 7-10 provides a completed form for face washing. Under the columns "What does the task routine hold?" the team marks any sensory feature that would be present in face washing. We have only completed one column because face washing is a simple task; with more complex tasks like meal preparation, the team might want to break it down into gathering supplies (column A), cooking the food (Column B), and serving the meal (column C). As you can see, there are many sensory features to face washing. We all have these sensory experiences during face washing; these features are not specifically related to the child of interest.

The next column, "What does the particular environment hold?" is reserved for additional comments related to the actual context for the target child's performance. In the example, the child needs to wash face at the classroom sink, which brings some additional sensory features to consider (e.g., there are paints on the school sink that you would not find at home on the sink).

So now the team has all the sensory analysis information they need to consider the sensory features of face washing performance. The final column, "What adaptations are likely to improve functional outcomes?" is reserved for the team's brainstorming. In the example, the team considered each sensory event in face washing and then came up with an idea to change that feature (e.g., if the splashing water is creating "light touch" arousal and interfering with the child's performance, then we can turn the water off). Each idea is to reconstruct the sensory experience toward the goal of improving the performance of face washing.

The team would never implement all the ideas at once, because then it would still be unclear what was interfering with face washing. The team would consider all the possibilities and select a likely candidate for interference, and then try that change to see what happens. During this process the team is vigilant about collecting data so they know which performance changes are related to which intervention options. When they keep track like this, they can also use their insights to support other task performance.

The usefulness of this process is in getting everyone to think about the sensory features of performance. Occupational therapy personnel cannot be with teacher, parents, and children all the time to offer this point of view, so materials and processes such as these infuse our wisdom into children's daily lives. When a team member understands the nature of our suggestions a little more clearly, then the team member will be more likely to implement our suggestions consistently, which is ultimately in the child's best interest. For example, a paraprofessional might think it is irritating to turn the water on and off for each child, delaying the time to get to lunch. However, if the paraprofessional understands that turning the water off will decrease the possibility of a child getting irritable, the paraprofessional becomes more motivated to implement the suggestion. The suggestion is no longer a mysterious and silly suggestion, but one that supports the paraprofessional's work and the child's outcome. If the child gets better at completing face washing, both the child and the paraprofessional are successful.

Table 7-4 provides additional material that can be used with teams. This table also provides rows for each sensory system; the columns represent daily life tasks. In each intersection, there are behaviors that one might observe during that life task; the behaviors are indicators of difficulty with that particular sensory system. This table provides another way for team members to link the child's sensory processing with performance in daily life. We are trying to help our colleagues (and parents) to derive meaning from the behaviors they observe from a sensory perspective.

Routine/task _____ Sensory characteristics		What does the task routine hold? A	B	C	What does the particular environ- ment hold?	What adaptations are likely to improve functional outcome?
Somato- sensory	light touch (tap, tickle)					
	pain					
	temperature (hot, cold)					
	touch pressure (hug, pat, grasp)					
	variable					
	duration of stimulus (short, long)					
	body surface contact (small, large)					
	predictable					
	unpredictable					
Vestibular	head position change					
	speed change					
	direction change					
	rotary head movement					
	linear head movement					
	repetitive head movement (rhythmic)					
	predictable					
	unpredictable					
Proprio- ceptive	quick stretch stimulus					
	sustained tension stimulus					
	shifting muscle tension					
Visual	high intensity					
	low intensity					
	high contrast					
	high similarity (low contrast)					
	competitive					
	variable					
	predictable					
	unpredictable					
Auditory	rhythmic					
	variable					
	constant					
	competitive					
	noncompetitive					
	loud					
	soil					
	predictable					
	unpredictable					
Olfactory/ Gustatory	mild					
	strong					
	predictable					
	unpredictable					

Task: A = _____
Components: B = _____
C = _____

Figure 7-9. Sensory components of task performance (Reprinted with permission from Dunn, W. (1991). The sensorimotor systems: A framework for assessment and intervention. In F. P. Orelove & D. Sobsey (Eds.), *Educating children with multiple disabilities: A transdisciplinary approach* (2nd ed.). Baltimore: Paul H. Brookes.)

Routine/task _____ Sensory characteristics		What does the task routine hold?			What does the particular environment hold?	What adaptations are likely to improve functional outcome?
		A	B	C		
Somato-sensory	light touch (tap, tickle)	X				turn water off to decrease splashing
	pain					
	temperature (hot, cold)	X				try alternative water temperatures
	touch pressure (hug, pat, grasp)	X				Pat face instead of rubbing cloth on face
	variable	X				Pat large face area
	duration of stimulus (short, long)	L				
	body surface contact (small, large)	L				Try washing one part only; begin w/ chin area
	predictable	X				
	unpredictable					
Vestibular	head position change	X				alter water source so don't have to bend head (e.g., in a pan or tub)
	speed change					
	direction change	X				keep head up so don't have down-up pattern
	rotary head movement					
	linear head movement	X				keep head up; if need arousal, place items on counter to encourage more head turning
	repetitive head movement (rhythmic)					
	predictable					
	unpredictable					
Proprio-ceptive	quick stretch stimulus					
	sustained tension stimulus					move objects to decrease head control requirements
	shifting muscle tension					
Visual	high intensity					
	low intensity					
	high contrast					
	high similarity (low contrast)	X			X other objects	use a dark wash cloth and light soap; use dark containers on a light counter; remove extra items from counter
	competitive	X			X on sink	
	variable				X counter changes day to day	
	predictable	X				
	unpredictable				X	
Auditory	rhythmic	X				prepare wet cloth; don't have running tap water; use tub instead of running water
	variable	X				

Figure 7-10. Sample completed form for analyzing sensory characteristics of face washing. (Reprinted with permission from Dunn, W. (1991). The sensorimotor systems: A framework for assessment and intervention. In F. P. Orelove & D. Sobsey (Eds.), *Educating children with multiple disabilities: A transdisciplinary approach* (2nd ed.). Baltimore: Paul H. Brookes.)

Routine/task _____ Sensory characteristics		What does the task routine hold?			What does the particular environ-ment hold?	What adaptations are likely to improve functional outcome?
		A	B	C		
Auditory	constant					
	competitive				X other students	move child to the bath-room alone
	noncompetitive	X				
	loud				X teacher's voice	provide physical prompts and decrease talking
	soft					
	predictable	X				
	unpredictable				X unplanned	
Olfactory/ Gustatory	mild	X				if arousal is needed, use strong smelling soap
	strong					
	predictable	X				
	unpredictable					

Task:	A = _____
Components:	B = _____
	C = _____

Figure 7-10 continued. Sample completed form for analyzing sensory characteristics of face wash-ing. (Reprinted with permission from Dunn, W. (1991). The sensorimotor systems: A framework for assessment and intervention. In F. P. Orelove & D. Sobsey (Eds.), *Educating children with multiple disabilities: A transdisciplinary approach* (2nd ed.). Baltimore: Paul H. Brookes.)

PROJECTING OUTCOMES TO FRAME THE INTERVENTION PLAN

The IEP, IFSP, and IHP processes require the team members to anticipate several levels of progress as part of their plans. Professionals who are providing best practice services engage in a collaborative process to hypothesize about desired long-term outcomes so they can frame the current intervention planning. The team routinely considers anticipated annual progress, since individualized planning documents require development of annual goals. Best practices also include long-range planning during which professionals and families consid-er what they "dream" and "fear" the child will be doing in adulthood. Long-term projections can include living, working, and social situations. The team discusses skills and supports for living a satisfying life; when children are older, they can participate in this process themselves. Two widely-used approaches are the COACH model (Giangreco, Cloniger, & Iverson, 1990) and the MAPS process (Vandercook, York, & Forest, 1989); be sure to find out about your setting's strategies and participate in them (see the references listed in this chapter).

For example, many parents of children with complex disabilities worry that there will be no one to care for their child when they grow older or die. It is important to provide an environment that supports the fam-ily members to express concerns such as these; the team can only address issues that are expressed. When par-ents are silently worried about a concern such as this one, it can contaminate current intervention planning (e.g., "what's the use….", or "we must provide *everything* possible so my child is 'cured' before I get too old…").

When the team projects long-term life outcomes, it becomes easier to determine what is relevant for cur-rent planning. In the example above, knowing that the parents are thinking about independent/supported liv-ing guides the team members to discussing issues in relation to the child's functional skill development for independent living. The team can also introduce the family to community supports that they might learn about so they feel ready for various transitions they will face.

Projecting outcomes also provides clarity about what might be appropriate or inappropriate for current intervention plans. For example, if the team of a young child projects that the child will use an augmentative

Table 7-4.

Examples of Observable Behaviors that Indicate Difficulty with Sensory Processing During Daily Life Tasks

	Personal Hygiene	Dressing	Eating	Homemaking	School/Work	Play
Somatosensory	Withdraws from splashing water Pushes wash-cloth/towel away Cries when hair is washed and dried Makes face when tooth-paste gets on lips, tongue Tenses when bottom is wiped after toileting	Tolerates a nar-row range of clothing items Prefers tight clothing More irritable with loose-tex-tured clothing Cries during dressing Pulls at hats, head gear, accessories	Only tolerates food at one temperature Gags with textur-ed food or uten-sils in mouth Winces when face is wiped Hand extends & avoids objects & surfaces (fin-ger food, uten-sils)	Avoids participa-tion in tasks that are wet, dirty Seeks to remove batter that falls on arms	Cries when tape or glue gets on skin Overreacts to pats, hugs; avoids such actions Only tolerates one pencil, type of paper, only wooden objects Hands extend when attempt-ing to type	Selects a narrow range of toys, textures similar Can't hold onto toys/objects Rubs toys on face, arms Mouths objects
Proprioception	Can't lift objects that are heavier such as a new bar of soap Can't change head position to use sink and mirror in same task	Can't support heavier items, e.g., belt with buckle, shoes Fatigues prior to task completion Misses when placing arm or leg in clothing	Uses external support to eat (e.g., propping) Tires before co-mpleting meal Can't provide force to cut meat Tires before completing foods that need to be chewed	Drops equipment (e.g., broom) Uses external support such as leaning on cou-nter to stir batter Has difficulty in pouring a glass of milk	Drops books Becomes uncomfortable in a certain position Hooks limbs on furniture to obtain support Moves arm and hand in repeti-tive patterns (self-stimulato-ry)	Unable to sus-tain movements during play Tires before game is complete Drops heavy parts of a toy/game
Vestibular	Becomes disori-ented when ben-ding over the sink Fails when try-ing to partici-pate in washing lower extremi-ties	Gets overly excited/distract-ed after bend-ing down to assist in putting on socks Cries when moved around a lot during dressing	Holds head stiffly in one position during mealtime Gets distracted from meal after several head position changes	Avoids leaning to obtain cook-ing utensil Becomes overly excited after moving around room to dust	Avoids turning head to look at persons or find source of sound After being transported in a wheelchair, more difficult to get on task Moves head in repetitive pat-tern (self-stimu-latory)	Avoids play that includes movement Becomes overly excited/anxious when moving during play Rocks exces-sively Craves move-ment activities
Visual	Can't find uten-sils on the sink Has difficulty in spotting desired item in drawer Misses when applying paste to toothbrush	Can't find buttons on patterned or solid clothing Overlooks desired shirt in closet or drawer Misses armhole when donning shirt	Misses utensils on the table Has trouble get-ting foods onto spoon when they are a similar color to the plate	Can't locate correct canned item in the pantry Has difficulty finding cooking utensils in the drawer	Can't keep place on the page Can't locate desired item on communication board Attends exces-sively to bright/ flashing objects	Has trouble with matching, sort-ing activities Has trouble locating desired toy on cluttered shelf

From Dunn, W. (1991). *The sensorimotor systems: A framework for assessment and intervention.* In F. P. Orelove & D. Sobsey (Eds.), Educating children with multiple disabilities: A transdisciplinary approach *(2nd ed.). Baltimore, MD: Paul H. Brookes.*

Table 7-4 continued.

Examples of Observable Behaviors that Indicate Difficulty with Sensory Processing During Daily Life Tasks

	Personal Hygiene	Dressing	Eating	Homemaking	School/Work	Play
Auditory	Cries when hair dryer is on Becomes upset by running water Jerks when toilet flushes	Is distracted by clothing that makes noise (e.g., crisp cloth, accessories)	Is distracted by noise of utensils against each other (e.g., spoon in bowl, knife on plate) Can't keep eating when someone talks	Is distracted by vacuum cleaner sound Is distracted by TV or radio during tasks	Is distracted by squeaky wheelchair Is intolerant of noise others make Overreacts to door closing Notices toilet flushing down hall	Play is disrupted by sounds Makes sounds constantly
Olfactory/ gustatory	Gags at taste of toothpaste Jerks away at smell of soap	Overreacts to clothing when it has been washed in a new detergent	Tolerates a narrow range of foods Becomes upset when certain hot foods are cooking	Becomes upset when house is cleaned (odors of cleansers)	Overreacts to new person (new smells) Intolerant of scratch-n-sniff stickers Smells everything	Tastes or smells all objects before playing

From Dunn, W. (1991). The sensorimotor systems: A framework for assessment and intervention. In F. P. Orelove & D. Sobsey (Eds.), Educating children with multiple disabilities: A transdisciplinary approach (2nd ed.). Baltimore, MD: Paul H. Brookes.

communication system as an adult, they can begin working on this outcome immediately. This projected outcome might guide the occupational therapist to work on adaptations for optimal positioning of the device, and on reaching and pointing to activate the device. The speech language pathologist might address vocabulary and phrasing for the device. The occupational therapist and speech pathologist might explore augmentative devices and switch options that lead to an adult setup. There would be a low demand for addressing oral control for talking, and so this would not be a priority for this child's plan (although there may be a need to address oral motor control for eating in another aspect of planning). The occupational therapist might decide not to emphasize head control, opting for biomechanical support so that the child can spend more time interacting with the augmentative device for talking and socializing.

We must also be sensitive to the family's coping abilities when projecting outcomes. In Case #1 (see Chapter 10), David is a very young infant; his mother is distressed due to David's highly aroused state and her inability to cope with his behavior. You will see in reading the case materials that the mother is resistant to therapist involvement at first; this is probably related to her inability to see past the day-to-day challenges she faces in caring for David. The therapists and the community nurse express their confidence in David's ability to learn to play and interact, and the mother eventually experiences some successes with David herself. During the initial distress period, the mother would not have been able to participate in a process to project outcomes for herself and David. However, as she began feeling more competent, this would be a good time to begin the projecting outcomes process.

Projecting outcomes is an emotional process and professionals must be prepared to deal calmly with the situations. When families project outcomes, they also must mourn the loss of the "child they dreamed they would" have, regardless of how much they love the child that "is". It is appropriate for people to be sad, angry, despondent, and even hopeful when they hear the dreams projected by the more informed members, such as the occupational therapist who has scientific reasoning knowledge to recognize the possibilities.

Take the risk to engage in these processes with families; it lets them know everyone is dedicated to their child's progress. There are a number of methods for projecting outcomes; find out what your agency uses and seek to participate.

PROGRAM EVALUATION COMPONENTS OF THE INTERVENTION PLAN

Occupational therapists include a method for evaluating the child's progress in the intervention plan and as part of the documentation. Best practice dictates that these evaluation features must be: easy to measure, measured in the natural context, and directly about desired performance. By designing evaluation criteria about performance, therapists ensure that they address the daily life and not the child demonstrating isolated skills. Additionally, when the evaluation criteria are imbedded in the natural environment, we can see the potentially positive effects of all the service approaches, not just those directed at restorative interventions (i.e., person variable focused). Chapter 8 provides detailed information on methods for charting and evaluating a child's progress as part of comprehensive documentation.

PROVIDING FOLLOW-UP AND DISCONTINUING SERVICES

We provide occupational therapy intervention services to develop functional performance that eliminates the need for continued service. Once the child has achieved service goals and maintains the desired performance, the team reviews the need for continued service (Muhlenhaupt, 1991). Children can achieve desired performance in all of the ways we have discussed in this chapter (i.e., by improving sensorimotor, cognitive, and psychosocial skills through adaptations in the environment and task demands to support performance and through changes in the places in which the child needs to perform). Occupational therapists are in an ideal position to recognize each child's functional abilities separate from the presence of a temporary or long-term disabling condition.

Sometimes parents are reluctant to discontinue services they see as supportive to their children. One reason this happens is that teams fail to point out to parents that the child has made significant progress and therefore does not **need** the same supports any more. This is **good** news; when we reduce services this means that the team is concluding that the child can function in a natural setting with peers without additional services. This good news message needs to be the first information the family receives.

Once the team introduces the idea that the child does not need particular services, then they can design a follow-up or contingency plan with the family. In this process, the team solicits the parents' fears and concerns regarding their child's vulnerabilities if services are discontinued. The team can then set criteria for each fear, and agree that if any of these criteria are met in the next period of time (e.g., the next school quarter), the professionals will immediately investigate and provide service support. If the quarter goes by and the child does not need additional supports, parents can see through the data that their child can indeed function independently of this support. When the family sees that the team is willing to serve their child, it is easier to recognize that it is the child's progress that leads to a reduction in services rather than the team's unwillingness to serve the child.

For example, if the parents are fearful that their child will slowly fall back to poor postural patterns and then get less and less seatwork completed, the team can monitor daily seatwork productivity and agree that if it drops below a critical level, they will reinitiate the postural control supports from the occupational therapist (see Chapter 8 for examples of progress monitoring data collection). When a quarter goes by without this happening, then the team, child, and parents have documented cause for celebration, and discontinuing services is a smooth transition.

SUMMARY

Best practice service provision is a complex process. When therapists are vigilant about listening, observing, and considering options, children and their support groups (i.e., families and teachers) receive the very best of occupational therapy wisdom. Using systematic steps to establish the process ensures that therapists will consider all factors when planning the best possible services for children, families, and other providers.

REFERENCES

American Occupational Therapy Association. (1987). *Guidelines for occupational therapy services in school systems.* Rockville, MD: Author.

American Occupational Therapy Association. (1989). *Guidelines for occupational therapy services in school systems.* Rockville, MD: Author.

American Occupational Therapy Association. (1999). *Occupational therapy practice guidelines.* Rockville, MD: Author.

Campbell, P. (1987a). Integrated therapy and educational programming for students with severe handicaps. In L. Goetz, D. Guess, & K. Stremel-Campbell (Eds.), *Innovative program design for individuals with sensory impairments.* Baltimore, MD: Paul H. Brookes.

Campbell, P. (1987b). The integrated programming team: An approach for coordinating professionals of various disciplines in programs for students with severe and multiple handicaps. *Journal of the Association for Persons with Severe Handicaps, 21*(2), 107-116.

Dunn, W. (1989a). Integrated related services for preschoolers with neurological impairments: Issues and strategies. *RASE, 10*(3), 31-39.

Dunn, W. (1989b). Occupational therapy in early intervention: New perspectives create greater possibilities. *American Journal of Occupational Therapy, 43*(11), 717-721.

Dunn, W. (1991a). Consultation as a process: How, when, and why? In C. Royeen. (Ed.), *School-based practice for related servies.* Rockville, MD: AOTA.

Dunn, W. (1991b). A comparison of service provision models in school-based occupational therapy services. *Occupational Therapy Journal of Research, 10*(5), 300-320.

Dunn, W., Brown, C., McClain, L., & Westman, K. (1994). The ecology of human performance: A contextual perspective on human occupation. In C. Royeen (Ed.), *The practice of the future: Putting occupation back into therapy.* Washington, DC: AOTA.

Dunn, W., Brown, C., & McGuigan, A. (1994). The ecology of human performance: A framework for thought and action. *American Journal of Occupational Therapy, 48*(7), 595-607.

Dunn, W., & Campbell, P. (1991). Designing pediatric service provision. In W. Dunn (Ed.), *Pediatric occupational therapy: Facilitating effective service provision* (pp. 139-160). Thorofare, NJ: SLACK Incorporated.

Giangreco, M., Cloninger, C., & Iverson, V. (1990). *C.O.A.C.H. microform: Cayuga-Onandaga assessment for children with handicaps: Version 6.0.* Burlington, VT: University of Vermont, Center for Developmental Disabilities.

Idol, L., Paolucci-Whitcomb, P., & Nevin, A. (1987). *Collaborative Consultation.* Austin, TX: Pro Ed.

Jaffe, E & Epstein, C. (1992). *Occupational therapy consultation: Theory, principles, and practice.* St. Louis, MO: Mosby.

Lyon, S., & Lyon, G. (1980). Team functioning and staff development: A role release approach to providing integrated educational services for severely handicapped students. *Journal of the Association for the Severely Handicapped, 5*(3), 250-263.

McDonnell, A., & Hardman, M. (1989). The desegregation of America's special schools: Strategies for change. *Journal of the Association for Persons with Severe Handicaps, 14*(1), 68-74.

Muhlenhaupt, M. (1991). Components of the program planning process. In W. Dunn (Ed.), *Pediatric occupational therapy: Facilitating effective service provision* (pp. 125-135). Thorofare, NJ: SLACK Incorporated.

NBCOT. (1997). *A national study of occupational therapy practice final report.* New York, NY: Professional Examination Services.

Rainforth, B., & York-Barr, J. (1997). Collaborative teams for students with severe disabilities. Baltimore, MD: Brookes.

Sternat, J., Messina, R., Nietupski, J., Lyon, S., & Brown, L. (1977). Occupational and physical therapy services for severely handicapped students: Toward a naturalized public school service delivery model. In E. Sontag (Ed.), *Educational programming for the severely and profoundly handicapped.* Reston, VA: Division of Mental Retardation.

Taylor, S. (1988). Caught in the continuum: A critical analysis of the principle of the least restrictive environment. *Journal of the Association for Persons with Severe Handicaps, 13*(1), 41-53.

Vandercook, T., York, J., & Forest , M. (1989). The McGill Action Planning System (MAPS): A strategy for building the vision. *JASH, 14*(3), 205-215.

8

Best Practices in Documentation

Jean Linder, MA, OTR, FAOTA
Gloria Frolek Clark, MS, OTR

INTRODUCTION

Documentation is the key to communicating the outcomes of occupational therapy services to other professionals, the family, the child (if appropriate), and involved agencies. As occupational therapists participate in the processes of referral, assessment, planning, implementation, and re-assessment, they collect an immense amount of information that must be reported efficiently and effectively. The therapist also continually manages additional information (e.g. results from other professional team members, the family's concerns, third-party payer inquiries, or medical and educational issues). Records and reports must reflect the quality of the intervention taking place. In a very real sense, documentation represents the quality of one's professional work; recording one's information, decision making and outcomes demonstrates the professional's willingness to be accountable for the work (Hopkins & Smith, 1993).

There are four main reasons for documenting one's work (adapted from the AOTA's Elements of Clinical Documentation, see Appendix B):

1. To provide a chronological, legal record of the child's level of performance, and detail the complete course of therapeutic intervention.

2. To facilitate communication among professionals, families, and community-based services that contributes to the child's care.

3. To provide an objective basis to determine the appropriateness, effectiveness, and necessity of the therapeutic intervention.

4. To reflect the practitioner's reasoning and professional decision-making.

Professional, agency, and governmental standards and regulations dictate the type of documentation and the time frames required for those agencies' services. It is the responsibility of the occupational therapist to know and meet those requirements. However, each therapist must select what is relevant to report from a vast amount of data collected from others involved with the child, direct observations, and individualized intervention activities across environments. It is also critical to consider the audience for which the documentation is intended (Hopkins & Smith, 1993). The type of documentation necessary for school-based therapy is not the same as required for a referring physician, a concerned parent, or a third-party payer. The occupational therapist must clearly understand the purpose of the documentation and communicate in an appropriate manner to those consumers. Documentation in all settings may include evaluation reports, intervention plans, record of contact, progress notes, discharge summaries, parent consent forms, and when applicable, physician's orders and billing records (Lewis-Jackson, 1994).

The purpose of this chapter is to introduce strategies for best practice documentation of occupational therapy services that therapists provide to children and families in community settings. Early intervention programs, public schools, and community-based health agencies are typical service providers for children with special needs. Ideally, occupational therapy services are provided in family homes, day care centers, classrooms, or any other natural environments for children.

REGULATIONS GUIDING DOCUMENTATION

Within school systems, the education agency must comply with state and federal regulations. The Individuals with Disabilities Education Act (IDEA 97) Parts B and C govern documentation procedures for eligible individuals of school-age or early childhood populations and infants and toddlers under the age of three years. The IEP is the legal document that guides special education resources, programs, and services for early childhood or school-age students and serves as an evaluation device in measuring the child's progress toward identified goals. For infants and toddlers under the age of 3, the IFSP provides documentation of services provided and progress on child and family outcomes. Other work settings (i.e. home health care agencies, clinics, and hospitals) have accreditation and regulatory standards to comply with as well. It is important for occupational therapists to learn about the laws and regulations for any setting that employs them. The appendices in this book contain federal legislation that mandates practice for children (i.e., IDEA 97, section 504 of the Rehabilitation Act of 1973, and a summary of the Americans with Disabilities Act of 1990). Chapter 9 summarizes this legislation.

DOCUMENTATION AS WRITTEN COMMUNICATION

Regardless of the regulatory or standards requirements, professionals must follow basic communication principles when recording findings, decision-making, plans, and effectiveness of services. The same communication principles from oral communication apply to documentation. These are a sense of respectfulness, clarity, and reciprocity in the communication process.

Respectful written communication involves using words that everyone will understand so that they will not need a "translator" to decipher comments. When professionals use jargon in reports it creates a barrier between themselves and others without this expertise, including professionals from other discipline as well as families. Instead of saying "the child demonstrates vestibular hypersensitivity," the therapist can report "Sam cries after swinging a very short time, and refuses to participate in tumbling in physical education class, suggesting that he is very sensitive to movement experiences". Using everyday words also contributes to reciprocity of written communication. When the reader understands, it is easier to formulate comments and questions.

As stated in Chapter 1, "person first" language also contributes to respectful written communication. Therapists say the child's name whenever possible, and say "the child" or "the student" when needed. We refer to the child's limitation or disability only when *absolutely* necessary for clarity of communication. It is not necessary to include the child's disability in statements about other functions; e.g., "The child with cerebral palsy will participate in the reading group." We reserve comments about a child's disability when we need to communicate about the impact of the condition on performance, e.g., "Sam needs a wedge for sitting to minimize the impact of his spasticity on sitting."

Professionals use active verbs in written communication to establish clarity. This means that professionals construct sentences in the following manner: "who did it," then "what did they do."

Passive form #1: The child was evaluated for cognitive abilities.

Passive form #2: The child was evaluated by the therapist for cognitive abilities.

Active form #1: The occupational therapist evaluated the child's cognitive abilities.

Active form #2: I evaluated the child's cognitive abilities.

In passive form #1, one must infer who did the evaluation; in passive form #2, one finds the "actor" imbedded in the sentence. Both active forms state who the "actor" is immediately, providing a context for the action to come. Some professionals and some settings prefer the more formal "the occupational therapist" rather than using a more personal reference (i.e., "I"); both active forms are acceptable for best practice documentation.

Several things contribute to reciprocity in written communication. As stated above, writing respectfully and clearly provides the opportunity for discussion about the documentation. Occupational therapists also generate a reciprocal communication when we relate all of our comments to the performance concern, and explain meanings and decisions in this context. When individuals solicit occupational therapy services, they want our professional expertise, but they primarily want their problem solved. If we, as therapists, communicate our expertise but do not link our insights to the original problem, we leave our communication partners to wonder what our insights have to do with anything that is relevant to them. It is inadequate to say, "Jackie has a postural control problem". Instead, say "the teachers have been concerned that Jackie cannot complete her seatwork in a timely manner. I observed Jackie during seatwork and found that her trunk muscles are not strong enough to hold her up in her chair."

Professionals also use data to support their decisions and recommendations as part of reciprocal communication. When occupational therapists take responsibility for explaining how we came to a decision, we make it possible for others to understand our reasoning and offer alternative interpretations. The interactions that occur while considering alternative interpretations enables the team to identify the exact nature of the performance problem and design a more effective program plan. Data collection, interpretation of the data, and good documentation open the door to problem-solving opportunities and also demonstrate our willingness to be accountable for our work.

DOCUMENTATION AS A METHOD TO ESTABLISH ACCOUNTABILITY

Occupational therapists are accountable for the services that they provide. The only way to make professional decisions and outcomes available for scrutiny is through the documentation process. Best practice dictates that when we design and implement intervention strategies, therapists must produce sufficient evidence to demonstrate that their efforts actually increased or improved the desired outcomes. Accountability for improved results is a major emphasis of IDEA 97, state legislatures, and health care systems. The questions to be answered are simple, yet can become challenging if one does not collect the appropriate data to answer these questions convincingly. Are the children we care for making progress in areas of priority to families? Does occupational therapy intervention make a difference in the daily lives of children with special needs and their families? Through ongoing assessment and documentation, those questions can be answered. "The problem is, I think, that we collect not too few, but rather the *wrong* data." (Deno, 1995, p. 358).

For example, a practitioner may have tried various intervention strategies and reported the child is "doing significantly better than the previous 4 weeks." One is then forced to ask which intervention strategy was most effective, and specifically how much improvement the child made in the performance area of interest. In best practice, the therapist would have recorded the strategies and responses and would have observed the impact of the strategies on the performance of interest, so that she could report "Andrew can participate in 5 minutes of the reading group when the staff provides touch cues during the discussion. He participates for 1 minute in the reading group when the staff provide oral cues for paying attention." In the second scenario, the therapist is reporting what the team tried and the impact of that trial strategy on the performance of interest (i.e., participating in reading group).

Ongoing assessment and documentation of progress toward identified goals makes therapists accountable for the right thing—improved performance in children's daily lives. Documentation of outcomes also allows schools and other service agencies to be accountable and to satisfy a community's reasonable question on how the system is performing (i.e., Are the children making progress? Is this service worth the dollars it costs?).

DOCUMENTING ASSESSMENT FINDINGS

Professionals use the initial assessment report to document the initial contact, background information, assessment results, meaning of the information from the discipline's perspective, and the projected outcomes of therapy. Occupational therapy assessment links assessment directly to intervention. As described in Chapter 6, assessment is an ongoing process of data collection to support clinical reasoning. Best practice suggests that professionals address the following issues when documenting assessment data:

- What is a child able to do, and how does the child perform in various occupational roles?
- How does the child's performance compare with peer performance?
- What does a child need to know or do in order to be successful as a member of a family, in a student role, as a friend, etc.?
- What intervention activities have a high probability of being successful?
- How will the team and child know the identified performance goals have been met?

For novices, it is sometimes helpful to use this list of questions to check written communication and outline oral reporting in order to ensure that all areas are covered.

The therapist records and interprets data from multiple and varied sources. Therapists must be careful not to fall in the trap of formal pre and post testing to measure the effectiveness of interventions (Deno, 1986). Intervention plans are the result of the functional assessment of a child's performance problem (e.g., cannot feed self independently, cannot organize classroom assignments, etc.). As professionals design interventions, they include a method to determine their effectiveness. Some agencies refer to this process as "progress monitoring," or ongoing assessment (Iowa Department of Education, 1991).

DOCUMENTATION THAT OUTLINES THE INTERVENTION PLANS

The team designs the intervention based on information from the functional assessment (including observation in the environment, interviewing significant individuals, conducting ecological assessments, reviewing records or collected data, and, when necessary, evaluation results; see Chapter 6). Intervention planning, implementation, and monitoring is a clinical reasoning process in which the professional conducts hypothesis-testing procedures. There is no way to guarantee that a particular intervention will succeed. Using clinical reasoning skills, the therapist forms several hypotheses as possible explanations for the child's performance difficulty. The intervention plan is an effort to test these hypotheses.

To design the intervention plan, the team identifies as many solutions to the hypotheses as possible, then chooses strategies that are feasible and acceptable. This documentation outlines both the intervention parameters (i.e., the special materials or equipment needed, frequency, setting, model of service, and persons responsible for carrying out the plan) and the parameters for monitoring the effectiveness of the intervention (i.e., the goal, criterion for success, measurement strategy, and decision-making rules). Such information is documented in the service section of the IEP and in individual intervention plans for other agencies (examples are given later in this chapter). Chapter 7 contains detailed information about the intervention planning process.

DOCUMENTING AND MONITORING PROGRESS FOR ACCOUNTABILITY

There are essential components and procedures for designing and implementing a systematic approach to monitor children's progress toward performance goals. This process simultaneously allows the team, system, and discipline professionals to demonstrate accountability for their work because an on-going assessment process yields objective data describing the child's rate of progress and level of performance in goal areas. The data collection and analysis system can be used to document a child's improvement or lack of improvement, and the team can then make decisions about the relative effectiveness of a therapeutic intervention and the need to change strategies to meet the goals. Fuchs (1989) cites studies that have demonstrated ongoing progress monitoring is associated with effective special education practices and improved outcomes for students.

SYSTEMATIC APPROACH TO ON-GOING DATA COLLECTION

Outcomes for the child are based on the team's decisions from comprehensive assessment. Occupational therapists offer a functional perspective to the performance problem articulated in the referral concern (see Chapter 5). From this initial picture of the child and the performance need, the team clearly defines targeted behaviors and establishes measurable goals and individualized interventions that they believe will support attainment of the target behaviors. Best practice directs teams to use this systematic approach so that there is a useful database for making service modifications, program modifications, and decisions to end therapy (Iowa Department of Education, 1991).

There are several steps to this systematic approach: setting goals that meet accountability standards, recording data (including graphing when possible), documenting the intervention plans, monitoring the intervention effectiveness, and making changes when data indicate the need to do so.

Setting Goals

It is necessary to write specific goal statements to communicate a clear understanding of the desired outcomes and to be able to make judgments about the child's progress. Goals enable the team to determine the relative effectiveness of an intervention or instructional program. Goal statements emerge from functional assessment data and have a direct relationship to the identified behaviors of concern. The team considers both the child's current level of performance as well as the intended outcome after intervention when developing a goal. Goal statements have four parts:

1. **The conditions under which the child must demonstrate behavior.** Conditions include many aspects of the context, such as:
    *   The timeline for completion (e.g., in 6 weeks).
    *   The setting(s) in which the child is to exhibit behavior (e.g., during snack time).
    *   The stimuli necessary to elicit the behavior (e.g., two verbal cues).
    *   Specific equipment or set-up that is necessary (e.g., using a weighted spoon and given a bowl of soft-textured foods).

2. **The behavior.** Identifying the specific behavior of interest is an essential part of goal writing. This targeted behavior must be observable, measurable, and specific. It is a description of the task to be performed. The behavior must be stated in a positive way so that the team and the child knows what is expected (e.g., the student will play with one peer, rather than the student will not hit anyone). When trying to reduce a negative behavior, it is better to record what the desirable behavior is that will replace the current negative behavior.

3. **The individual.** Identify by name the student expected to meet these goals.

4. **The criterion.** State the level of behavior that is acceptable. When setting the criterion, remember to be ambitious, yet realistic. Research cited in Fuchs and Shinn (1989) indicates that the ambitiousness of the goal was associated with better growth in skills. The goal takes into account the child's current levels of performance and reflects a level of improvement that would reduce or eliminate the performance problem. Professionals can use various performance standards to establish the appropriate criterion; here are some examples:

    Peer performance (child's behavior approximates a typical peer in the setting)

    Criteria for next environment (what the child has to master to participate in the program of interest)

    Adult expectations (parent, teacher, employer)

    School policy/standards

    Developmental norms

    Local norms

    Professional judgment

Table 8-1.

Sample Progress Monitoring Process for Signe

Outline of tasks	Signe's plan
Behavior	Signe is a 4 1/2 year old child who has difficulty remaining seated. She runs around the room, knocking over toys and books
Goal	In 30 weeks, during group time, Signe will remain seated in her "assigned" space for 10 minutes, without prompts or cues, for 4 out of 5 consecutive school days.
Hypothesis for observed behavior	If Signe's difficulty remaining seated for 10 minutes is due to her body's need to seek sensory input, then providing Signe with a sensory diet enriched in movement and proprioceptive activities should improve this behavior.
Intervention plan	1. Change environment to support more opportunities for movement and proprioceptive activities. 2. Educate educational staff about sensory processing theory. 3. Provide occupational therapy service weekly within the classroom to promote Signe's ability to modulate sensory input.
Measurement strategy	Teacher or paraprofessional will collect data in the classroom setting during group time using a stopwatch to record the time. If Signe moves out of the designated area, timing will be stopped and that time recorded on the chart.
Decision-making plan	• Teacher and occupational therapist will review data every 4 to 6 weeks. • If three or more consecutive data points are above the goal line, we will continue with the intervention plan and adjust the criteria (i.e., criteria could be raised or estimated time of completion shortened). • If three or more consecutive data points are below the goal line, we will change the intervention strategy. • If neither of the rules apply, we will continue with the current intervention plan.

When occupational therapists work in natural environments such as a preschool, school, or community job-site, it is beneficial to observe peers. This performance is usually the "expected" performance that parents, teachers, or employers desire. By including expected performance in the goal statement, we form a direct link between current performance and expected performance. The child is also aware of the expectations and desired behavior.

Tables 8-1 and 8-2 contain two examples of goals a team wrote using these standards.

Recording Data Using Graphs

Although there are many ways to record data, a graphed, visual presentation of data is frequently easier for community-based teams because they can review a lot of data very quickly and see the relationships between the interventions and the impact on performance simultaneously. When time is of the essence, reading lengthy reports can be cumbersome.

A chart or graph is a visual method that allows the professionals to display a large quantity of data in a systematic manner. This allows the viewer to analyze actual student performance and compare this performance to the expected student performance. It promotes decision-making, since the viewer can easily determine if the intervention is promoting student performance. When data indicate that interventions are not supporting change, the team can modify the intervention immediately. The most important graphing decision is to determine how to display data on the chart or graph so team members can easily make decisions.

We will illustrate two methods for displaying data in this chapter. This will enable the novice to begin and then branch out to more complex graphing strategies when needed. In the first method, we recorded the rate of behavior. In the second method, we recorded the acquisition of the various sub-skills of the goal behavior.

Table 8-2.

Sample Progress Monitoring Process for Geoff

Outline of tasks	Geoff's plan
Behavior	Geoff is working on skills for independent living, including eating in a public restaurant and managing money.
Goal	In 20 weeks, Geoff will be able to "purchase a meal at a fast food restaurant" by completing each sub-skill and the criteria established
Hypothesis for observed behavior	If Geoff had the opportunity to go to a fast food restaurant each week, he could learn to purchase food independently using his Epson communicator.
Intervention plan	Provide training and opportunities for Geoff in a natural community setting to experience purchasing food.
Measurement strategy	Teacher, occupational therapist, or speech language pathologist will collect data on each sub-skill once a week on an outing to the restaurant.
Decision-making plan	Teacher will examine data weekly. Once a month, teacher, occupational therapist, and speech language pathologist will meet to determine progress toward the goal. Intervention or goal criteria may be modified accordingly.

Method 1: Geoff's chart (Figure 8-1) lists various sub-skills that Geoff must master in order to meet his goal of purchasing a meal. For this graph, the days are marked across the bottom of the graph, but on the vertical axis, we place the sub-skills in sequence.

The team and Geoff have identified six sub-skills, or milestones, to be mastered over a period of 20 weeks in order for Geoff to purchase a meal independently. This technically means that in order for Geoff to meet his goal, he will have to master 1.5 sub-skills by 5 weeks (first quarter), 3 sub-skills by 10 weeks (second quarter or half-way point), 4.5 sub-skills by 15 weeks (third quarter) and 6 sub-skills by 20 weeks. The team writes down the sub-skills on the graph and designates these arbitrary intermediate targets with a "quarter-star" to serve as a progress checkpoint to Geoff and the team. In reality, some sub-skills may require more time than others to achieve so the stars are only guides for determining adequate progress toward the goals.

Geoff's graph illustrates that he needed a lot of physical and verbal prompts at first. The graph also shows that Geoff achieved the 4th sub-skill before others, a reminder that people don't always learn life tasks sequentially. By week 11, Geoff had mastered 4 sub-skills, which was above the 3 needed to suggest he is making progress. The last two sub-skills took longer for Geoff to master, but he still met his goal in the 20-week period.

Method 2: Signe's chart (Figure 8-2) reflects the number of minutes (or seconds, initially) that Signe was able to remain seated with her peers. Therefore, we set up the graph with minutes on the vertical axis and days on the horizontal axis. The bottom of this particular graph provides a place to record the actual data, and then the teacher or therapist can graph the actual time on the graph above as a data point. This team also decided that Signe could achieve this level of performance in approximately 30 weeks; they recorded the dates across the bottom of the chart.

During comprehensive assessment, the team recorded that Signe could remain seated for 3 seconds. Signe's peers sat for 8 to 15 minutes during group time. During goal setting, the team decided that they wanted her to sit for 10 minutes within the next 30 weeks. The team member graphs the current performance on the left side of the graph and the desired performance at the 30-week mark and draws a line that connects Signe's baseline data of 3 seconds to the expected goal of 10 minutes. Look at Figure 8-1 to see the straight diagonal line that the team drew to indicate the desired progress (i.e., the "aim" line). The aim line reflects the rate of growth that must occur for Signe to meet her goal. Now the graph is set up to provide the occupational therapist, as well as other team members, with a visual representation of Signe's desired rate of progress toward her goal over time.

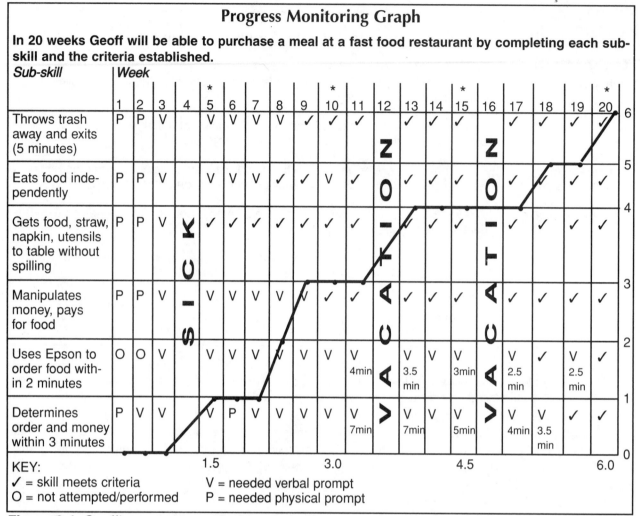

Figure 8-1. Geoff's progress monitoring graph. (A cooperative effort by the Iowa Area Education Agencies, Local School Districts, and Department of Education.)

The teacher and therapist plot Signe's performance each week and can see when she is on track, and when she is ahead or falling behind the desired outcome. The graph illustrates that after vacations, Signe's performance drops below the targeted level of performance, but that she recovers quickly. She meets her goal prior to 30 weeks and maintains this performance for several weeks, indicating stability of this behavior in her repertoire.

Monitoring the Effectiveness of the Intervention

Research supports progress monitoring as an essential aspect of problem-solving (Fuchs, 1989). Performance data should be collected and documented on a regular and frequent basis to provide objective data regarding the individual's progress towards the goals. "Progress monitoring is not an optional luxury to be used when time permits. Instead, it is a necessary part of every effort to change student performance" (Iowa Department of Education, 1991, p. 29).

There are several questions to answer when deciding the measurement strategy (i.e., how to monitor the intervention as it relates to the goal). Table 9.3 contains Signe and Geoff's measurement strategies. These include:

1. What materials are necessary? This may include the type of paper the child will use for writing and the toys needed for sharing with peers.

Progress Monitoring Graph

In 30 weeks, during group time, Signe will remain seated in her assigned space for 10 minutes, without prompts or cues given, for 4 out of 5 consecutive school days.

Began Intervention (at Week 2)   Changed Intervention (at Week 6)

Day	Wk1	Wk2	Wk3	Wk4	Wk5	Wk6	Wk7	Wk8	Wk9	Wk10	Wk11	Wk12	Wk13	Wk14	Wk15	Wk16	Wk17	Wk18	Wk19	Wk20	Wk21	Wk22	Wk23	Wk24	Wk25	Wk26 (MET)	Wk27	Wk28 (MONITOR)	Wk29	Wk30
M	5	10																								10				
T	0	3	20	30	30	45		1	2.5	5	4		2	5	4			2	4	6	8	8		6	8	10	10		10	10
W	0	8																								10				
Th	3		30	28	30		30	2	2.5	3			4	5	5			4	7	8	10	8		8	10	10	10			
F																														

*numbers before Week 6 are in seconds, numbers after Week 6 are in minutes.

Figure 8-2. Signe's progress monitoring graph. (A cooperative effort by the Iowa Area Education Agencies, Local School Districts, and Department of Education.)

2. What setting will the data be collected in? This should be the setting in which the concern occurs; however, it may be the environment in which the problem is most traumatic or occurs more frequently.

3. How frequently will data be collected? Data need to be collected frequently (at least once a week for most behaviors). The data collection methods must be simple, cost-effective, and sensitive to small changes in the individual's performance. The more frequently data is collected, the sooner decisions can be reached regarding the success of the intervention.

4. How much data will be collected during each measurement session? Sometimes it is appropriate to collect data during one or more observations during each measurement session.

Making Decisions Based on Data

To assist in making decisions about the effectiveness of an intervention, it is important that the decision-making plan be clearly documented. This plan allows for the systematic interpretation of the individual's performance trends with regard to progress toward the identified goal. (There are various rules for modification of interventions or goals that will be covered in the next section.) The team constructs the decision-making plan prior to the implementation of the intervention in best practice service programs.

The team makes decisions about the child's progress based on a review of the data. There are three options for data-based decision-making:

1.   Continue with current intervention.
2.   Modify intervention or criteria.
3.   Discontinue current intervention or services.

We have illustrated these options within Signe's and Geoff's progress monitoring plans.

In standard practice, team members can become frustrated with the rigidity of intervention plans that are only linked to the IEP process, because these are designed for annual review. In best practice, therapists design data collection procedures along with intervention plans so that there is a continuous flow of information throughout the year.

In best practice, the team identifies the criteria for the child's successful performance. These criteria are documented as part of the intervention plan (as described here). Service modifications, program modifications, and decisions to discontinue services are based on these specific criteria. Many times the team will anticipate a child's readiness to move into more independent work (e.g., in the regular classroom without supports) and include criteria about the stability of the child's behaviors in inclusive settings to ensure success across time. IDEA 97 requires that the IEP include a description of how a parent will be regularly informed about the student's progress, which includes progress on IEP goals and the extent to which the child is expected to meet goals. Therapists must make systematic decisions when considering modifications or discontinuation of the child's intervention program. The team must review all the information available and collect any new information that might aid in the decision-making process. We must make decisions about the nature of the changes, and then design and implement a plan for implementing the changes.

Review All of the Existing Information and Collect Additional Information as Necessary

It is helpful to keep several questions in mind when gathering information for decision-making:

Has the child met the program goals? This information is readily available as part of the child's current files; team members can review this together.

Is the current level of performance sufficient to meet the demands and expectations of present and subsequent environments? In the school system it is very helpful to know about teacher expectations, classroom rules, and the curriculum when making decisions about a child's capability to succeed.

What kind of supports are the child, family, or teachers receiving for successful attainment of current goals, and what kind of support will be needed if services are discontinued?

Make a Decision About the Appropriateness of a Change or Exit Recommendation

The team compares what they know about the child's current performance in relation to the established goal. This is done to make decisions about the effectiveness of the intervention and need for the expertise of occupational therapy services, as well as the affect of the anticipated demands of a new setting. If the child has not met the standards for performance in a particular classroom, the decision would be to continue services and make appropriate modifications in the program, intervention, or environment. If the child has met all the established goals and there is no further need requiring the expertise of occupational therapy, the child is discontinued from occupational therapy services and the team records the decisions and factors. This way, if the child begins to have difficulty, services can be reinitiated quickly based on past successful interventions. A therapist must be able to justify and convey thoughtful decisions surrounding any change in services so those questions about the changes can be answered accurately. For instance, the anticipated demands of a new setting may bring about a change in service level. Appropriate data collection and accurate documentation along the way will support your professional decisions.

Formulate and Document a Transition Plan

Once the team has made a decision for a change in program or services, the team develops an action plan with timelines to ensure a smooth transition. If discontinuation of any services is recommended, the team sets in place the necessary supports and resources to assist the family or school personnel with both the transition and the indicators of ongoing success or difficulty. This way, if a child begins to struggle, the team can intervene quickly, and if the child is successful independently, the team can rejoice with the child and family.

CONCLUSION

Best practice documentation provides a mechanism for professionals to take responsibility for their work. Team members collaborate in program design, implementation, and data collection to evaluate effectiveness. Professionals can feel great satisfaction from knowing services truly make a difference in the daily lives of children with special needs and their families. When professionals design and implement interventions without documentation to support the process or decision making, professional responsibilities are not met, decision-making is thwarted and professional knowledge cannot develop. As J. D. Green (1992, p.15) said in regard to the documentation of services, "There will be a sense of a job well done, and this is the best possible reward."

SUGGESTED READINGS

American Occupational Therapy Association (1997). *Occupational therapy services for children and youth under the individuals with disabilities education act.* Bethesda: Author.

Dunn, W. (1991). *Pediatric occupational therapy: Facilitating effective service provision.* Thorofare, NJ: SLACK Incorporated.

Clark, G. & Coster, W (1999). Evaluation/problem-solving and program evaluation. In J. Case-Smith (Ed.), *Occupational therapy: Making a difference in school system practice.* Bethesda, MD: AOTA.

Clark, G., & Linder, J. (1999). *Assessing student performance: A problem-solving process.* Unpublished manuscript.

Clark, G., & Miller, L. (1996). Providing effective occupational therapy services: Data-based decision-making in school-based practice. *American Journal of Occupational Therapy, 50,* 701-708.

Heartland Area Education Agency 11. (1998). *Program manual for special education.* Johnston, IA: Author.

Young, M. (1998). The intervention-based model of evaluation. *School System Special Interest Section Quarterly, 5*(2).

REFERENCES

American Occupational Therapy Association (1994). *Elements of clinical documentation (revision).* Bethesda, MD: Author.

Deno, S. (1986). *Formative evaluation of individual student programs: A new role for school psychologists. 15*(3), 358-374.

Deno, S. (1995). School psychologist as a problem solver. In Thomas & Grimes (Eds.), *Best practices in school psychology-III* (471-483). Washington, DC: The National Association of School Psychologists.

Farlow, L., & Snell, M. (1994). *Making the most of student performance data.* Washington, DC: American Association on Mental Retardation.

Fuchs, L. (1989). Evaluating solutions, monitoring progress and revising intervention plans. In M. R. Shinn (Ed.), *Curriculum-based measurement: Assessing special children.* New York, NY: Guilford Press.

Fuchs, L., & Shinn, M. (1989). Writing CBM IEP objectives. In M. R. Shinn (Ed.), *Curriculum-based measurement: Assessing special children.* New York, NY: Guilford Press.

Green, J. D. (1992). How to use your documentation and not let it use you. In C. Royeen (Ed.), *School-based practice for related services.* Bethesda, MD: American Occupational Therapy Association.

Hopkins, H., & Smith, H. (1993). *Willard and Spackman's Occupational therapy* (8th ed) (pp. 387-390). Philadelphia, PA: Lippincott.

Individuals with Disabilities Education Act Amendments of 1997. Pub. L. No. 105-17, 34 C.F.R.

Iowa Department of Education. (1991). *Understanding components of the problem-solving process.* Des Moines, IA: Author.

Lewis-Jackson, L. (1994). Third-party billing in public schools. *AOTA School System Special Interest Section Newsletter, 1*(1), 4-6.

CHAPTER 9

Impact of Federal Policy on Services for Children and Families in Early Intervention Programs and Public Schools

Ellen Mellard, MS, OTR

INTRODUCTION

Services for children and families have been dramatically and positively impacted over the past 25 years by federal legislative actions, regulations, and case law. These actions have resulted in more consistent and comprehensive services to children and families and have changed the scope of occupational therapy practice. Prior to 1975, very few occupational therapists worked in public schools, but now (according to a 1995 AOTA survey) schools are the most common work setting for OTR's.

There have been many federal policies effecting health and education services to children beginning in the 1800's and evolving to current laws and policies (Hanft, 1988 for a review). This chapter will focus on current laws, regulations, and resources guiding occupational therapy practice when serving children and families; specifically, the Education of the Handicapped Act (EHA), IDEA 97, the Americans with Disabilities Act (ADA), and the Rehabilitation Act.

Best practice dictates that occupational therapy personnel familiarize themselves with the laws and regulations that govern their practices. By knowing what the laws and regulations say, occupational therapists can advocate for services within the appropriate parameters for the service agency and in support of the intent of the laws. Sometimes administrative structures can become cumbersome in an attempt to meet the letter of the law and may lose track of the spirit of the law. When occupational therapists know what the laws actually say, they are in a stronger position to advocate for a child's and family's behalf to provide the most appropriate service plan. Appendices E, F, and H contain copies of the IDEA 97, Section 504 of the Rehabilitation Act, and a summary of the ADA, respectively.

EDUCATION OF THE HANDICAPPED ACT

Before the EHA was enacted in 1975 (Pub. L. No. 94-142), children with disabilities were not receiving adequate educational programs to meet their needs. Many children with disabilities were entirely excluded from public schools, with estimates of up to 1,000,000 children being denied access to free, appropriate, public education with their peers. Many families were forced to find services for their child with a disability outside of the public school system at their own expense and often a distance from their home. Many other children went through the public school undiagnosed and had an unsuccessful experience because of their disability. Children were excluded who were not ambulatory, not toilet trained, or unable to feed themselves or speak. The EHA was a landmark piece of legislation designed to rectify these inequities and provide federal funds to state education agencies (SEAs) and LEAs. Some of the provisional highlights of Pub. L. No. 94-142 were:

- There would be free, appropriate, public education for all children with disabilities (FAPE).
- LEAs would provide special education and related services, including occupational therapy, to meet the unique educational needs of students with disabilities.
- Education must be provided in the least restrictive environment (LRE).
- Written annual IEPs would be designed for all students receiving specialized services.
- LEAs would provide due process rights for parents related to identification, evaluation, and placement procedures for their children.

SEAs and LEAs had until 1980 to fully implement this legislation and provide free, appropriate public education to all children without losing federal funds for education. Children ages 5 to 21 were included in this act. Each state's Department of Education defined who was considered handicapped.

Related services were defined as transportation, developmental, corrective, and other supportive services as may be required to assist a handicapped child to benefit from special education. These included: speech pathology, audiology, psychology, occupational therapy, physical therapy, adaptive PI, early identification (assessment), medical services for diagnosis/evaluation only, school health, social work, parent counseling/training, and transportation.

Occupational therapy was defined as assisting in the development of underlying skills that are prerequisites for academic learning and vocational training: fine and gross motor, organizing and using materials appropriately, interacting with peers appropriately, increasing coordination, and daily life skills. Examples of students excluded from therapy included those with a temporary disability (muscle injury, fracture), a disability that doesn't interfere with a student's education, or a student that has received maximum benefit from therapy services. LEAs and Special Education Cooperatives began hiring occupational therapists as related service providers to enable children with disabilities to benefit from regular and special education.

Major Principles of the EHA

Turnbull (1986) summarized the major principles of the EHA as follows.

Zero Reject

No child with a disability can be excluded from public education. This policy ensures that children with disabilities are entitled to the same educational services and programs as other children. It also goes one step further, by ensuring that all children with disabilities have equal opportunities to develop their own capabilities. Thus, schools must provide programs and facilities for each student to meet his or her needs. Individual strengths and needs must be assessed student by student, not by diagnosis or handicapping condition.

Nondiscriminatory Evaluation

Congress recognized that discrimination, through the misuse of testing and inappropriate classification, presents a major obstacle to receiving a free and appropriate education (U.S. Senate Report, 1975). The EHA therefore requires the public schools to assure that testing and placement of children with disabilities will not be racially or culturally biased.

Multidisciplinary evaluations are required and must be administered in the child's native language, or (in the case of a child with a hearing loss) in their mode of communication, unless it is clearly not feasible to do so. Procedural safeguards entitle parents to notice of the school's actions, a fair hearing, and the right to appeal. Access to professional records is also granted.

Testing procedures require that all personnel, including occupational therapists, use assessments that will give the student a fair and unbiased chance to perform to the best of his or her ability.

Individualized and Appropriate Education

The EHA provides for appropriate education by requiring that education be individualized. This is achieved through the IEP, as developed by the student's teacher and parents, the student, a representative of the public school, and other individuals chosen by the parents or school. The IEP must include statements addressing the following:
- Present levels of education performance
- Annual goals and short-term instructional objectives
- Specific educational services to be provided, as well as how much the student can participate in regular education
- Projected dates for services
- Criteria, evaluation procedures and timelines for determining whether or not the IEP objectives are met [20 U.S.C. 1402 (19)]

Appropriate education is also protected by the requirement of placement in the least restrictive program. This means having the opportunity to interact and learn with able-bodied children, to the extent possible. An "appropriate" education under EHA is one that results from a process of non-discriminatory evaluation, IEP development, and placement in the least restrictive program.

In 1982, the U.S. Supreme Court further clarified "appropriate" education to mean giving students with disabilities the same opportunities as other students (Board of Education v. Rowley). This, however, does not mean the best education, or one designed to help the child reach his or her maximum potential. Occupational therapy services in the school system, therefore, are not intended to help a student develop his or her full potential, but should assist the student in benefiting from special education.

Another landmark U.S. Supreme Court decision, addressing appropriate education with regards to related services, was made in 1984 (Irving Independent School District v. Tatro). This decision distinguished between related and medical services. A medical procedure, such as catheterization, that can be provided by parents and educational personnel with minimal training would be considered a related service under EHA.

Least Restrictive Environment

This provision ensures that children with disabilities have the right to placement in an integrated or "regular" educational environment, if appropriate for the individual student. This does not depend on whether the school can conveniently place the student in a regular classroom, or whether the teachers or other students find the placement acceptable. Students with disabilities also have a chance to participate in extracurricular activities, such as sports, recreation, clubs, field trips, lunch, recess, and transportation on the school bus.

The principle of the "least restrictive" placement rests on whether the education is appropriate for the individual student. This varies from student to student, depending on the severity of the disability and individual learning and coping styles. For example, not all students with the diagnosis of cerebral palsy are mentally retarded or have severe physical limitations.

Procedural Due Process

These provisions give families and advocates the right to protest how the state or local educational agencies educate the student. Two previously discussed court cases, PARC (1971, 1972) and Mills (1972) set the precedent for establishing the following rights under the EHA:
- Access to all relevant school records
- Independent educational evaluation by a qualified examiner not employed by the school
- Written notice in the parent's native language for any change or initiation in the identification, evaluation, or placement of the student;
- Assignment of a parent surrogate, if the child's parents are unavailable;

- Opportunity for an administrative hearing before an impartial officer, with appeal to the SEA or state or federal courts, if necessary [20 U.S.C. 1415 (b) (1)].

EDUCATION OF THE HANDICAPPED AMENDMENTS OF 1986 (PUB. L. NO. 99-457)

In the mid 1980s, it became clear that Pub. L. No. 94-142 needed to be more comprehensive, and so the federal government enacted the EHA amendments, i.e., Pub. L. No. 99-457. There were two critical features of these amendments:

1) Part H: Federal Incentive Program for Infants and Toddlers
2) Amendment of section 619 of EHA, which extended all requirements to 3 to 5 year olds

These amendments expanded Pub. L. No. 94-142 to provide special education and related services to preschool children with disabilities, ages 3 to 5 (Part B) (i.e., extend services to include 3 to 21 year olds, rather than the original 5 to 21 year range). Occupational therapy now became available for preschool children with disabilities. It also stated that services could be provided for children from birth to 3 years (Part C). Table 9-1 provides a comparison of Parts B and C of this legislation.

These amendments also provided incentives for early intervention services, Part H, for children from birth up to age 3. Part H provided financial incentives to the states to provide systems of intervention and family support services to enhance the development of infants and toddlers. This was a voluntary program on the part of the states that agreed to implement services to infants and toddlers if they received the federal money. Congress recognized the need to start services earlier in order to minimize the effects of a disability, as well as to decrease costs to society.

This legislation had four equally important purposes:

- Develop and implement a statewide, comprehensive, coordinated, multidisciplinary, interagency program of early intervention services for infants and toddlers with disabilities and their families.
- Facilitate the coordination of payment for early intervention services from federal, state, local, and private sources (including public and private insurance coverage).
- Enhance the states' capacity to provide quality early intervention services, and expand and improve existing early intervention services being provided to infants and toddlers with disabilities and their families.
- Enhance the capacity of state and local agencies and service providers to identify, evaluate, and meet the needs of historically under-represented populations, particularly minority, low-income, inner-city, and rural populations (34 CFR 303.1).

(Taken from 19th Annual Report to Congress: Section IV; U.S. Department of Education, 1997.)

The implementation of Part H services was not the responsibility of any one agency, but of many different agencies, therefore interagency coordination and collaboration was critical.

Sixteen services are considered Early Intervention Services. They are:

- Assistive Technology Services
- Audiology
- Family Services Coordination
- Family Information and Counseling
- Health Services
- Medical Services for Evaluation
- Nursing Services
- Nutrition Services
- Occupational Therapy
- Physical Therapy
- Psychological Services
- Social Work Services
- Special Instruction
- Speech Language Pathology
- Transportation
- Vision

In this legislation, occupational therapy is one of 10 primary services and can stand alone as a service. A child and his or her family could receive any combination of services in order to meet the needs of their child and the needs of the family to improve the child's developmental skills.

Table 9-1.

Comparison of Part B and Part C of IDEA

	Part C	Part B
Age	Birth up to age 3	Age 3 to 21
Referral	Parent, doctor, neighbor, etc.	Parent, teacher
Timelines	Evaluation and IFSP must be completed in 45 calendar days	Evaluation and IEP must be developed in 40 school days
Documents	Individual Family Service Plan (IFSP)	Individual Education Plan (IEP)
Emphasis	Enhancing the family's ability to meet the needs of their child as well as enhancing the development of the child	Meeting the educational needs of the child
Eligibility	Delay in 1 or more of these developmental areas: Cognitive Physical Communication Social or Emotional Adaptive 1. If discrepancy of 25% or more between chronological age after corrections for prematurity and developmental age in any one area or 2. 1.5 standard deviation or more below the mean in any one area 3. Delays of at least 20% or at least one standard deviation below the mean in two or more areas 4. Clinical judgment of the multidisciplinary team 5. Established risk for developmental delay such as children diagnosed with a mental or physical condition that has a high probability of resulting in developmental delay	Child with a disability who is in need of special education services Eligibility is determined by each state Example of Kansas eligibility: 1. The response of the presenting problem or behaviors of concern to general education interventions indicates the need for intense or sustained resources 2. The resources necessary to support the child to participate and progress in the general education curriculum are beyond those available in the general education curriculum, or appropriate activities 3. Evidence of a severe discrepancy in peer performance in the area(s) of concern 4. The presence of an exceptionality is substantiated by convergent data from multiple sources including general education interventions, record review interview, observation and tests. A preponderance of the data must support the eligibility of a child as a child with an exceptionality.
Services	Early intervention services Assistive technology Audiology Family services coordination Family information and counseling Health services Medical services for evaluation Nursing services Nutrition services Occupational therapy Physical therapy Psychological services Social work services Special instruction Speech-language pathology Transportation Vision	Special education services means specially designed instruction to meet the individual needs of a child. Special education includes modification of regular instructional program, adaptive physical education, vocational education and community based instruction. *Related services include:* Assistive technology services and Instruction Audiology Counseling services Early identification and assessment Medical services for diagnostic purpose Occupational therapy Orientation and mobility Parent counseling and training Physical therapy

Table 9-1 continued.

Comparison of Part B and Part C of IDEA

	Part C	Part B
Services		Psychological Services Recreation School Health Services Social Work Services Speech/Language Pathology Special Transportation Transition Services
Natural Environments	Services shall be provided in the natural environment in which the child is found. This includes home and community settings where children without disabilities participate	To the maximum extent appropriate services for children with disabilities shall be provided in the "least restrictive environment"
Occupational Therapy	Occupational therapy is a primary service	Occupational therapy is a related service that helps identified students benefit from special education.

The requirement for this Part H system are different from the Part B system. Part H requires that IFSPs be in place 45 calendar days from the referral date. (These 45 days include weekends and holidays.) The Part B (3 to 21 year olds) system allows for 40 school days, which only includes the days school is in session. Congress made the timeline shorter for infants and toddlers, recognizing that time is critical for very young children and services should be implemented as soon as possible. Other comparisons of the Infant Toddler Early Intervention System and the School-Aged System (Part B) can be found in Table 9-1.

IDEA AMENDMENTS (1997) PUB. L. NO. 105-17

With the reauthorization of IDEA, legislators made significant changes in the laws provisions; it was enacted into law on June 4, 1997. Stakeholders studied, discussed, and eventually came to agreement regarding changes in the law resulting in passage with the following highlights:
- Having high expectations for children with disabilities and ensuring their access in the general curriculum to the maximum extent possible.
- Strengthening the role of parents.
- Coordinating the other local, state, and federal school improvement efforts to ensure that special education is a service for children, rather than a place where they are sent.
- Providing appropriate special education, related services, aids, and supports in the regular classroom whenever appropriate.

The focus of these amendments is on improving results for children with special education needs, not just providing services. Changes that were made which are most relevant to occupational therapists practicing in school systems were changes to the IEP and changes in evaluations.

Changes to the Individualized Educational Program

Muhlenhaupt, Miller, Sanders, & Swinth (1998) summarized the 10 most critical changes to the IEP process with the implementation of 1997 IDEA:

1. The *present levels of performance* section must now include a statement of how the child's disability specifically affects involvement and progress in the general curriculum.

2. The occupational therapist must now *relate the child's disability to how it affects the child's involvement in the general education curriculum*. In order to do this, the occupational therapist must be familiar with the general education curriculum and have observed the student in the educational environment where the student is having difficulty.

3. The *IEP now needs to include measurable annual goals and benchmarks* or short-term objectives that address the needs of the student; this means that the annual goals must reflect behavior that can be measured, is able to be monitored and is meaningful. Benchmarks or short-term objectives that may be used must be measurable and based on a logical breakdown of the annual goal.

4. Progress towards completion of the annual goals must be *reported as frequently as the progress of peers without disabilities* in the school system (i.e., if the elementary school where you are seeing children sends out reports every 4 and a half weeks for regular education students, then you must also report the progress on the IEP goals that frequently).

5. The *frequency, duration, and location of the services* and modifications provided must be included on the IEP.

6. The child's *technology needs* (if any) must be addressed on the IEP.

7. The *regular education teacher* (and appropriate related-service providers at the request of the parent or school) is expected *to attend meetings* and participate in IEP development and revision.

8. A *statement of the special education, related services, and supplementary aids and services for the child are written on the IEP.*

9. If the IEP team determines that the child will not participate in a state-wide or district-wide evaluation, the *team must write justifications for not testing the child* and describe the methods that will be used to evaluate progress in place of those tests.

10. Transition services are addressed beginning at age 14, and by age 16, a statement of transition services, including a statement of interagency responsibilities, must be added.

Changes in Evaluation

The information gathered during an evaluation must include information about the child's abilities and any discrepancies between abilities and the environment; in other words, the information must include discrepancies between the child's performance abilities and the expectation of the general education curriculum and classroom. In the past, many occupational therapists relied almost exclusively on standardized testing with minimal information of how the information from this testing relates to a student's performance in regular education. IDEA 97 reinforces the need for the occupational therapist to be familiar with the regular education curriculum, to observe the student in the classroom and other school environments, and from this information, to create a plan for those adaptations and services needed to design a program for the student.

There is an emphasis on reduction of unnecessary testing. Team members may use existing data first, including classroom-based assessments. If the team, including the parents, believes that no further data are needed to determine continued eligibility for special education, then a 3-year re-evaluation will not be necessary.

There is also an emphasis on greater parental involvement in evaluation and re-evaluation.

Personnel Standards

Some of the definitions of personnel were revised or clarified in the IDEA 97. AOTA provided testimony on the regulations that focused on assurance that only qualified personnel would provide the services defined in IDEA 97.

The definition of qualified OT personnel is "any state-approved or recognized certification, licensing, registration, or other comparable requirements. This would mean that if occupational therapy personnel are licensed in the state by a Board of Healing Arts or a Medical Board, then that licensing would be the minimum personnel standard required to provide occupational therapy services in schools.

The use of paraprofessionals is also included in the regulations. The regulations allow use of paraprofessionals and assistants only if they are appropriately trained and supervised, and that the use of these personnel be consistent with state law. This is the first time that occupational therapy assistants have been included in the regulations.

SECTION 504 OF THE REHABILITATION ACT OF 1973

Section 504 of the Rehabilitation Act of 1973 forbids discrimination against any person with a disability in programs and activities, public and private, that receive federal funding. Many people consider this act as the first civil rights law for people with disabilities. The purpose of this law was to prevent intentional or unintentional discrimination against persons with disabilities. This applies to state and local governments, colleges and universities, schools, child care centers, recreation programs, libraries, and clinics that receive federal financial assistance. This section covers any person who has a physical or mental impairment that substantially limits one or more major life activities, has a record of such an impairment, or is regarded as having such an impairment. A major life activity refers to self-care, walking, seeing, hearing, speaking, breathing, learning, and working.

The regulations for both Section 504 and for EHA became effective in 1977, but Section 504 is much less known and implemented, and has been largely disregarded by school districts until recently. This disregard was due in part to no funding being attached to this law, making implementation difficult.

Section 504 is extremely broad. It covers individuals with wide-ranging conditions such as asthma, alcohol and drug addiction, cancer, and the HIV virus.

Students who are receiving treatment for chemical dependency may qualify for protection under Section 504, and knowledge that a student is receiving treatment should initiate a referral to discuss a student's eligibility and needs.

The implementation of this law is the responsibility of regular education agencies. An occupational therapist may become involved in providing services for a student under Section 504 regulations. Students with disabilities may be eligible for Section 504-related services whether or not they qualify for special education services. Table 9-2 compares components of Section 504, ADA, and IDEA 97—including referral, evaluation, meetings, and placement.

THE AMERICANS WITH DISABILITIES ACT (ADA)

ADA was passed in 1990 for the purpose of prohibiting discrimination solely on the basis of disability in employment, public services, and accommodations. ADA is also considered a civil rights law for persons with disabilities. ADA has a broad definition of disability, which includes physiological disorders or conditions, loss affecting one or more of the body systems, or any mental or psychological disorder (i.e., mental retardation, emotional or mental illness, and specific learning disabilities). It covers employment, public services, public accommodations and services operated by private entities (includes day care centers, nursery, elementary, secondary, undergraduate, or post-graduate private school or other places of education), and telecommunications. Any public entity with 50 or more employees must develop a written plan setting forth the necessary steps to undertake structural changes necessary to achieve program accessibility. This was to have been completed by July 1992.

Public schools must comply with ADA in their services, programs, or activities, including those that are open to the public. This includes accessibility to parents and other community members for such school events as graduation, parent teacher organization meetings, plays, and sporting events.

All schools must have a plan on file that describes any barriers to accessibility, as well as the modifications needed to make buildings and facilities accessible.

New information was released in 1998 by the Federal Access Board on Titles II and III of ADA for accessibility in new construction and alterations of facilities designed for children. This final rule allows exceptions to various ADA Accessibility Guidelines (ADAAG) requirements based solely on adult dimensions. These exceptions are for drinking fountains, rest rooms, and fixed or built-in seats and tables for buildings or portions of buildings that will be used by children aged 12 and younger. Prior to these exceptions, many of the modifications made in elementary schools were designed for adults and not appropriately scaled down for younger children.

Occupational therapists may participate when looking at modifications to community and school facilities. Often times, individualized modifications must be made to restrooms and playgrounds for children. The occupational therapist, along with other team members, must consider a number of factors when making modifications (including ADA specifications, safety, durability, and ease of use).

Table 9-2.

Comparison of Laws

Issues	IDEA	ADA	Section 504
Purpose	To provide federal financial assistance to states to ensure free appropriate public education for students with disabilities.	To prohibit discrimination against individuals with disabilities.	To prohibit discrimination against individuals with disabilities in programs and activities, public and private, that receive federal funds.
Type	Education Act	Civil Rights Law	Civil Rights Law
Responsibility	Special Education	Public & Private Schools	Regular Education
Funding	State, Local and Federal	Public & Private	State and Local (no federal funding)
Administrator	Special Education Director	Requirement for school districts of 50 or more employees (suggest to use 504 coordinator)	Section 504 Coordinator
Free Appropriate Public Education (FAPE)	Yes, requires FAPE to students covered under IDEA	Yes, requires FAPE to students covered under 504	Provides additional protection in combination with 504 and IDEA but does not directly provide FAPE
Eligibility	Child with a disability who is determined to be eligible in one or more of 10 categories and who is in need of special education	Child with a physical or mental impairment that substantially limits one or more major life activities; has a record of such an impairment	Child with a physical or mental impairment that substantially limits one or more of the major activities of such individual; a record of such an impairment; or being regarded as having such an impairment
Evaluation/ Placement	Comprehensive evaluation of child's cognitive, behavioral, physical, and developmental factors is required Completed by multidisciplinary team that includes parents Requires reevaluations every 3 years. (Team\ determination)	Information must be gathered from a variety of sources in the area of concern and decisions are made by a group knowledgeable about the student, evaluation data, and placement options Requires periodic reevaluations.	Does not specify evaluation and placement procedures; specifies provision of reasonable accommodations for eligible students across education activities and settings.
Procedural Safeguards	Requires written notice to parents in regards to identification, evaluation, and placement and parent right to participate on the team.	Requires written notice to parents in regards to identification, evaluation, and placement.	Provisions for complaint procedures, public notice, and hearings.

OTHER CHILDREN'S INITIATIVES

Medicaid

Title XIX of the Social Security Act included the passage of Medicaid, which is the largest federal program providing funding for services to individuals with developmental disabilities. The federal government provides partial funds to the states, which provides for medical, social, psychological and health services to families and individuals meeting income eligibility criteria. The Early and Periodic Screening, Diagnosis, and Treatment program (EPSDT) provides for medical, dental, vision, and health intervention. (This includes occupational therapy services in early intervention programs, schools, clinics, and hospitals.) Medicaid will only pay for direct intervention provided by qualified therapists and does not pay for consultation.

Many early intervention and school programs access Medicaid funds for related services to help supplement program costs. Occupational therapists in these settings will be required to complete Medicaid forms and submit documentation in order to receive these funds. It is imperative that therapists make decisions about which children require occupational therapy services and what those services will look like based on best practices in the field and the collective wisdom of the team, rather than based on a child's Medicaid eligibility or possibility of additional funds.

Developmental Disabilities Assistance and Bill of Rights Act

This act protects the rights of children and adults with developmental disabilities and includes four programs: basic state grants for planning, protection and advocacy, university-affiliated facilities, and special projects. One of the most visible of these is the UAP (University-Affiliated Program). These programs are affiliated with a university or college, and provide interdisciplinary training to prepare professionals (including occupational therapists) to work with individuals with developmental disabilities.

SUMMARY

A number of key pieces of legislation have shaped and continue to shape the practice of occupational therapy for children. Occupational therapists should be proactive as legislative and regulatory actions are taken by federal and state governments. It is the responsibility of occupational therapists to become involved in the design, modification, and implementation of laws that both affect the practice of occupational therapists as well as the lives of the children and families that they serve.

An additional responsibility for the occupational therapist and other team members is to assist families in accessing and coordinating services that they are entitled to by law. Occupational therapists must continually strive to be informed of ever-changing laws and regulations.

REFERENCES

Board of Education v. Rowley. (1982). 458 U.S. 176, 102 S..Ct. 3034, 73 L. Ed, 2d 690.

Hanft, B., (1988). The changing environment of early intervention services: Implications for practice. *American Journal of Occupational Therapy, 42*(11), 724-731.

Irving Independent School District v. Tatro. (1984). 104 S. Ct. 3371, 82 L. Ed. 2d 664.

Mills v. D. C. Board of Education. (D.D.C. 1972). 348 F. Supp 866.

Muhlenhaupt, M., Miller, H., Sanders, J., & Swinth, Y. (1998). Implications of the 1997 Reauthorization of IDEA for school-based occupational therapy. *AOTA's School System Special Interest Section Quarterly, 5*(30).

Pennsylvania Association for Retarded Children (PARC) v. Commonwealth of Pennsylvania. (E.D. Pa 1971, 1972). 334 F. Supp, 1257, 343 F. Supp 279.

Turnbull, R. (1986). *Free appropriate public education: The law and children with disabilities.* Denver, CO: Love Publishing Company.

U.S. Department of Education. (1997). *Nineteenth annual report to Congress on the implementation of the education of the handicapped act.* Washington, DC.

U.S. Senate. (1975). *Report accompanying Pub. L. No. 94-142* (No. 94-168) (pp. 26-29). Washington, DC: U.S. Government Printing Office.

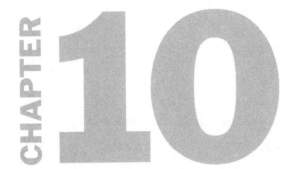

10.

Case Studies Applying Best Practices in Early Intervention and Public Schools

Ellen Mellard, MS, OTR
Winnie Dunn, PhD, OTR, FAOTA

INTRODUCTION

We have proposed many strategies for thinking, organizing, and documenting your work on behalf of children and families in this book. These ideas about how to implement best practice are merely conceptual and theoretical if we cannot also show you how it will look in actual practice. The purpose of this chapter is to illustrate best practices as they occur with children, families, and other service providers in actual community settings and situations. The children's stories in this chapter are the ones you will be able to tell as you practice; they are the stories we can tell because we have and are practicing. When you are learning and we are teaching you concepts, we fall prey to using "perfect" examples. This strategy has a useful function, because it allows teacher and learner to focus on the *idea*, or point of the story, as the salient place for attention. However, after we study concepts, we must be able to use them with the flexibility and generalization required by human beings as they live their lives, which is never (nor would it be desirable to be) perfect. The nuances that make our decision making complicated are also what make the practice of occupational therapy an interesting and intimate endeavor. We must be *vigilant* in practice to notice what might support or hinder a positive outcome; it does not matter how theoretically brilliant our recommendations are if families, teachers, and children don't use them because some contextual feature prohibits implementation. The artful dance of practice lies in a therapist's ability to stay *relevant* to the child and family's lives.

CHAPTER ORGANIZATION AND STRUCTURE

We have organized the chapter to facilitate your learning and practice. We present 8 children of all ages with a variety of performance needs and a charter school as summarized on Table 10-1. We have tried to emphasize different aspects of the practice process with the different children so you will have examples of all aspects of practice (e.g., initial referrals, changing services, dismissing services, differing presenting performance problems, various levels of resources in families, and school personnel). We have also only completed one target goal for each child as an illustration of the direction of the therapist's and team's thinking; these are not

Table 10-1.

Case Studies in This Chapter

Case #	Name	Age	Performance Need	Page #
1	David	2 months	Irritability interferes with daily routines, including feeding	159
2	Ted	32 months	Transition from infant toddler services to school services	172
3	James	3 years	Eating and talking - Using hands during play	177
4	Peter	5 years	Play appropriately with peers — Manage self in classroom	183
5	Derek	10 years	Integration with peers in school	191
6	Cameron	12 years	Transition to middle school	201
7	Sarah	16 years	Reintegration after head injury	205
8	Tammy	19 years	Transition to work life	209
9	Westwood Charter School		Improve student's success	214

complete plans for the children. We encourage you to "complete" the child's record by creating other goals and documentation plans as rehearsal for your own service.

You will notice that we have altered the margins in this chapter. We have done this to enable you to make notes in the margin. You will see that we made notes on the first case study to provide a model. We encourage you to make the same type of notes on other children and then compare them with colleagues in class; the discussions you have will be an important part of your learning. Table 7-1 summarizes the main concepts from other chapters; use this table to make notes on the cases for yourself. This is the best way to practice, and therefore learn best practice concepts. Take this reference table with you on fieldwork experiences and identify the presence of these ideas in discussions and documentation in these sites; talk to practicing therapists about how they implement these ideas in practice. These strategies enable these ideas to become part of your routine thinking.

There are two types of fonts in the text portion of the children's stories.

The indented and italicized sections represent excerpts from the child's report/record.

The remaining text represents our discussion about what is happening and our hypotheses about the meaning of these actions and information in the story. We are trying to show you our metacognitive processes (i.e., how experienced therapists are thinking through the problems of the case). Many times novices watch experts, and marvel at the expert's skills, but remain unclear how the expert got to the solution or the options. We want to illustrate how we have traversed the territory from the referral/performance problem to our suggestions and recommendations about how to proceed toward a more satisfying outcome. The outside column is for identifying the processes at work in the stories (i.e., what clinical reasoning, what practice models, what philosophies, etc., are at work in the story). We hope all of these formatting cues help you to develop your own strategies for clinical reasoning.

CASE #1 – DAVID (2 MONTHS OLD)

Pre-Assessment Process

Referral: The Neonatal Intensive Care Unit (NICU) referred David to the Part C Infant Toddler Program upon dismissal due to complicating conditions of prematurity and generally being at risk for developmental problems.

The Infant Toddler Program is part of a network of federally mandated Part C of IDEA programs. These programs are for children 0 to 3 years old who have a developmental disability and their families. The Part C Coordinator of the local program assigned David's case to an occupational therapist with expertise in sensory processing and a speech-language pathologist with oral motor and feeding expertise. The therapist requested records from the NICU and David's pediatrician. The records provided information on David's birth history.

History: David was born at 28 weeks gestation weighing 2 pounds, 10 ounces. In the first 5 days of life, he suffered initial prolonged hypoxia followed by several short periods of hypoxia. No seizures, infections, or intraventricular bleeds occurred during his 2-month intensive care unit stay. David was born to a single teenage mother who was working to complete her general equivalency diploma (GED). She lives with her mother in one town and occasionally sees David's father who lives in another town 20 miles away. David's maternal grandmother is the other most available caretaker of David. The father is occasionally involved with David but has made infrequent trips to the NICU to visit. The NICU, where David has been for the first 2 months of his life is 50 miles from the homes of the parents. The father is also trying to complete high school graduation requirements.

A nurse from the county health department is making weekly home visits to the mother's home to aid in the transition from the hospital and to monitor the use of the apnea monitor, feeding issues, and general care issues. In addition, she has been supporting the mother in trying to complete her high school degree requirements as well as finding employment during the mother's pregnancy.

Due to the welfare-to-work program, this young mother has only 60 months of total lifetime welfare benefits before these benefits run out. She is also dealing with the pressures of completing her GED requirements, finding a job, and caring for a premature baby.

David was referred at 2 and a half months of age. This gives him an adjusted age that is less than the age of birth. David was "screaming" several hours a day, inconsolable most of the time, and unable to enjoy or complete feedings. Changes in formula did not help. Subsequent laboratory tests and x-rays suggested no physical reason for David's irritability. There is growing concern on the part of the county health nurse and the physician regarding the stress on this young mother as a result of lack of sleep and lack of family support.

Scientific Reasoning Information

Record Review for Assessment

Pre-Assessment Hypothesis

Chronic irritability and feeding difficulties in the absence of medical problems could indicate poor modulation of sensory input. Since David's irritability was affecting both the mother and those around her, the therapist decided that the mother, the maternal grandmother, and the county health nurse should be part of the evaluation process. Since this mother's concern was that her son was "inconsolable" and difficult to feed, David would be seen in his home at a feeding time as well as at a time when he cries uncontrollably.

Even though this mother was stressed due to David's difficulties, she was not extremely receptive to having David evaluated by the Infant Toddler Program. It is easy for young professionals to interpret this mother's hesitancy as being irresponsible about supporting David, when in fact it likely reflects that she feels anxious or even fearful. This mother probably does not know what occupational therapy is or what an occupational therapist could do to help her situation. Parents are sometimes hesitant to get involved with additional government programs that they may see as intrusive in their lives. Since the county health nurse had a relationship with this mother before David was born, she was instrumental in convincing this mother that it would be a good idea to get additional help for her and her son.

Assessment Plan

When the therapist completes a review of the initial data, then she can plan the assessment. In David's case, the county health nurse and the NICU nurse provided significant historical information and discussed family concerns with the therapist in a telephone conversation. The occupational therapist and speech-language pathologist decided to employ several methods to investigate the reasons for irritability, including an extensive sensory history, observation of responses to handling, feeding, and movement, as well as determination of developmental level in postural and motor skills. David's age (3 months, or 0 months adjusted age), and unpredictable state necessitated that much of the data would have to be gathered from parent interview and observation of David.

The mother expressed frustration concerning David's feeding difficulties and irritability and a need for help in finding child care for David while she is completing the requirements for her GED. The county health nurse is currently assisting the mother in finding quality infant care in the community.

The occupational therapist and speech-language pathologist together scheduled to see the infant and mother at home during a feeding time when the father was also available. This approach to teaming for evaluations is often employed in early intervention programs. It promotes a more transdisciplinary approach to evaluation and intervention and allows the professionals to collaborate regarding the "whole" infant and family.

The therapists use the Infant Toddler Sensory Profile (Figure 10-1) to collect information, and they interview both the parent(s) and primary caretakers, as viewpoints may differ. This may generate positive interaction between the parents, thus reducing the anxiety, guilt, or blame surrounding a difficult situation. If an objective discussion can be main-

---

Sensory Integration Practice Model

Family-Centered Care Philosophy Implemented

Narrative Reasoning

Interagency Collaboration Philosophy Implemented

Skilled Observation and Interview Assessment Strategies. Therapist is blending developmental, biomechanical, and sensory integration knowledge.

Participation Philosophy Implemented

Family-Centered Care Philosophy Implemented

Sensory Integration Practice Model

Infant Toddler Sensory Profile

Winnie Dunn, PhD, OTR, FAOTA, with Debby Daniels, MS, CCC
July 1999 – Research Version

Child's Name: ___David_____   Birthdate: _____
Person Completing Form: _____   Date: _____

Instructions: Please check the response that best describes your child's behavior. Add any additional comments in the space after each category. If you are unable to comment because you have not observed the behavior, or feel that it's not applicable to your child, please draw an 'X' through the number for that item.

Please do not leave any spaces blank.

If your child is 6 months old or younger, only complete the white line items.

Use the following key to mark your responses:
1. *Always*: when presented with the opportunity, the child responds in the manner **every time**, 100%.
2. *Frequently*: when presented with the opportunity, the child **usually** responds in this manner, at least 75% of the time.
3. *Occasionally*: when presented with the opportunity, the child responds in the manner approximately 50% of the time.
4. *Seldom*: when presented with the opportunity, the child **usually doesn't** respond in this manner, less than 25% of the time.
5. *Never*: when presented with the opportunity, the child **never** responds in this fashion, 0% of the time.

SP Item	General Processing	Always	Freq.	Occ.	Seldom	Never
1	My child's behavior deteriorates when the schedule changes.	X				
2	My child has difficulty getting to sleep and is easily awakened.	X				
3	My child is irritable.	X				
4	My child is unaware of people coming in and out of the room.					X
	Auditory Processing					
5	I have to speak loudly to get my child's attention.					X
6	My child is distracted or has difficulty eating in noisy environments.	X				
7	My child seems oblivious to continuous noise in the environment (such as TV, stereo).					X
8	My child enjoys making sounds with his/her mouth.				X	
9	My child takes a long time to respond even to familiar voices.				X	
10	My child ignores me when I am talking.					X
11	My child finds ways to make noise with toys.					
12	My child prefers to play with noisy toys					
13	My child refuses to play with musical toys.					
14	It takes a long time for my child to respond to his/her name when it is called.					
	Visual Processing					
15	My child enjoys looking at moving or spinning objects (ceiling fans, toys with wheels or other moving parts, floor fans, etc.).					X

Figure 10-1. Infant Toddler Sensory Profile for David (research version).

SP Item	Visual Processing	Always	Freq.	Occ.	Seldom	Never
16	My child avoids eye contact with his/her caregiver.			X		
17	My child enjoys looking at shiny objects.					X
18	My child recognizes all faces the same way (strangers, parents, caregivers, grandparents, siblings, etc.)					X
19	My child startles at his/her reflection in a mirror.					
20	My child avoids looking at toys.			X		
21	Busy picture books are distracting for my child.					
22	My child refuses to look at books with me.					
23	My child enjoys looking at his/her reflection in a mirror.					
24	My child requires more support for sitting than other children the same age (infant seat, pillows, towel roll, etc.)			X		
25	My child becomes distressed when placed on his/her back to change diapers.		X			
26	My child enjoys physical activity (bouncing, being held up high in the air).				X	
27	Riding in the car upsets my child.				X	
28	My child resists having his/her head tipped back during bathing.	X				
29	My child cries or fusses whenever I go to move him/her.	X				
30	My child enjoys rhythmical activities such as swinging, rocking or car rides.			X		
31	My child is easy to move about because she/he doesn't seem to notice position change.					X
32	My child refuses to participate in roughhousing.					
33	It takes a lot of roughhousing for my child to react.					
	Tactile Processing					
34	My child seems unaware of wet or dirty diapers.					X
35	I have to touch my child to gain his/her attention.					X
36	My child becomes agitated when having his/her hair washed.	X				
37	My child resists being held.	X				
38	My child resists being cuddled.	X				
39	Unpredictable changes in the bath water temperature upset my child.					
40	My child avoids contact with rough/cold surfaces (squirms, arches, cries, etc.).					
41	My child enjoys playing with his/her food.					
42	My child becomes very upset if he/she has messy clothing, face or hands.					
43	My child seeks opportunities to feel vibrations (stereo speakers, washer, dryer, etc.).					

Figure 10-1 continued. Infant Toddler Sensory Profile for David (research version).

SP Item	Tactile Processing	Always	Freq.	Occ.	Seldom	Never
44	My child enjoys splashing during bath time.					
45	My child uses his/her hands to explore food and other textures.					
46	My child gets upset with extremes in room temperature (hotter, colder).					
47	My child becomes anxious when walking or crawling on certain surfaces (i.e. grass, sand, carpet, tile)					
	Oral Sensory Processing					
48	My child notices changes in the textures of his/her foods.					
49	My child licks/chews on nonfood objects.					
50	My child refuses all but a few food choices.					
51	My child mouths objects.					
52	My child resists having his/her teeth brushed.					
53	My child is unaware when food or liquid is left on his/her lips.					
	Taste/Smell Processing					
54	My child enjoys bitter, sour, and/or spicier foods than most children of the same age.					
55	My child likes to smell nonfood objects.					
56	My child likes to smell foods.					
57	My child refuses to try new foods.					
58	My child chooses foods with strong flavors (e.g., lemon, pepper, ethnic spices).					

Figure 10-1 continued. Infant Toddler Sensory Profile for David (research version).

Standardized Test and Interview Assessment Strategy

tained, the process of gathering pertinent information can be therapeutic. Quality interviewing skills need to be employed. An example might be "Can you describe a typical feeding?", "What calms your baby when he is upset?", "What does your baby like or dislike?", etc. When you ask open-ended questions in this way, you will be able to gain more information, as well as not be judgmental or more directive in your questioning. When you ask questions that can be answered with a yes or no, parents often feel that by answering no, their baby and perhaps they themselves are not being successful.

Skilled Observations Assessment Strategy

The parent(s), primary caretakers, and therapists observations of responses to handling, feeding, and movement are recorded. In this case, the therapist also interviewed the county health nurse, as she has had frequent contact with the mother and baby. These observations will include changes in state (ranging from calm to irritable), changes in emotional responses (ranging from joy to fright), changes in postural responses (ranging from decreased to increased tone; flexion to extension; approach to avoidance, etc.), and also what techniques the child uses to calm or excite when he finds himself at one or more of these extremes.

Contextual Assessment

The assessment process is ongoing, and for a very young infant the therapist will probably just be able to gain some preliminary information using standardized evaluations, structured observations, and parent interview. Often times, the therapist must make repeat appointments to the family's home to gain more complete information due to the infant's sleep/wake patterns, any medical difficulties the infant may have at the time of the initial evaluation, and the infant's response to handling by a stranger. In this case, differing environmental or contextual features that may be affecting David's feeding and irritability would also be assessed.

Findings and Interpretation

The evaluation data gained on David was both formal and informal and from multiple sources (i.e. record review, observation, interview, and standardized evaluation). A more formal evaluation of an infant such as David would not yield the quality and quantity of information gained from a more informal interview and observation of David and his family. This more informal approach is also less invasive for families who are already in a vulnerable and scary position and typically dealing with multiple members of the medical community.

Sensory Integration Practice Model

Developmental Practice Model

The mother's impression as summarized on the Infant Toddler Sensory Profile (see Figure 10-1) indicates that David's biobehavioral state is often very highly aroused, and he is vulnerable to frequent episodes of sensory overload. Sudden touch or movement, position changes, or any noise seem to result in startle responses and intense crying. He is extremely difficult to calm and has few strategies to calm himself (e.g., he does not suck on his fingers, hand, or a pacifier). During the observation he made several attempts to get his hands to his mouth but each attempt resulted in a total extension pattern which reflexively moves his hands away from rather than towards his face and mouth. Once calm, the mother knows of no specific clues as to how to maintain that calm, or what might "set him off" the next time.

Family-Centered Care Philosophy Implemented

The mother's impressions as well as other key people in David's environment are very important considerations in this case. (These people would include the maternal grandmother and the county health nurse.) The father chose not to attend the evaluation session in the home. It is important for the therapist to listen carefully to all caregivers in order to formulate some conclusions regarding the infant, the task, and the contextual features that are most consistent and most important in designing an intervention. You will recall that the evaluation was scheduled at a normal feeding time because this was a particularly difficult time for the mother. Feeding time did prove to be difficult, and thus provided an opportunity to discuss methods for interrupting the cycle of escalating irritability and calming the child. For example, as David became more irritable, the mother became more tense; as everyone relived this stressful situation, they were able to recall all the strategies they have tried to calm David. An interview question outside of the context would not be a successful strategy to gath-

Coping Practice Model

Context Data Worksheet	
Physical	**Code**
Grandmother's home	s
Cluttered environment	b
Large TV which is always on	b
Mother does not have a car	b
Social	
Grandmother assists as caretaker	s
Father is not involved	b
Little support from former peer group	b?
Cultural	
Mother is a teenager trying to complete GED requirements	
Mother is hesitant to get involved with I-T program	b
Temporal	
David is a newborn	
David is irritable and has feeding problems which are likely to be acute in nature	
Code: s=supporting factor; b=barrier to performance; ?=could be either a support or barrier	

Figure 10-2. David's context data worksheet.

er this important information. This provided an excellent opportunity for the therapist to gather more information, and to point out to the parents that their strategies are not the cause of the problem. It is important for the therapist to consider all contextual features of the individual's situation. (Figure 10-2). The therapists may consider all potential contextual features that may be a supporting factor; a barrier to performance could possibly be either.

Narrative Reasoning

David does not seem to enjoy cuddling, even during breastfeeding. He initially settles, begins to squirm, and then arches his back and begins crying. The mother describes his quickly escalating crying as "panic screaming". David does quiet, although he remains partially stiff, when held vertically over the mother's shoulder while being bounced and walked. The mother and grandmother disagree about whether or not David calms to or enjoys minor roughhousing in the form of firm patting on the back or buttocks, knee bouncing in a supported sitting position, or linear (heel to head) rocking prone over knees. David's grandmother feels that David enjoys these kinds of play. The grandmother also feels David maintains a more organized state following these kinds of play. David's mother feels that he has a delayed reaction to these sessions, becoming even more irritable and less consolable an hour or so later.

Contextual Assessment

Narrative Reasoning

It is not uncommon to receive conflicting reports. Grandmothers may want their grandchildren to be more awake and interactive and play. Mothers may be more interested in their child calming and sleeping so that she is able to accomplish all of her other tasks.

David objects strenuously when placed on his stomach, and prefers being held and carried with his head in a vertical position. He goes to sleep only when walked and bounced in a ver-

Pragmatic Reasoning

Scientific Reasoning	Narrative Reasoning	Pragmatic Reasoning	Ethical Reasoning
Problem Definition: "screaming" uncontrolled crying inconsolable feeding difficulties 1. Increase duration of night time sleeping 2. Improve feeding & eating *Procedural Reasoning:* Use of sensory profile Tactile, vestibular, and auditory input – David's response to touch, pressure, and proprioception was positive: he calmed	Mother: David becomes more irritable after roughhousing Grandmother: David enjoys this kind of play and feels he is more calm or organized afterwards	Scheduling of appointments - during feeding - just prior to fussy times Incorporating calming activities into feeding, diapering routines Recognizing that this mother must be successful immediately in order to continue	Decrease number of professionals working directly with family

Figure 10-3. David's worksheet to outline clinical reasoning data.

All Aspects of Clinical Reasoning

Sensory Integration Practice Model

tical position, but usually wakes and cries immediately when placed in any other position (prone, supine, or sidelying) in his crib. He sleeps for 2 or 3 hours when held close to the mother's or grandmother's chest.

Using clinical reasoning, (Figure 10-3), the therapist is able to consider each of the four aspects outlined in Chapter 5. Given all of the observations above, the therapist concluded that the tactile, vestibular, and auditory inputs are most difficult for David to process. Tactile system problems are manifested in his difficulty with cuddling and poor tolerance for nipple and food textures. Vestibular problems are manifested in his intolerance for gravitational stimuli from various body positions (prone and supine) and his rigidity about desiring only the vertical position. His extreme reactions (screaming) to unexpected sounds led to a conclusion of auditory sensitivity. David responded positively to touch pressure and proprioception when he calmed to firm patting and holding; he also calmed with some vestibular stimuli while in the vertical position (i.e., bouncing).

Children such as David may also demonstrate delays in postural and motor development that can be misread as only postural and motor concerns. The therapist needs to be cautious when interpreting this assessment information. These patterns can also be produced when the child responds abnormally to sensory stimuli. Children who are hypersensitive to sensory input frequently withdraw from the environment to minimize contact (flexed positions), or their over-reaction leads to frequent and exaggerated movements to alert to each new stimulus as it becomes available (e.g., pushing away or orienting toward stimuli). This leads to an imbalance in overall movement patterns, inhibits development of co-contraction for stability in trunk and limb joints, and prevents development of rotation in both trunk and limbs. In David's case, he is orienting and pushing away so frequently that he has been unable to develop appropriate postural control. David is prohibited from engaging the environment in a goal-directed manner (parents, toys, etc.), due to the combination of his hypersensitivity to the sensory stimuli that becomes available and the resulting imbalance in postural reactions, which in turn keeps him from developing more advanced motoric, perceptual, and cognitive skills, such as playing and eating.

Program Planning

David's team consisted of the mother, grandmother, county health nurse, speech-language pathologist, referring pediatrician, and the occupational therapist. The father was invited to the Individual Family Service Planning meeting at the mother's home. A letter was sent and a phone call was made to the father's home with no response.

Many fathers feel left out of the care of their young children. In this case, because David's father and mother did not have a good relationship before David was born, David's father did not spend time with the mother during her pregnancy and did not spend time with David when he was in the NICU. Because he is the father, it is the responsibility of the Infant Toddler Program to notify him of meetings and program plans even if he does not respond. The team decided to continue to send information and make themselves accessible to the father. At some future point in time, the father may be more available to participate.

When considering the pattern of performance strengths and concerns and the expressed needs of the family, the team developed an Individual Family Service Plan (IFSP) for David and his family. The first priority or outcome was to increase the duration of nighttime sleeping in order to enable David to interact more appropriately during waking hours (play exploration); this also would allow his mother to be more rested, thus having more personal resources to care for David while continuing her education. The second outcome focused on reducing the stress generated during mealtime and improving feeding and eating. A related outcome may be to enhance the mother's ability to nurture and interact with David (socialization) (Figure 10.4). The therapist may use the data summary worksheet to consider sensorimotor, cognitive, and psychosocial factors when considering activities of daily living, work/productive activity, and play/leisure performance. Exact details for the therapist will still be contained in more detailed evaluation data summaries.

Because the assessment included the mother and grandmother, the therapist's interpretation of findings occurred throughout the assessment interview and observation. Strengths were noted in David's performance. Because the feelings of incompetence as a parent are so strong in families that include a child with sensory sensitivities, it is especially important for the therapist to note when any family member has initiated or responded in a way that enhanced interaction. (i.e., "When you hold him over your shoulder like that and bounce, he seems much happier and is able to look over and give Grandma a smile"). In order to facilitate parental confidence and increase socialization, the therapist incorporates examples of alternative positioning and handling techniques that use variations of sensory input that could be introduced during play and self-care. The therapist explains the evidence to support these options with other children like David.

Developmental Practice Model

Interagency Collaboration Philosophy Implemented

Pragmatic Reasoning

Family-Centered Care Philosophy Implemented

Coping Practice Model

Use of Evidence and Providing Choice Philosophy Implemented

Person Variables	Activities of Daily Living	Work/Productive Activity	Play/Leisure Performance
Sensorimotor	David's irritability & inconsolability interfere with sleeping & feeding.		David is easily over-stimulated during play & becomes fussy. Startles easily, over-responsive to sound!
Cognitive	David is overly aroused by sounds, movement & some tactile input.	Mother is trying to complete GED. Time management.	
Psychosocial		-Mother is disorganized has difficulty coordinating David's care and continued work on GED. -Mother is unable to consider multiple tasks.	David is not yet smiling, responsively which does not give mom positive feedback.

Figure 10-4. David's data summary worksheet.

Example of how we inform parents regarding evidence for Evidence-Based Practice.

Researchers in therapy procedures have demonstrated that children like David have an easier time interacting with other people and accepting food items when we make sure that David's nervous system can stay calm and does not have to work to keep his body organized (e.g., Royeen & Lane, 1991; Crott, Giesel, & Hoffman, 1998; Vergara, 1993; Evans-Morris & Dunn-Klein, 1987). If these strategies sound good to you, we will keep track of his responses to see if they work for David as they have worked for others.

David needed to develop a larger repertoire of self-regulatory strategies so that he could engage the environment more frequently in a goal-directed way. The therapist decided to design an intervention approach that incorporated the sensory qualities and physical properties of objects and tasks, and the inherent characteristics of the environment. Figure 7-5 is a worksheet for outlining therapeutic interventions using the Ecology of Human Performance conceptual framework. One must remember that sensory experiences and reactions are difficult to conceptualize because therapists observe only reactions to stimuli, which are motoric in nature, demonstrating the intimate relationship between input and response (Dunn, 1990, a and b). Additionally, motor actions produce sensations for the individual and must be considered in this framework.

In David's case, the therapist wanted to provide appropriate sensory input in order to establish and maintain an organized state for functional performance. Since proprioception and vertical bouncing are strengths, these would form the basis for the intervention plan. One would not want to begin the program plan by directing input toward poorly processing sensory channels, because goal-directed behavior would then be difficult.

Sensory Integration Practice Model

One of our colleagues has suggested that we look at children's responses to sensory information by considering how fast they respond to particular events. Her research has shown that there are patterns of responding associated with particular daily life challenges (see Dunn, 1997; Dunn & Brown, 1997). In David's case, he is responding very quickly to touch and move-

ment; that is probably why he gets overloaded and irritable so quickly. In these works, Dr. Dunn suggests that we select strategies that are less likely to overload the child. We know that certain kinds of movement and touch are calming (Kandel, Schwartz, & Jesell, 1994), and so I am suggesting activities that have these features in them for you to try with David. These ideas have been tested with preschool and school-aged children, so we need to watch to see if it also works with David, since he is still so young. Would it be all right with you for us to try this strategy?

We are giving Mom the evidence we have so she can make an informed decision as we work with David.

For example, David presently reacts to the horizontal position by becoming upset and losing postural control. Use of this position as the primary form of input would immediately trigger these "fight or flight" reactions, leaving the nervous system even more poorly equipped to interact with the environment. Any introduction of an undeveloped sensory parameter must be incorporated into intense use of strongly developed parameters.

David's mother's priorities are best addressed through the use of supervised therapy; a home program to initially decrease sensory sensitivity and then increase functional interaction with the environment will be most useful for David. Other priorities for the mother included obtaining respite and completing her GED. The team agreed that the county health nurse would continue working on these outcomes while the occupational therapist would focus on David's participation in daily life and the speech-language pathologist would address the feeding concerns. The occupational therapist will provide consultation to the speech-language pathologist, so that there is only one primary provider in the home. Although both the occupational therapist and speech-language pathologist have expertise in feeding, the team decided that the speech-language pathologist would be the primary implementor in David's case. Because home programs require a significant personal commitment from the parents, or mother in this case, the therapist assists the mother in choosing the best time for her to begin the program. The grandmother and county health nurse should also be included in the development of a parent-implemented program. Variables to consider include: a non-stressful time for the mother, a time when concentrated attention can be devoted to the intervention and when another team member can be available for support and feedback. It is important for the mother not to feel incompetent in dealing with her baby and to experience success very early.

Target Outcome 1

David will remain quiet and calm during interactions when we play and feed David (i.e., with his mother and grandmother).

When working in Early Intervention Services, the goals are written from the family's perspective and do not have the same features as a measurable goal on an IEP.

The therapist might measure this by interviewing the care providers or observing a session in a home visit.

Margin notes:

Example of Evidence-Based Practice Discussion

Establish/Restore Intervention

Establish/Restore Intervention

Participation Philosophy Implemented

Family-Centered Care Philosophy Implemented

Coping Practice Model

Performance	Establish/Restore	Alter	Adapt	Prevent	Create
Mother wants David to sleep more consistently.	Vertical bouncing during play to increase arousal during wake time and stimulate calming after this play.	Wrap David and let him sleep wherever he begins to indicate sleepiness.	Turn TV off or down as you approach rest periods.	Wrap David tightly in blankets for resting, and do this while David is calm.	
Mother and grandmother want David to remain calm during their playtime together.	Carry David around while talking to him and touching him.		Dress David in tight clothing for play.		

Figure 10-5. David's worksheet for outlining therapeutic interventions.

Establish/Restore
Intervention

Sensory Integration
Practice Model and
Developmental
Practice Model

Intervention Approach (Using clinical reasoning to formulate an intervention approach.)

Activities to decrease over-responsiveness to sensory input.

Intervention Procedures (Examples that prepare the system for functional tasks in other target objectives.)

a. Use joint compression by stabilizing the body and limbs proximal and distal to the limb joints and pressing the joints together gently for 3 to 5 seconds. This could be done after diapering, or prior to a position change when you know David might become irritable.

b. Introduce tactile sensations while David is being bounced gently in a vertical position with head supported; this pairs an acceptable stimulus with one that is more difficult for David to process. An example of a tactile sensation would be gentle rubbing of David's back.

c. Prepare mouth before each feeding. Rub roof of mouth and gums with light pressure. Use finger or nipple; do it quickly before David can react negatively.

As you can see, these procedures illustrate the therapist's use of both the developmental and sensory integration knowledge bases. This is an appropriate choice of practice models considering David's age, the family's concerns, and the presenting behaviors that interfere with his performance.

Figure 10-5 provides an example of a completed Intervention Plan form, using this first Target Outcome. All of the Target Outcomes would be written out in this same manner on David's complete Intervention Plan.

Since David spends most of his time in a highly aroused state, rhythmic input is preferred because it is more calming. Pairing of rhythmic input with a well-functioning sensory component will be a good place to start. Secondly, one would want to increase the intensity of a strong sensory component and begin pairing that input with sensory experiences that are more pleasurable for David.

Outcome

David received speech therapy services 2 times weekly for the first 3 weeks and 1 time weekly until age 1. The occupational therapist attended two of the first home visits with the speech therapist and then began phone consultation with the mother weekly, as well as consulting with the speech therapist weekly. At 6 months, the team will formally review David's progress and update goals. The team anticipated that this young mother may have difficulty remembering to follow through with these suggestions and visits; therefore, the therapists made a videotape of strategies that were helpful in calming David as well as strategies for more successful feeding to be left with the mother. Each time a new strategy was introduced and successful, they added it to the videotape. This videotape also provided a record of the positive changes that David was able to make. This videotape became the property of the mother so that she could keep it as a record of David's development. When the mother and visiting therapists had a more consistent schedule for interventions, David was able to sleep for longer periods of time and eat with less difficulty. The mother was then much more receptive to the therapist's visits and continuing suggestions for intervention.

CASE #2 – TED (32 MONTHS OLD)

Pre-Assessment Process

Referral: The Infant Toddler Program made a referral to the Early Childhood Special Education Program (Part B) when Ted was approximately 32 months of age. The referral was part of the transition process between Infant Toddler Programs (Part C of IDEA) and School-Aged Programs (Part B of IDEA).

Ted has been receiving early intervention services since 12 months of age, when his pediatrician referred him with a diagnosis of cerebral palsy.

History: Ted was the product of an uncomplicated full-term pregnancy that resulted in a long and difficult labor and delivery. At delivery it was noted that the cord was wrapped twice tightly around Ted's neck, and he had to be resuscitated to begin respiration. Apgar scores were one, three, and eight within 30 minutes. Ted was released from the hospital with no complications. In the first 3 months of his life, no particular concerns arose from either the family or the pediatrician. At his 12-month check-up, Ted's mother expressed some concern about tightness in his extremities, apparent difficulty coordinating the use of his eyes, and lack of head and trunk control. The pediatrician advised that there may be complications with Ted's motor development and made the referral to the local Infant Toddler Program. Ted has been receiving occupational and physical therapy in his home since his initial IFSP was written at 13 months of age.

Pre-Assessment Hypothesis

Ninety days prior to Ted's third birthday, the Family Service Coordinator from the Infant Toddler Program, Ted and his family, and representatives from the Preschool (Part B) team sit down to discuss the transition process and decide what assessments need to be conducted. As part of this process, Ted's family may visit the various programs available for children once they turn 3 years of age.

Children who have spastic cerebral palsy often have difficulty interacting with the environment because movement is restricted. Although sensorimotor components of performance are an obvious area for further investigation, it will be more important to focus on Ted's ability to perform functional life tasks. It is likely that Ted will require adaptations in task parameters and/or environmental variables (e.g., a positioning device) to perform some functional life tasks. Assessment data must include all of these components to enable the development of a comprehensive program plan.

Assessment Plan

The Transdisciplinary Play-Based Assessment (TPBA) is an appropriate tool for a child like Ted because it can assess all of the various domains. The Assessment Team members will include the school psychologist, speech-language pathologist, occupational therapist, physical therapist, and the early childhood special education teacher. Ted will be evaluated in one of the center-based classrooms at a time when most of the team members can be present. The evaluation will be facilitated by the occupational therapist, since function in daily life will be the primary area of concern. This early childhood team has decided to minimize standardized testing and use the TPBA format to gain more qualitative information regarding the child in all domains, such as his play skills, his interaction skills with peers, and his interaction skills with his parents.

Many states are now requiring that team members observe preschool-aged children in the home setting as part of comprehensive assessment. This requirement enables the team to be certain about the children's behaviors in a very familiar setting, and not just settings that professionals construct for them. For Ted, the therapist will join a home-based worker during a regular visit to obtain the necessary information.

The requirements to qualify for early childhood special education services are determined by each state's Department of Education, but often include criteria such as a child must have scored at least 1.5 standard deviations below the mean in at least one domain or have a team decision based on clinical judgment that deems the child in need of special education services. With the TPBA, the team can make this determination.

Findings and Interpretation

The team conducted the assessment in the early childhood classroom with both parents present, as well as a peer. The TPBA assessed cognitive, language, sensorimotor, and social-emotional skills. This format allowed the child to engage in self-directed play activities with a play facilitator. It also provided information across many developmental domains, so that intervention strategies can be designed directly from the information obtained. Ted is easily engaged with materials in the classroom.

Ted appeared very interested in toys and tried to get to them even if they were out of his reach. In the supported sitting position, he was inconsistently able to reach and attempted to grasp objects presented. He was able to hold objects, although he demonstrated no voluntary release. While he was unable to get an object to his mouth in a supported sitting position, he was able to put his mouth on toys when placed in a side-lying position on the floor. His visual skills exceed his manipulative skills, which is a common pattern to observe in children such as Ted. He visually pursues a lost toy, moves a toy towards his mouth when it's placed in his hand, and makes attempts to retrieve a toy out of reach.

Ted rolls back-to-side, demonstrates functional head control in supported sitting, and when pulling to sit. Trunk control was not functional in supported sitting, meaning Ted has trouble holding his own body upright. This in turn makes it impossible for him to manipulate objects or watch friends, although he can do some independent propped sitting.

Ted eats solids from a spoon, opens his mouth in anticipation, demonstrates adequate lip closure on the cup but is not able to hold his own cup, or get finger foods to his mouth.

Ted enjoys all forms of motion, tactile experiences, and appears visually alert. Ted tracks and focuses on slow moving or fixed objects or toys, although occasionally his eyes cross.

Ted maintains eye contact inconsistently with toys and objects, but maintains better eye contact with faces. Ted responds to auditory stimuli by orienting to and turning toward the sound.

Ted demonstrated difficulty in all areas of assessment. I observed abnormal muscle tone throughout his body, with increased extensor tone noted in the lower extremities (i.e., his legs are stiff in the straight position) and increased flexor tone in the upper extremities (i.e., his arms are stiff in the bent position). The right side of his body is also tighter than the left side. When on his back (supine) and stomach (prone), Ted's head and trunk pull backward. Ted was not able to engage with objects and people in either supine or prone postures. In a supported sitting position (i.e., a chair with high sides and pillows around him), Ted used head control for orienting to auditory and visual input and was able to maintain his head in a midline position. In the supported sitting position, Ted attempts to reach and grasp small toys. When I moved Ted's arms and legs, (i.e., passive range of motion) his joints moved within normal limits, but when Ted participated in moving (i.e., active range of motion), his muscles that bend the limbs (i.e., flexion) and pull limbs toward the body (i.e., adduction) were tight. Ted demonstrated automatic patterns of movement associated with earlier development (i.e., persistent reflex patterns including the Moro, flexor withdrawal, tonic labyrinthine, asymmetrical and symmetrical tonic neck reflexes—the right side patterns were more pronounced, and palmar grasp).

Ted's physical status was the most obviously compromised area of development, and his parents expressed the most concern about his physical capabilities. In order for Ted to be able to explore his environment and be more mobile, the therapist recommended that the family obtain a power wheelchair. The Infant Toddler Program had just begun to explore this possibility with the family and other funding agencies. The program coordinator contacted State Special Health Services Office, United Cerebral Palsy, and the Make a Wish Foundation to find funding for a wheelchair. The team also recommended that Ted attend a seating clinic at a nearby teaching hospital and have a team of professionals make recommendations as to the type of wheelchair and modifications that would best support Ted's functional skill development.

Ted's physical limitations needed to be addressed in a way that would emphasize Ted's strengths while planning for his needs. During the home visit, the therapist asked the family about the strategies they were already using that they had learned through early intervention services as well as problem-solving themselves. Since this family has been receiving early intervention services, they are familiar with the terminology and behaviors the team was observing during the play-based assessment. It is important to make sure you use explanations that the family understands. In the previous report, the therapist defined any formal terminology right in the report. This is a good strategy to support the family to learn words like "supine" while still using clear communication (see Chapter 9).

The team also wants to facilitate open dialogue in the evaluation staffing, so they post a large piece of newsprint on the wall. The assessment team began talking about Ted's strengths as well as Ted's "next steps". They record their comments on the newsprint so everyone can see what is being said. This allows for a visual "picture" of Ted and helps all team members, including the family, see the whole child. This open process also sends the family a message that these professionals are willing to share openly about Ted, they care about figuring out what is going on, and the family can participate just like everyone else. When teams communicate separately and then report to families, families don't feel invited to participate (see Chapter 1).

We want to use a strategy today that makes sure that everyone feels comfortable participating. The writing in early intervention and preschool services indicates that when we use these strategies, families are more likely to join in the planning (see Salisbury & Dunst, 1997; Turnbull, Blue-Banning, Turbiville, & Park, 1999).

Program Planning

After the evaluation staffing (described above), the team scheduled the IEP meeting for a week later. Team members from the Infant Toddler Program, the parents, and the early childhood special education team attended the meeting. Based on the results of the evaluation, the team asked the family to prioritize the "next steps" for Ted. The parents' priorities were to:

a. Increase Ted's ability to move actively in all positions so he can interact with toys and people.

b. Develop skills in reach-grasp-release and object manipulation so Ted can play and learn self-care skills.

c. Increase eating skills and independence in eating.

d. Increase social skills for play and interaction with people.

The team then designed measurable annual goals at this IEP meeting and discussed placement options regarding what type of services would best meet Ted's goals.

The team decided that Ted would attend a community preschool program three mornings each week with paraprofessional support. Because Ted's goals addressed function, the team also decided to include occupational therapy service. The occupational therapist would visit Ted at home two times monthly and would visit Ted at the preschool weekly.

Because of Ted's movement challenges, both in the whole body and in his mouth, the team also included physical therapy and speech-language therapy at the preschool and solicited an early childhood special education teacher to visit the preschool to provide curricular support.

(The priority area we selected was to develop skills in reach-grasp-release and object manipulation so Ted can play and learn self-care skills.)

Target Outcome 1

Ted will activate the 4" press switch to make the bear dance within 30 seconds of the toy being presented (within a 36-week school year).

Intervention Approach (Using clinical reasoning to formulate an intervention approach.)

Encourage arm and hand movement to the front through use of toys and activities that Ted enjoys, provide positions to encourage use of the hands, and provide sensory input to support reach and grasp.

Intervention Procedures

It is critical to use positions that enhance arm and hand function throughout the day if Ted is going to develop skills for interaction with the environment. Since the evaluation revealed that Ted is most capable in the supported sitting position, we selected this position to facilitate arm and hand functioning first. Supported sitting reduces the effort of maintaining postural control, freeing Ted to explore arm and hand use.

The literature suggests that it is very important to address upright postures, such as sitting, with children like Ted. This is because being upright encourages other functions such as socialization and interacting with objects (Brogren, Hadders-Algra, & Forssberg, 1996; Green, Mulcahy, & Pountey, 1995; Larnet & Ekberg, 1995; Myhr, Von-Wendt, Norrlin, & Randell, 1995; and Noronha, Bundy, & Groll, 1989).

For example, by placing Ted's hands in a forward position and encouraging him to knock over a stack of blocks, he can begin to enjoy a game with minimal assistance. The therapist showed the preschool staff and family how to get Ted situated with support, so Ted had the best possible opportunity for interaction. The therapist then worked with the paraprofessional to teach him how to play with Ted on the floor. This play was directed at getting Ted to begin weight-bearing with his arms. When Ted can hold himself up with one arm, he can shift weight, begin to rotate, and then have a bigger world available because he will be less restrained by the adapted chair and able to reach farther into space.

At home, the therapist addressed eating and playing. She helped Mom select foods Ted could hold at first and showed her how to help Ted without doing it for him. She also explained and demonstrated play activities from preschool.

Outcome

Ted received the services as recommended on the IEP. The occupational therapist provided supervision of the paraprofessional one time weekly initially until routines were established and the regular preschool teacher had a better understanding of how to modify the curriculum in order for Ted to participate. The therapist included Ted's peers in these discussions so they also would understand how to include Ted in activities. This included becoming familiar with Ted's adaptive equipment (a power wheelchair, an adapted classroom chair, augmentative communication device, ankle foot orthoses (AFO), and an adapted playground swing). The therapist encouraged the other children to try out these devices so they would understand how they worked.

The occupational therapist continued home visits two times monthly to continue working on eating and play skills in the home. This provided an easier transition for the family, who had been receiving all home-based services. It also provided the opportunity for carryover in the environment that Ted needs to use his skills.

CASE #3 – JAMES (PRESCHOOLER)

Pre-Assessment Process

Referral: The parents referred James to a local early education program that serves children 3 to 5 years of age. The parents' major concerns at the time of the referral were poor oral motor skills for eating and talking and difficulty with eye-hand coordination during play. Parents were also concerned about James' lack of speech and their difficulty understanding what he was saying. James was 3 years old at this time.

In this case, the parents were concerned about James' development, as they saw differences between James and other children his age. They began calling community agencies to find a program where they might be able to receive some help. James' mother found out about preschool screenings and scheduled James for one (see Child Find information in Chapter 5).

History: The pregnancy was apparently normal and the labor was long but not significant. James was a large baby (over 10 pounds) and apparently post-term by 2 to 3 weeks. Early developmental milestones were delayed. He sat at 1 year, pulled to stand at 16 months, and walked at 22 months. James' mother noted frequent choking and gagging problems when she introduced solids in his diet. The parents managed these concerns by thinning foods, making smaller bites, and taking extra time during feeding. The parents both described James as a rather clumsy child who is motivated to try anything and persists until he can accomplish the tasks.

Pre-Assessment Hypothesis

Results from the screening suggest that James is delayed in his development, but there seem to be some key areas of concern that need particular attention during the assessment. James seems to be having his most significant difficulties in activities that require organization of movement, or motor planning. It will be important to record evaluation data in such a way that the team knows not only whether James can perform a task, but to carefully document the way that he approaches tasks and how he performs. This information will help the team formulate effective strategies.

It is also important to note that the parents have demonstrated insight in relation to James. They have been able to target James' functional needs themselves, which led them to seek assistance, and have already made some adaptations for James. The team needs to capitalize on their wisdom and perspectives throughout the assessment.

Assessment Plan

Because the family's major concerns were about oral motor skills and eye-hand coordination, the school district screening director assigned the speech-language pathologist, early childhood special education teacher, and the occupational therapist to conduct the assessment. These professionals met to plan their strategy and decided that the early childhood special education teacher would facilitate the play-based assessment, the occupational therapist would serve as the parent facilitator, and the speech-language pathologist would videotape the assessment. This allowed all team members to obtain information about James at the same time without duplicating assessment items. It is also a more holistic approach to assessment that allows team members to observe the child in a natural play environment. In addition to the play based assessment, the occupational therapist and speech-language pathologist conduct an oral examination. The occupational therapist also evaluated James' postural reflexes and obtained a sensory history from the parents in their home.

This occupational therapist and speech-language pathologist often team up to assess and provide intervention for children with oral motor issues. The occupational therapist in this situation was primarily concerned with the variability and functional use of James' suck, swallow, and breath synchrony. Frequently, children who have low normal muscle tone demonstrate difficulty coordinating the use of various body components, such as are required to make a seal, suck, swallow, and then breathe in-between events. Poor oral motor synchrony can compromise development of orchestrated movements for eating and talking, but can also be a sign of more general difficulties with movement organization and planning. The occupational therapist will need to be attentive to these possibilities during the play-based assessment.

Findings and Interpretation

The team combined data from all of their assessment methods to gain insights about James.

Gross Motor: James moves through his environment with a wide base of support (i.e., feet wide apart) and high guard stance (i.e., arms above shoulders). He demonstrates difficulty in balance, especially when moving quickly, and demonstrates difficulty in planning and controlling skilled gross motor patterns. For example, James was unable to adjust his course when toys were in his path, so he fell over them.

James is having difficulty even with simple patterns of movement like running and stopping. It is common for parents to seek help during this age period because their child has become more mobile and is frequently the victim of mishaps. The children have many more scrapes, cuts, bruises, and sometimes broken bones, because of their inability to plan and organize their movements within and around their environment. Additional information such as this can be gained during history taking.

Fine Motor: James demonstrates an immature grasping pattern (i.e., he holds objects with a fisted hand instead of with fingers), and he is not yet using a pincer grasp (i.e., holding small objects between finger and thumb tips). He enjoyed playing and building with blocks and putting puzzles together, but had difficulty in both problem-solving (e.g., rotating objects to make them fit) and reproducing structures from a model. He is just beginning to use a crayon or marker, holding it with his entire hand. He accurately reproduced a horizontal and vertical line but was unable to draw a circle or cross. James did not visually monitor his hands during these fine motor tasks. James is farsighted and wears glasses to correct this; he also intermit-

tently wears a patch for strabismus (cross-eyedness). These factors may be contributing to his poor visual monitoring of fine motor activities.

James is also having trouble organizing movements with his hands. An additional complication here is his poor use of visual monitoring; when children watch their hands, they obtain further information about how their hands work and what their capabilities are. James is probably not profiting from sensory feedback from his eyes or his hands (visual, tactile, and proprioceptive), and therefore cannot construct accurate and reliable maps of his body. His clumsiness in fine motor movement may be due to his lack of accurate sensory information from which to plan his approach to the task. Erhardt (1990) provides evidence and information about these processes that can be used for Evidence-Based practice; she combines developmental, sensory, and postural knowledge and applies this knowledge to the practical performance problems that children such as James have.

Oral Motor: The speech-language pathologist and occupational therapist conducted an oral exam while James ate a snack of crackers, cheese, apple sauce, and juice in a cup. James had difficulty maintaining lip closure around the cup and the spoon that is needed for efficient eating and drinking. Food stayed in the middle of his mouth, reducing opportunities for chewing; his tongue was not moving food around. He also did not demonstrate rotary chewing, a more mature way to break up food in the mouth. James also displayed reverse swallowing or gulping especially while drinking (i.e., liquid pushed forward instead of back in mouth). James had difficulty initiating swallowing patterns following chewing or sucking; food often collected in his cheeks during eating, which he would still have in his mouth well after the meal/snack ended. He was unable to move the food into a position for swallowing. James used breathing patterns functionally during chewing activities, but he had difficulty synchronizing breathing during drinking or sucking.

He also demonstrated breathing difficulties during fine motor tasks. James frequently holds his breath, apparently to increase body stability for control of arms and hands. James tends to get winded easily during gross motor activities that require either strength or endurance.

James' verbal language has a breathy quality to it, as though he does not always have enough air to complete a sentence or string of sentences. He takes small breaths while speaking, but they are not always at the end of phrases or sentences, so it is hard to understand what he says.

The problems noted in the oral motor examination also indicate difficulty with organizing movement in relation to task demands. Breathing is such an automatic task for most of us; we do not consider that it takes coordination to breathe in relation to an activity. James could not coordinate breathing with talking, eating, or performing fine motor tasks. Difficulty with the sequencing, timing, and orchestration of any movement patterns is a primary characteristic of dyspraxia, or the inability to organize and plan new motor acts.

Postural Mechanisms: James demonstrates low normal muscle tone and has difficulty initiating and maintaining adequate joint stability, especially in the jaw, neck, shoulders, and hips. Primitive automatic motor responses (i.e., the asymmetrical and symmetrical tonic neck patterns) continue to occur when James moves. These automatic responses interfere with James' goal-directed movements, which then compromises development of more mature and organized movement patterns (e.g., postural rotation, protective responses, and righting and balance reactions). The result is poor quality of movement.

The presence of primitive postural reflexes limits James' ability to mobilize body parts in isolation from the trunk or head. It is difficult to know whether the presence of these primitive patterns is a causal or effect factor. If these primitive patterns dominated James' early movement attempts, they could have limited his movement experiences, leaving him with a small movement repertoire. On the other hand, with poor motor planning skills, James may have been unable to overcome the effects of the primitive reflex patterns to develop more mature patterns of movement. It is likely that both scenarios contributed to his present condition.

Sensory Processing: Mother reports that James is somewhat sensitive to food and clothing textures, and seems to react to textures and temperatures on his hands (e.g., hands get messy and he doesn't like it, but can't get them wiped without help). However, his responses to sensory experiences in daily life are generally the same as other children. He likes to be moved about in the air and bounced.

There seems to be poor sensory support for James' motor planning. He may be able to process movement stimuli, but not touch input that contributes to one's body map. The motor planning process is dependent on accurate and reliable maps of the body (Cermak, 1993 provides good review of the evidence about the role of praxis in performance).

In summary, James is demonstrating mild delays in development. His poor ability to organize patterns of movement in all activities suggests that James has motor planning problems, sometimes called developmental dyspraxia. It may be helpful for James to be seen by a pediatric neurologist to either confirm or rule out other CNS disorders, since James' movement organization problem is so pervasive.

It is possible that James has mild cerebral palsy. A pediatric neurology consultation could help to confirm or deny this possibility for the parents. This diagnosis will not significantly alter the program planning strategies for the team, since their observations of his performance will form the basis for intervention in any case. A specific diagnosis is sometimes very important to families; sometimes a specific diagnosis makes programs or community resources available to a family. For example, if James does indeed have a mild form of cerebral palsy, his family will have access to the resources of United Cerebral Palsy or the state program for children with special health care needs. A differential diagnosis is also useful in those cases where a family trend may be present, or when the disorder may have new or different manifestations as the child grows. In some cases, the occupational therapist may accompany the family and child to the appointment with a specialist when seeking a diagnosis or guidance on intervention. The occupational therapist can be a filter or interpreter of the physician information. Many families are quite intimidated by these experiences with the medical community, and it is often helpful for the therapist to ask questions the family might be too overwhelmed or intimidated to ask and then respond to the family's questions after the appointment.

Program Planning

Following the assessment, the team met with the family to discuss findings and establish an IEP. The team was careful to avoid professional jargon, as it can be intimidating and confusing for families entering a service system for the first time. Sometimes colleagues forget, so team members must be vigilant with each other on the family's behalf. For example, during James' IEP meeting, the speech-language pathologist reports her assessment information and uses the term "dyspraxia" without explanation. So the early childhood education teacher asks the speech-language pathologist to explain dyspraxia to her and the rest of the team. This releases the family from either staying confused or having to ask. Many families do not feel comfortable asking the "professionals" to explain what they are saying. The teacher's strategy enables the parents to understand the information being shared with them without them having to ask themselves. Team members discussed their findings by describing the quality of James' performance in all areas, since the quality of his performance was the cornerstone of the parents' concerns and the need for intervention.

James' formal diagnosis would qualify or reject him from particular community services. The team felt that James' performance warranted a label of either mild cerebral palsy or developmental dyspraxia. The diagnosis of cerebral palsy is a medical diagnosis, and is more familiar to both third party insurance companies and public school programs. Developmental dyspraxia is less familiar to payers, and therefore requires more justification to be deemed eligible for funding. The family wanted to know everything they could about James' condition, and so they decided to pursue the possibility of a diagnosis of mild cerebral palsy through the services of a pediatric neurologist. This referral would provide the parents with an additional source of information. In this case, James' family had insurance options available to them. Various federally supported programs have different eligibility criteria than do local programs or public school programs. Knowledge of eligibility criteria is essential for appropriate and adequate intervention planning.

Additionally, the occupational therapist would play a key role in James' service provision process, with several areas targeted for intervention:

a. Increase the use of mature postural control mechanisms and gross motor planning skills for effective movement within the environment and increased participation in age activities and with peers.

b. Improve oral motor skills for eating and talking.

c. Improve eye-hand coordination and manual dexterity for learning, self-care, and play.

Target Outcome 1

James will transition among learning centers within 2 minutes 75% of the time so he can participate with peers in classroom activities within 36 weeks.

Intervention Approach

Provide strong proprioceptive input during activities to increase sensory support for functional movement.

Intervention Procedures

James seeks and enjoys intense movement experiences, so utilizing movement with heavy work in activities that require planning a sequence of steps will promote better performance and more interest and motivation for the activity. As James receives the sensory input during active movement, his brain will be able to establish more mature body maps for use in planning motor behaviors.

The therapist also introduced the use of unstable surfaces and alternate positions during visual motor and fine motor activity, such as sitting on a Therapy Ball (Abilitations, Atlanta, GA) or Hop A Roo (Southpaw Enterprises, Dayton, OH), sitting on a T-stool (Southpaw Enterprises, Dayton, OH), or sitting on a gel-filled cushion. Each of these options allows increased feedback from small postural movements that occur while James is sitting. However, by practicing these postural shifts during table-top activities, James must incorporate postural control into his performance schema. If the therapist only practiced postural control in an isolated therapy setting (e.g., on the Therapy Ball), she would not be taking responsibility for making sure that this background skill would be available to support performance.

In addition, the therapist and teacher collaborated to design a center in the preschool classroom that all the children could choose. This center included equipment such as large therapy balls, obstacle courses made of hoops, tables and rocker boards, and balls. These activities are useful for all children James' age and also provide opportunities for social interaction.

Outcome

James did not have mild cerebral palsy. The team had to provide detailed documentation about what developmental dyspraxia is and how it was adversely affecting performance and development. Because James was interested in exploring, the therapeutic enhancements of the preschool program were very helpful for him. When it was time for James to transition into public school, the family had involved James in tumbling and swimming, and with consultation from the occupational therapist, the first grade teacher, physical education teacher, and music teacher were able to provide a successful environment for James. The occupational therapist routinely met with each subsequent set of teachers to support James' transition each year.

CASE #4 – PETER (KINDERGARTEN)

Pre-Assessment Process

Referral: The kindergarten teacher referred Peter for a comprehensive evaluation at age 6 due to her concerns regarding Peter's behavior in the classroom, difficulty understanding and following directions, and difficulty with fine motor tasks and using playground equipment.

Peter had struggled in kindergarten and his teacher had discussed his difficulties at the collaborative team meetings held each month. These collaborative team meetings are an opportunity for regular education teachers, special education teachers, related service personnel, and administrators to discuss individual children who may be having difficulties. In this particular school, the principal hires a substitute teacher who assumes duties for each of the regular education teachers for about 45 minutes at a time. This enables the regular education teacher to discuss her concerns about the children in her classroom with a team of professionals. This is sometimes referred to as the pre-assessment or problem-solving process (see Chapter 5).

After the team first discussed Peter, the school psychologist observed him in the classroom and made some recommendations to his teacher for modifying instructions during transitions and giving him more time. Peter was not able to make any significant change with this instructional adaptation so the team decided that they should refer him for a comprehensive evaluation. In addition, the parents were concerned about Peter's readiness for the more structured first grade curriculum.

In this school, the school psychologist coordinates the comprehensive evaluation. The first step is gaining the signed parent permission to evaluate Peter. After the parent signs this, the school psychologist sends out an assignment sheet based on the preassessment team's discussion that describes the focus for the assessment process. This sheet also gives the date all evaluation needs to be completed, as well as a staffing date to meet with the parents and discuss the results of the evaluation (Figure 10-6).

History: Peter is the oldest of two boys. The pregnancy, labor, and delivery were unremarkable. His mother described Peter as an alert and active baby with a mind of his own, but she had no concerns about his development, since he achieved major milestones within expected ages. Peter had attended a church-sponsored preschool two mornings each week since the age of 4. The preschool teacher did mention, and the mother also noticed when she was a parent helper in the preschool, that Peter had difficulty following directions, staying on task, and participating in fine and gross motor activities. Both the teacher and the mother felt that by the time Peter reached the more structured kindergarten program, he would be more mature and respond to this increased structure.

Peter also becomes easily upset by unfamiliar environments, the presence of many people in close proximity, or changes in schedule. The coping inventory revealed that Peter had difficulty with "internal resources" in relation to physical and affective states remaining stable for him; he seemed to react to "Material

---

Comprehensive Evaluation Team Assignment Sheet

Consent for an evaluation has been granted regarding:

Student's Name: _____Peter_____ DOB: _____

School: _____ Grade: _____ Teacher: _____

Parent's Name: _____

Address: _____ Phone: _____

Reason for Referral : ___Peter has difficulty understanding and following directions and also has problems ___
_____ with fine motor skills with playground equipment _____

School Psychologist's Name: _____

Dates for Testers to Begin Evaluation: ___November 1999 _____

Tester's Name	Evaluation/Test to be Given:	Date Needed
OT, psychologist	Observation/Student Interview	Dec 99
Psychologist	Social History/Student History	Dec 99
Speech pathologist	Contextual language sample	Dec 99
	Hearing	
	Vision	
	Academic Achievement Test:	
Special educator	Woodcock Johnson Psychoeducational Tests	Dec 99
	Rating Scales:	
OT, Teacher	School Function Assessment	Dec 99
Parents, OT	Sensory Profile	Dec 99
	Intelligence Test:	
Psychologist	Kaufman Assessment Battery for Children	Dec 99
	Other:	
OT	Teacher interview	Dec 99

The appropriate evaluation team member should then provide a photocopy of Written Summary of Classroom Observation Form, Achievement Test Results, Description of Speech and Language needs, Behavior Rating Scale Summary, and a Written Summary of the Social History, PT and OT needs, HI or VI needs to the School Psychologist by the date needed.

Remarks: _____
_____
_____

Figure 10-6. Comprehensive evaluation team assignment sheet.

and Environmental Support" (an external resource) negatively when situations were unexpected. Peter occasionally struck out at people when they invaded his space or would also crawl under the table to avoid contact. Both the parents and the classroom teacher observed that Peter often chose to hang back before and during transitions to new activities, and that these were particularly difficult times for him. Peter has also cried for no apparent reason while riding the bus to and from school, while playing on the playground, and sometimes while spending time in the mall or at a restaurant with his family. He has infrequently demonstrated mild outbursts of temper at transition times, during free play on the playground, and one time on the bus. Parents noted these behaviors are more significant at home when there is a sudden change in plans of the normal routine.

Information from both parents, as well as the classroom teacher, helped define the kind of sensory input and situations that lead to poor coping, over-arousal, and "fight or flight" behaviors. It appeared that unexpected light touch, moderate to intense background noise, unpredictable movement of children in his vicinity, as well as unfamiliar situations were most likely to negatively affect his ability to maintain attention to tasks and remain in control of his own behavior. The therapist will need to follow up on these hypotheses.

As the conversation progressed, it became apparent that his family has understood his sensitivity to certain situations, and has approached his behavior in different ways. Peter's mother has taken responsibility for protecting Peter from situations which he perceives as threatening, whereas Peter's father has believed that Peter needs to "act right" in all situations and that Peter's mother is "too soft" on Peter. The classroom teacher has been reluctant to implement strategies, such as allowing Peter more time to make transitions or allowing him to redefine or not participate in some directed activities, as she feels this would show favoritism and/or would be unequal treatment that the other children would see as unfair.

This is an interesting case, because we see the adults responding differently to Peter. From a coping frame of reference, we would have to consider the coping strategies of each important person in Peter's life before we would know how to proceed with planning. For example, teachers sometimes feel that making accommodations for an individual student would be seen as unfair by the other students. This is especially true for students who do not have an obvious physical disability but may be perceived as just "misbehaving" or being "non-compliant". The occupational therapist can play an important role in explaining the nature of sensory processing difficulties and how they affect a student's behavior and learning. The therapist could also provide an in-class lesson for the other students regarding how different people respond differently to sensory input. Once the therapist shares this information and teachers and students understand, they become more able to recognize Peter's behaviors as coping responses related to his processing ability; then they can have alternative ways to support him to be more adaptive.

Pre-Assessment Hypothesis

Both the classroom teacher and the parents provided information that suggested possible sensory sensitivities and motor planning problems. It is common for early motor milestones, such as walking, to occur within the normal age expectations. Children with motor planning problems can sometimes use motor skills in free-play situations. But as the child has to problem-solve using his movement abilities, his performance breaks down. Many times these children are bright enough to manipulate situations to minimize their use of motor planning and to cope with their situation the best they can. Peter recognizes what needs to happen, and so uses his cognitive abilities to tell others what to do. This leads family members and other care providers to believe that the child can do things that he may not be able to do. However, the child is unable to use those same skills when they are required in directed learning or play situations that require organization and planning on the spot.

Assessment Plan

The occupational therapist decided to follow-up on these hypotheses by first observing Peter in the classroom during transition times, during a fine motor activity, and on the playground. The Certified Occupational Therapy Assistant (COTA) would assist in this assessment by doing the observation on the playground. The OTR would also consult with Peter's teacher regarding their observations. The occupational therapist also decided that after these observations, she would ask the teacher to complete the *School Function Assessment* and the parents to *complete the Sensory Profile* in order to obtain more complete information regarding Peter's sensory sensitivities and school performance strengths and concerns.

The COTA assists the OTR in assessing a student after the COTA has demonstrated competency on whatever portion of the assessment she will be doing.

The OTR and COTA must partner in the development of the COTA's competency in completing portions of the assessment. The OTR is ultimately legally responsible for all aspects of the occupational therapy process. In this case, the OTR and COTA have biannually watched videotapes of children together to discuss what they observe and record. This process enables them to maintain consistency in their data collection.

Findings and Interpretation

As part of the interdisciplinary assessment, the occupational therapist and the COTA observed Peter in several settings, administered the School Function Assessment with the help of the teacher, obtained a Sensory Profile from parents, and administered the short form of the Bruininks Oseretsky Test of Motor Proficiency.

A summary of the assessment information suggests strengths in some aspects of school performance, and difficulties with processing touch and movement and organizing and executing gross and fine motor movements (motor planning) when trying to produce work. Peter also demonstrated hypersensitivity for sensory input, poor coping with internal resources related to body functions, and good coping related to human support.

Since sensory defensiveness was an unfamiliar term to the parents, the occupational therapist took extra time during the interpretation to define the term and describe the ramifications of sensory defensiveness in Peter's behavior. The Bruininks Oseretsky Test of Motor Proficiency results also suggest difficulty coordinating and timing in both gross and fine motor movements. These findings are confirmed in the observations of Peter's movement patterns throughout the school.

The School Function Assessment is a measure of children's performance during life tasks at school. The teacher reported that Peter has difficulty with recreational movement, manipulation with movement, and using materials. He struggles more than other children to complete tasks and is not always happy with his own performance. He also had difficulty with the behavior regulation and social interaction categories; the teacher reported that she has to mediate a lot of interaction experiences with Peter.

The teacher is identifying Peter's difficulties with task performance, and they also relate to his difficulty with manipulation and movement. His difficulties are also showing up as he tries to negotiate socialization experiences. This is a common correlation for children who have poor motor planning.

It is important to remember, when using standard scores from any test, that you must combine this information with other test data, skilled observations, and actual performance at school, home, and within the community to determine an accurate picture of the child. Some school districts have eligibility guidelines based on students' performance on standardized measures as well as their performance in the educational setting. Students could potentially "qualify" using test scores alone, but if their school performance is not affected, they would not qualify for Occupational Therapy Services as part of IDEA. Making links between assessment data and behaviors observed by the referral parties is an important responsibility of the therapist.

Because this evaluation was part of a comprehensive evaluation in a public school, the therapist combined standardized testing to establish eligibility with skilled observation to identify intervention planning data. It is the responsibility of the occupational therapist in the schools to report assessment findings in relation to facilitating or compromising school-related performance. When a school-based occupational therapist identifies a problem that is not affecting classroom performance, a suggestion to look into other community resources is appropriate. They can include swimming, gymnastics, martial arts, and art programs, or may include a referral to an occupational therapy program in another agency. Care must also be taken to identify these non-school-related occupational therapy needs; it is not the school district's responsibility to pay for services that are not educationally-related.

Although the therapist has a professional responsibility to inform families about identified needs, it is also important to delineate for them school-related needs from other needs that they may choose to act upon using family resources. For example, the issue of family counseling came up during a discussion with the mother, due to her frustration managing Peter's outbursts and the different parenting styles between the mother and father. The occupational therapist noted their struggles to cope with Peter, and reminded herself to suggest a referral to a local pediatric psychologist with whom she had worked on a similar case. She would suggest this to the team as an outside referral.

Program Planning

The evaluation staffing included the parents, all members of the evaluation team, the school principal, and the kindergarten teacher. In some cases, team members may send a copy of their evaluation results to the meeting with another team member as it may not be possible to attend every meeting. In other cases, the team members may collaborate on their reports to focus on a more integrated interpretation. Although it is typically preferable to have team members present, sometimes a decreased number of professionals can be more conducive to parent participation because a large number of staff can be overwhelming to the parent. It is useful to send reports to families for review and questions too. This facilitates discussion at the meeting rather than reporting on test results.

The team reported performance area strengths in overall cognitive ability and language. They expressed concern in Peter's social domain and learning skills. After all areas of strengths and concerns were fully discussed, the team went on to discuss possible placements for Peter in school next year. The team members felt that a fall placement in a regular first grade classroom with the least number of students would be best with support from the occupational therapist and the consulting special education teacher.

The occupational therapist would provide expertise to:

a. Collaborate with staff to support Peter's ability to manage successfully at school.

b. Increase tolerance and use of sensory input to increase attention to learning, socialization, and play performance.

c. Increase postural control and motor planning so that Peter can manage his body within the classroom environment.

Target Outcome 1

Peter will complete 90% of seatwork assignments before lunch each day by the end of the school year (i.e., 36 weeks).

Intervention Approach (Using clinical reasoning to formulate an intervention approach.)

Provide environmental adaptations to accommodate problem areas during stressful activities, to provide a graded sensory program to increase Peter's ability to process input, and to provide parents and teachers with adaptive and restorative strategies.

Intervention Procedures

Since everyone was struggling to cope with Peter's ways of interacting and expressing interest in understanding this, the occupational therapist recommended a reading from the occupational therapy literature on the Coping Frame of Reference. She also provided an adult coping inventory for the parents and teacher so that they could gain insights about their styles in relation to Peter (see Williamson & Szczepanski, 1999).

The first grade teacher began to implement some of the strategies to minimize Peter's hyperexcitability. Because the bus ride and the lunchroom were two of the most difficult environments for Peter, the teacher and occupational therapist collaborated to identify some successful strategies for these particular situations. They met weekly during the teacher's scheduled planning time.

The teacher and occupational therapist designed a progress monitoring plan (see Chapter 9) for Peter's rides on the school bus to prevent him from getting kicked off the bus. Table 10-2 contains a summary of this plan. The therapist and teacher approached the bus driver about assigning

Table 10-2.

Sample Progress Monitoring Process for Peter

Outline of Tasks	Peter's plan
Behavior	Peter hits, screams, fights with others and gets out of his seat on the bus.
Goal	By the end of September, Peter will sit, keep his hands to himself and have neutral or positive engagements with others during the entire bus ride to school.
Hypothesis for Observed behavior	Peter has low sensory thresholds and therefore is very sensitive to sensory experiences that others may not notice, such as brushing up against him. He overreacts to these events in comparison to others.
Intervention plan	*Collaborate with bus driver to adapt Peter's bus seating to minimize inconsequential bumping that may set him off. *Discuss clothing options with family that will reduce Peter's ability to notice sensory experiences (e.g., tighter clothing).
Measurement strategy	Therapist and teacher will provide bus driver with cards for marking Peter's behaviors for the day. Bus driver will complete card each morning and hand it to the teacher who greets the bus. Teacher will chart the frequency of Peter's positive and negative behaviors daily.
Decision-making plan	Teacher and therapist will review Peter's data weekly. When Peter demonstrates 5 consecutive days of 0 negative and at least three positive behaviors, we will consider the plan complete and the goal met. If Peter's negative behaviors remain present and the same or more for 3 days, the teacher and therapist will meet with the bus driver and construct a new plan.

a front seat for Peter, to minimize the amount of space he would have to negotiate getting to his seat and to decrease the amount of inadvertent bumping and shoving that he would have to cope with during the trip. They introduced the data collection strategy, and agreed on the frequency for review. The bus driver agreed that this would be a manageable plan.

The teacher and therapist decided to introduce Peter to the lunchroom in a graded manner. Initially, Peter would be allowed to eat his lunch with one or two of his classmates just inside the lunchroom at a separate table. As he tolerated it, they would add children to the table, and then begin moving the table closer to the others until he would be fully integrated.

The family requested more information on strategies they could employ at home. The occupational therapist described Peter's needs in relation to activities that occur within the home. Bath time was always a challenge, so they discussed why this activity was difficult for Peter and created strategies for managing this time. For example, rubbing Peter lightly with a towel would upset him, due to his sensitivity for light touch. A better strategy would be to press the towel firmly into his skin to dry him after his bath. Other strategies were developed as the parents identified problem situations.

The occupational therapist also designed a direct service intervention program to increase Peter's tolerance for sensory input. She planned many experiences that would allow Peter to explore the nature of his own sensory input, and create adaptive responses to these stimuli. She also emphasized increasing the range and complexity of stimuli that Peter could manage, since natural life environments provide unpredictable amounts and types of stimuli. The occupational therapist joined the class during a body awareness period once a week to provide intervention, since Peter was in a first grade that emphasized exploratory and developmental aspects of learning. Many of the strategies the therapist used were slowly incorporated into Peter's classroom day as the teacher began to understand what Peter needed; having the therapist in the classroom providing intervention was very helpful in this process. The occupational therapist also designed a supervised therapy program with the physical education teacher to increase Peter's tolerance for movement.

Outcome

Once the teachers and family understood Peter's behaviors and their meaning in relation to his attempts to cope with situations, they all began to come up with ideas. They would share their ideas at the quarterly meetings they held to review Peter's program and identify the next steps for Peter. Eventually, Peter began to participate in idea generation and was able to ask for changes when he needed them to remain calm and in control of himself. He began competing in video chess on the computer; this manner of playing chess still capitalizes on the cognitive challenge without requiring quick or precise motor movements, and so Peter was successful and developed a new set of friends from this activity.

CASE #5 – DEREK (4TH GRADE)

Pre-Assessment Process

Referral: Derek moved into the school district over the summer with an existing IEP. He is 10 years old and has been receiving special education services since his 3rd birthday, when he was diagnosed as having autism. Derek's current IEP includes occupational therapy services that have been directed towards improving his fine motor skills. The team meets prior to the start of school so that services can be in place on the first day of school. Derek's mother has brought a videotape of Derek to this meeting so Derek's team could learn more about him prior to school starting. Derek's mom describes him as a child who has a good memory, can recite information, and enjoys building and drawing. She also describes Derek as being a social isolate who has difficulty communicating and engaging with his peers as well as adults, has difficulty with any change or transition, and has limited foods that he will eat.

Autism has a number of characteristics, including poor modulation of sensory input. Derek's prior school had not addressed these sensory issues, but rather chose a developmental and cognitive approach to intervention. The occupational therapist was providing standard practice when addressing Derek's difficulties with fine motor and writing skills, which supported the curricular goals the team had established for Derek. This approach would not be considered best practice because it takes a more narrow view of Derek. Derek's social and self-help skills are likely affected by sensory processing difficulties, and none of these areas are addressed on the current IEP.

The team decided to implement Derek's current IEP until further assessment could be completed and a new IEP could be developed. The only change that the team made in the current IEP was to have Derek enrolled in the regular fourth grade classroom as opposed to a self-contained classroom. Individual team members would then have time to get to know Derek and assess Derek's skills, as well as the current demands of the curriculum and environment. The fourth grade teacher was quite concerned about how Derek would do in her classroom, although she was receptive to having Derek as a student. The team decided to recommend a paraprofessional for the fourth grade classroom to assist in implementing Derek's IEP.

History: Derek lives with his mother and older sister. The family has just moved to the community from a neighboring school district. Derek's father sees him occasionally, as he finds Derek's behaviors difficult to deal with. Derek has been enrolled in a self-contained special education classroom since kindergarten, with limited inclusion in the regular education classroom.

Derek is functioning at approximately a second grade level in most academic areas. He has required one-to-one assistance to complete academic tasks, but this strategy supported the team's goals of academic progress.

Derek's mother wants Derek to have friends, but she is quite concerned about Derek being included in the fourth grade classroom. She is particularly concerned about how Derek will get along with other students and how students will react to and get along with Derek. She also expressed concern about Derek's difficulty with schedule changes and his limited diet choices.

Pre-Assessment Hypothesis

Derek's parents are changing their ideas about what they want for Derek's school experience. It appears that everyone was more focused on his academic performance early on, but now the parents seem more focused on socialization and daily life. This is a common shift in priorities as families watch their children grow and see that there are other important aspects to their child's life, in addition to academic performance. The team needs to support the old plans, as well as the transition to a new focus.

The information from Derek's current IEP, as well as information from Derek's mother, suggests that Derek's patterns of responding to sensory events may be interfering with his ability to interact with peers appropriately, to participate in school activities appropriately, to make changes in the schedule, and to eat a varied diet. The team, including Derek's mother, decide that if some of these sensory issues could be sorted out and understood, Derek would have a more successful and positive experience in fourth grade.

Assessment Plan

The team decided that Derek's mother should complete the *Sensory Profile Caregiver Questionnaire* as part of the assessment process. The occupational therapist would score this assessment. The team would view the videotape of Derek both at home and at his previous school for additional information. The teacher, paraprofessional, and occupational therapist would complete the School Function Assessment (SFA). This would help identify in a more global manner any part of the school day or school curriculum that was particularly difficult for Derek. The school psychologist would do additional classroom observations, the speech-language pathologist would do both classroom observation and direct one-on-one assessment, and the regular classroom teacher would determine where Derek is functioning in the curriculum.

Findings and Interpretations

Derek had difficulty with auditory processing and tactile (i.e., touch) processing. He also has difficulty with oral sensory processing (i.e., textures, tastes, and temperatures in the mouth area). Derek prefers to drink six to eight drink boxes each day and eat a minimal amount of solid foods. The solid foods he prefers are macaroni and cheese or french fries.

Derek played parallel to his peers, interacting infrequently. If peers attempted to enter or change Derek's play, he become upset and sometimes screamed, flapped his hands, or struck out at the peer. He frequently lined up small objects or stacked blocks to make an elevator. He also preferred to draw elevators on paper. Derek clearly prefers interaction with adults. He frequently hums to himself when engaged in a self-directed activity. During isolated play, he appears to be oblivious to voices and sounds around him.

Derek communicates in a variety of ways, including gestures and nonverbal communication, as well as some phrases that are repetitive in nature. At times, adults provide a verbal cue to facilitate Derek to use his words when he wants or needs something. Derek also has difficulty with situations that are unpredictable, such as on field trips or days on which there are "special programs". An increase in screaming or hitting was noted on these days.

On the School Function Assessment, Derek performed like other peers in cognitive performance tasks, but had difficulty with peer interactions and behavioral responses. This indicates his need for control over situations. He responds better to accommodations (i.e., changing the environment or task) for manipulation tasks than to assistance (i.e., someone helping him); he rejects another person trying to show him how to do something, particularly when they try to guide him through the task. This is consistent with other observations that Derek does not like to have his hands messy or for others to touch his hands, which limits the teachers' ability to provide physical prompting during new tasks. He also needed more assistance or accommodations when there were unpredictable situations in the classroom. The teacher also reported that Derek had difficulty making transitions to new tasks, demonstrating perseverance (i.e., repeating the same behavior over and over when it is no longer useful) behaviors at these times.

On the Sensory Profile, Derek's scores were variable, with some in the typical range and others below the typical response range. He tends to actively avoid sensory experiences, especially unfamiliar ones (Figure 10-7).

The team observed Derek over all school environments for the first 3 weeks of school. The School Function Assessment provided information regarding Derek's ability across all school settings. The combination of these two strategies ensures that the team considers overall performance and not a "good" or "bad" day.

Derek's sensory processing abilities are consistent with the "Sensation Avoiding" category (see Dunn, 1997). Many of Derek's behaviors seem to be the result of Derek needing to control or avoid potentially unfamiliar sensory input. However, there are also some indications of poor modulation of input, as Derek sometimes appears oblivious to auditory input and generates his own sounds. If these behaviors are interpreted from a neuroscience viewpoint, it is Derek's way of managing incoming auditory input to maintain an appropriate level or arousal.

Figure 10-7a. Sensory profile caregiver questionnaire (Page 1). (Reprinted with permission from The Psychological Corporation.)

SENSORY PROFILE

Winnie Dunn, Ph.D., OTR, FAOTA

Caregiver Questionnaire

Child's Name: DEREK Birth Date: ______ Date: ______

Completed by: MOTHER Relationship to Child: ______

Service Provider's Name: ______ Discipline: ______

INSTRUCTIONS

Please check the box that **best** describes the frequency with which your child does the following behaviors. Please answer all of the statements. If you are unable to comment because you have not observed the behavior or believe that it does not apply to your child, please draw an X through the number for that item. Write any comments at the end of each section. Please do not write in the Section Raw Score Total row.

Use the following key to mark your responses:

- **ALWAYS** When presented with the opportunity, your child always responds in this manner, 100% of the time.
- **FREQUENTLY** When presented with the opportunity, your child frequently responds in this manner, about 75% of the time.
- **OCCASIONALLY** When presented with the opportunity, your child occasionally responds in this manner, about 50% of the time.
- **SELDOM** When presented with the opportunity, your child seldom responds in this manner, about 25% of the time.
- **NEVER** When presented with the opportunity, your child never responds in this manner, 0% of the time.

THE PSYCHOLOGICAL CORPORATION®
A Harcourt Assessment Company

Figure 10-7b. Sensory profile caregiver questionnaire (Page 2). (Reprinted with permission from The Psychological Corporation.)

Sensory Processing

Item			A. Auditory Processing	ALWAYS	FREQUENTLY	OCCASIONALLY	SELDOM	NEVER
	L	1	Responds negatively to unexpected or loud noises (for example, cries or hides at noise from vacuum cleaner, dog barking, hair dryer)			X3		
	L	2	Holds hands over ears to protect ears from sound			X3		
	L	3	Has trouble completing tasks when the radio is on			X3		
	L	4	Is distracted or has trouble functioning if there is a lot of noise around			X3		
	L	5	Can't work with background noise (for example, fan, refrigerator)			X3		
	H	6	Appears to not hear what you say (for example, does not "tune-in" to what you say, appears to ignore you)			X3		
	H	7	Doesn't respond when name is called but you know the child's hearing is OK				X4	
	H	8	Enjoys strange noises/seeks to make noise for noise's sake		X2			
			Section Raw Score Total	24				

Comments

Item			B. Visual Processing	ALWAYS	FREQUENTLY	OCCASIONALLY	SELDOM	NEVER
	L	9	Prefers to be in the dark			X3		
	L	10	Expresses discomfort with or avoids bright lights (for example, hides from sunlight through window in car)			X3		
	L	11	Happy to be in the dark			X3		
	L	12	Becomes frustrated when trying to find objects in competing backgrounds (for example, a cluttered drawer)				X4	
	L	13	Has difficulty putting puzzles together (as compared to same age children)			X3		
	L	14	Is bothered by bright lights after others have adapted to the light			X3		
	L	15	Covers eyes or squints to protect eyes from light			X3		
	H	16	Looks carefully or intensely at objects/people (for example, stares)				X4	
	H	17	Has a hard time finding objects in competing backgrounds (for example, shoes in a messy room, favorite toy in the "junk drawer")				X4	
			Section Raw Score Total	30				

Comments

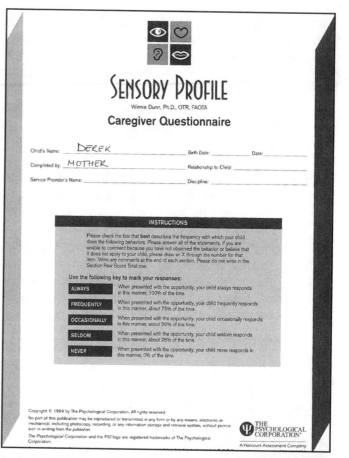

Figure 10-7c. Sensory profile caregiver questionnaire (Page 3). (Reprinted with permission from The Psychological Corporation.)

Item			C. Vestibular Processing	ALWAYS	FREQUENTLY	OCCASIONALLY	SELDOM	NEVER
→	L	18	Becomes anxious or distressed when feet leave the ground				X4	
→	L	19	Dislikes activities where head is upside down (for example, somersaults, roughhousing)				X4	
→	L	20	Avoids playground equipment or moving toys (for example, swing set, merry-go-round)				X4	
→	L	21	Dislikes riding in a car				X4	
→	L	22	Holds head upright, even when bending over or leaning (for example, maintains a rigid position/posture during activity)				X4	
→	L	23	Becomes disoriented after bending over sink or table (for example, falls or gets dizzy)					X5
→	H	24	Seeks all kinds of movement and this interferes with daily routines (for example, can't sit still, fidgets)				X4	
→	H	25	Seeks out all kinds of movement activities (for example, being whirled by adult, merry-go-rounds, playground equipment, moving toys)				X4	
→	H	26	Twirls/spins self frequently throughout the day (for example, likes dizzy feeling)				X4	
→	H	27	Rocks unconsciously (for example, while watching TV)				X4	
→	H	28	Rocks in desk/chair/on floor				X4	
			Section Raw Score Total			45		

Comments

Figure 10-7d. Sensory profile caregiver questionnaire (Page 4). (Reprinted with permission from The Psychological Corporation.)

Item			D. Touch Processing	ALWAYS	FREQUENTLY	OCCASIONALLY	SELDOM	NEVER
☼	L	29	Avoids getting "messy" (for example, in paste, sand, finger paint, glue, tape)		X2			
☼	L	30	Expresses distress during grooming (for example, fights or cries during haircutting, face washing, fingernail cutting)		X2			
☼	L	31	Prefers long-sleeved clothing when it is warm or short sleeves when it is cold		X2			
☼	L	32	Expresses discomfort at dental work or toothbrushing (for example, cries or fights)	X1				
☼	L	33	Is sensitive to certain fabrics (for example, is particular about certain clothes or bedsheets)	X1				
☼	L	34	Becomes irritated by shoes or socks		X2			
☼	L	35	Avoids going barefoot, especially in sand or grass			X3		
☼	L	36	Reacts emotionally or aggressively to touch		X2			
☼	L	37	Withdraws from splashing water		X2			
☼	L	38	Has difficulty standing in line or close to other people		X2			
☼	L	39	Rubs or scratches out a spot that has been touched		X2			
☼	H	40	Touches people and objects to the point of irritating others			X3		
☼	H	41	Displays unusual need for touching certain toys, surfaces, or textures (for example, constantly touching objects)			X3		
☼	H	42	Decreased awareness of pain and temperature			X3		
☼	H	43	Doesn't seem to notice when someone touches arm or back (for example, unaware)			X3		
☼	H	44	Avoids wearing shoes; loves to be barefoot			X3		
☼	H	45	Touches people and objects			X3		
☼	H	46	Doesn't seem to notice when face or hands are messy			X3		
			Section Raw Score Total			42		

Comments: Derek does better if we stick to a set routine for personal hygiene.

Item			E. Multisensory Processing	ALWAYS	FREQUENTLY	OCCASIONALLY	SELDOM	NEVER
👁		47	Gets lost easily (even in familiar places)			X3		
🏃		48	Has difficulty paying attention				X4	
👁	L	49	Looks away from tasks to notice all actions in the room				X4	
👂	H	50	Seems oblivious within an active environment (for example, unaware of activity)			X3		
🧍	H	51	Hangs on people, furniture, or objects even in familiar situations			X3		
🧍	H	52	Walks on toes			X3		
☼	H	53	Leaves clothing twisted on body			X3		
			Section Raw Score Total			23		

Comments

Figure 10-7e. Sensory profile caregiver questionnaire (Page 5). (Reprinted with permission from The Psychological Corporation.)

Item			F. Oral Sensory Processing	ALWAYS	FREQUENTLY	OCCASIONALLY	SELDOM	NEVER
	L	54	Gags easily with food textures or food utensils in mouth					X5
	L	55	Avoids certain tastes or food smells that are typically part of children's diets		X2			
	L	56	Will only eat certain tastes (list:_____)			X3		
	L	57	Limits self to particular food textures/temperatures (list:_____)		X2			
	L	58	Picky eater, especially regarding food textures		X2			
	H	59	Routinely smells nonfood objects			X3		
	H	60	Shows strong preference for certain smells (list:_____)		X2			
	H	61	Shows strong preference for certain tastes (list:_____)		X2			
	H	62	Craves certain foods (list:_____)			X3		
	H	63	Seeks out certain tastes or smells (list:_____)				X4	
	H	64	Chews or licks on nonfood objects					X5
	H	65	Mouths objects (for example, pencil, hands)			X3		
			Section Raw Score Total	36				

Comments

Modulation

Item			G. Sensory Processing Related to Endurance/Tone	ALWAYS	FREQUENTLY	OCCASIONALLY	SELDOM	NEVER
		66	Moves stiffly					X5
	H	67	Tires easily, especially when standing or holding particular body position				X4	
	H	68	Locks joints (for example, elbows, knees) for stability					X5
	H	69	Seems to have weak muscles				X4	
	H	70	Has a weak grasp			X3		
	H	71	Can't lift heavy objects (for example, weak in comparison to same age children)				X4	
	H	72	Props to support self (even during activity)			X3		
	H	73	Poor endurance/tires easily				X4	
	H	74	Appears lethargic (for example, has no energy, is sluggish)				X4	
			Section Raw Score Total	36				

Comments

Figure 10-7f. Sensory profile caregiver questionnaire (Page 6). (Reprinted with permission from The Psychological Corporation.)

Item			H. Modulation Related to Body Position and Movement	ALWAYS	FREQUENTLY	OCCASIONALLY	SELDOM	NEVER
		75	Seems accident-prone				X4	
		76	Hesitates going up or down curbs or steps (for example, is cautious, stops before moving)				X4	
	L	77	Fears falling or heights				X4	
	L	78	Avoids climbing/jumping or avoids bumpy/uneven ground				X4	
	L	79	Holds onto walls or banisters (for example, clings)				X4	
	H	80	Takes excessive risks during play (for example, climbs high into a tree, jumps off tall furniture)				X4	
	H	81	Takes movement or climbing risks during play that compromise personal safety				X4	
	H	82	Turns whole body to look at you				X4	
	H	83	Seeks opportunities to fall without regard to personal safety				X4	
	H	84	Appears to enjoy falling				X4	
			Section Raw Score Total	40				

Comments

Item			I. Modulation of Movement Affecting Activity Level	ALWAYS	FREQUENTLY	OCCASIONALLY	SELDOM	NEVER
	L	85	Spends most of the day in sedentary play (for example, does quiet things)		X2			
	L	86	Prefers quiet, sedentary play (for example, watching TV, books, computers)			X3		
	L	87	Seeks sedentary play options			X3		
	L	88	Prefers sedentary activities			X3		
	H	89	Becomes overly excitable during movement activity			X3		
	H	90	"On the go"				X4	
	H	91	Avoids quiet play activities				X4	
			Section Raw Score Total	22				

Comments

Item			J. Modulation of Sensory Input Affecting Emotional Responses	ALWAYS	FREQUENTLY	OCCASIONALLY	SELDOM	NEVER
		92	Needs more protection from life than other children (for example, defenseless physically or emotionally)			X3		
	L	93	Rigid rituals in personal hygiene			X3		
	H	94	Is overly affectionate with others			X3		
	H	95	Doesn't perceive body language or facial expressions (for example, unable to interpret)				X4	
			Section Raw Score Total	13				

Comments

Figure 10-7g. Sensory profile caregiver questionnaire (Page 7). (Reprinted with permission from The Psychological Corporation.)

Item			K. Modulation of Visual Input Affecting Emotional Responses and Activity Level	ALWAYS	FREQUENTLY	OCCASIONALLY	SELDOM	NEVER
👁	L	96	Avoids eye contact				X4	
👁	H	97	Stares intensively at objects or people			X3		
👁	H	98	Watches everyone when they move around the room			X3		
👁	H	99	Doesn't notice when people come into the room				X4	
			Section Raw Score Total			14		

Comments

Behavior and Emotional Responses

Item			L. Emotional/Social Responses	ALWAYS	FREQUENTLY	OCCASIONALLY	SELDOM	NEVER
♡		100	Seems to have difficulty liking self (for example, low self-esteem)			X3		
♡		101	Has trouble "growing up" (for example, reacts immaturely to situations)			X3		
♡		102	Is sensitive to criticisms			X3		
♡		103	Has definite fears (for example, fears are predictable)			X3		
♡		104	Seems anxious			X3		
♡		105	Displays excessive emotional outbursts when unsuccessful at a task			X3		
♡		106	Expresses feeling like a failure			X3		
♡		107	Is stubborn or uncooperative			X3		
♡		108	Has temper tantrums			X3		
♡		109	Poor frustration tolerance			X3		
♡		110	Cries easily			X3		
♡		111	Overly serious			X3		
♡		112	Has difficulty making friends (for example, does not interact or participate in group play)			X3		
♡		113	Has nightmares					X5
♡		114	Has fears that interfere with daily routine					X5
♡		115	Doesn't have a sense of humor			X3		
♡		116	Doesn't express emotions				X4	
			Section Raw Score Total			56		

Comments

Easily upset when his routine is disrupted.

Figure 10-7h. Sensory profile caregiver questionnaire (Page 8). (Reprinted with permission from The Psychological Corporation.)

Item			M. Behavioral Outcomes of Sensory Processing	ALWAYS	FREQUENTLY	OCCASIONALLY	SELDOM	NEVER
🔊		117	Talks self through tasks			X3		
👁		118	Writing is illegible			X3		
👁		119	Has trouble staying between the lines when coloring or when writing			X3		
♡		120	Uses inefficient ways of doing things (for example, wastes time, moves slowly, does things a harder way than is needed)			X3		
♡	L	121	Has difficulty tolerating changes in plans and expectations		X2			
♡	L	122	Has difficulty tolerating changes in routines			X3		
			Section Raw Score Total			17		

Comments

Item			N. Items Indicating Thresholds for Response	ALWAYS	FREQUENTLY	OCCASIONALLY	SELDOM	NEVER
🏃		123	Jumps from one activity to another so that it interferes with play				X4	
👄	H	124	Deliberately smells objects			X3		
👄	H	125	Does not seem to smell strong odors					X5
			Section Raw Score Total			10		

Comments

FOR OFFICE USE ONLY

ICON KEY		THRESHOLD KEY		SCORE KEY	
🔊	Auditory		Neither low nor high	1	Always
👁	Visual	L	Low	2	Frequently
🏃	Activity Level	H	High	3	Occasionally
👄	Taste/Smell			4	Seldom
🧍	Body Position			5	Never
→	Movement				
✋	Touch				
♡	Emotional/Social				

Figure 10-7i. Sensory profile summary score sheet. (Reprinted with permission from The Psychological Corporation.)

Factor Summary

Instructions: Transfer the child's score for each factor to the column labeled Factor Raw Score Total. Then plot these totals by marking an X in the appropriate classification column (Typical Performance, Probable Difference, Definite Difference).*

Factor	Factor Raw Score Total	Typical Performance	Probable Difference	Definite Difference
1. Sensory Seeking	60 /85	85——63	62——55	54——17
2. Emotionally Reactive	47 /80	80——57	56——48	47——16
3. Low Endurance/Tone	36 /45	45——39	38——36	35——9
4. Oral Sensory Sensitivity	23 /45	45——33	32——27	26——9
5. Inattention/Distractibility	24 /35	35——25	24——22	21——7
6. Poor Registration	27 /40	40——33	32——30	29——8
7. Sensory Sensitivity	16 /20	20——16	15——14	13——4
8. Sedentary	11 /20	20——12	11——10	9——4
9. Fine Motor/Perceptual	9 /15	15——10	9——8	7——3

*Classifications are based on the performance of children without disabilities (n = 1,037).

Section Summary

Instructions: Transfer the child's score for each section to the Section Raw Score Total column. Then plot these totals by marking an X in the appropriate classification column (Typical Performance, Probable Difference, Definite Difference).*

Sensory Processing	Section Raw Score Total	Typical Performance	Probable Difference	Definite Difference
A. Auditory Processing	24 /40	40——30	29——26	25——8
B. Visual Processing	30 /45	45——32	31——27	26——9
C. Vestibular Processing	45 /55	55——48	47——45	44——11
D. Touch Processing	42 /90	90——73	72——65	64——18
E. Multisensory Processing	23 /35	35——27	26——24	23——7
F. Oral Sensory Processing	36 /60	60——46	45——40	39——12
Modulation				
G. Sensory Processing Related to Endurance/Tone	36 /45	45——39	38——36	35——9
H. Modulation Related to Body Position and Movement	40 /50	50——41	40——36	35——10
I. Modulation of Movement Affecting Activity Level	22 /35	35——23	22——19	18——7
J. Modulation of Sensory Input Affecting Emotional Responses	13 /20	20——16	15——14	13——4
K. Modulation of Visual Input Affecting Emotional Responses and Activity Level	14 /20	20——15	14——12	11——4
Behavior and Emotional Responses				
L. Emotional/Social Responses	56 /85	85——63	62——55	54——12
M. Behavioral Outcomes of Sensory Processing	17 /30	30——22	21——19	18——6
N. Items Indicating Thresholds for Response	10 /15	15——12	11——10	9——4

*Classifications are based on the performance of children without disabilities (n = 1,037).

Program Planning

Derek's team (which consisted of the occupational therapist, special education teacher, regular education teacher, school psychologist, and speech-language pathologist) decided to focus on increasing interactions with peers in controlled situations as well as increasing Derek's ability to communicate, since this is a core skill for socialization at his age. The team also decided to honor Derek's need to control sensory input (i.e., sensation avoiding) as they constructed their plans so that Derek would remain available to learn (i.e., he would not burst out in response to unfamiliar input).

This team took a broader view of Derek's performance needs at school, including socialization and communication as critical areas of emphasis, rather than only addressing the curricular educational needs to learn (e.g., math, reading, writing). This is also occurring because the parents are ready to expand their view of Derek's needs and life.

The occupational therapist on a team such as this must also see the role of occupational therapy in this broader view and offer expertise to all aspects of this program. It is common for students with autism to respond differently to sensory events in daily life, and this is an area of expertise for occupational therapy. This viewpoint offers the team a way to approach Derek's socialization and communication needs in a completely different manner, while also giving the parents some ways to understand Derek's behavior as a coping strategy (i.e., he is keeping new stimuli from occurring by fleeing situations or by acting out to limit participation). In a program such as this one, the team must be vigilant about collecting data so they can adjust the program based on Derek's responses. Remember, the team's goal is for Derek to socialize, not to "improve sensory processing".

Target Outcome 1

Derek will work with two peers on an assigned classroom task for 30 minutes without striking out, hand flapping, or screaming (in 36 weeks).
Benchmarks:
- One peer for 10 minutes in 9 weeks
- One peer for 30 minutes in 18 weeks
- Two peers for 15 minutes in 27 weeks

Intervention Approach

The team decided to include students from Derek's fourth grade classroom in the intervention. In addition, they discussed the sensory supports they would make available to Derek in order to honor his need to control sensory input throughout the day.

Intervention Procedures

Derek's mother gave permission to implement the *Circle of Friends* approach, which helped identify students in Derek's classroom who would be willing to assist in the implementation of Derek's program. The teacher and students discussed activities that the students thought Derek could participate in. The teacher and paraprofessional selected two students to actively engage with Derek on a consistent basis. The teacher and paraprofessional trained these students to give Derek feedback when he was making inappropriate noises in the classroom. They would tell Derek that "the noises you are making make it hard to get work done. You need to go to the library". They also learned to ask Derek if they could join his play and then proceed to copy what Derek was doing with similar materials. This gained Derek's interest and honored his need for familiarity, which increased Derek's ability to be more participatory with the other students.

The teacher seated Derek at the far end of the aisle (to reduce random contact with objects and other children passing by) in a pod of four desks facing one another. One of the peers who had agreed to assist Derek sat next to him. The quiet area was directly to Derek's right, making it more available to him when he needed it.

The team identified "getaway places" both in the classroom and in other parts of the school building. If Derek needed a place to control sensory input, he was allowed to go to the "quiet" area of the classroom where students would go to read. This area included a clawfoot bathtub with pillows in it and bean bag chairs, enabling students to construct an environment that supported their bodies and provided the amount of sensory input that was comfortable (e.g., how many pillows piled underneath and on top of you, laying on the bean bags or sitting on them). In addition, Derek was allowed to go to the library to re-stack books when he needed to stand and move. Stacking books provides input to support postural control and organize body scheme information because the weight of the books activates the proprioceptive receptors, which contribute to one's sense of self (see Chapter 6).

The paraprofessional in the classroom moved around the room to assist any of the students who needed help. She did not sit next to Derek unless the task was not suitable for a peer to help him. This was critical for Derek's socialization; if he had an adult hovering all the time, students would not have an interest or need to interact with Derek, and vice versa.

The occupational therapist provided handouts (see Chapter 6) for team members, including the regular education teacher, regarding the impact of sensory processing difficulties on performance, and suggested ways to structure activities to support children like Derek.

Derek's collaborative team initially met each week to plan Derek's program and make modifications. After 6 weeks, they agreed that they had worked out all the inconsistencies and could touch base monthly.

Outcome

Derek's tantruming and screaming decreased over the first few months. Derek's interaction with the two targeted peers increased and Derek accepted directions, assistance, and even began initiating interactions with each of them. The next step would be to include several more peers in a structured manner in Derek's program.

Derek used the "quiet" area of the classroom frequently and eventually was able to return to his desk after spending brief periods in the quiet area. Derek was becoming aware of his own internal signals and acting in his own behalf to get needs met. This is a critical skill for transition to middle school.

The team decided to increase the sensory features of his school routines. They provided a weighted blanket for Derek to lay across his legs while seated at his desk and added weight to his writing utensils. They asked him to wear a backpack with heavy books in it when transitioning among rooms and activities and designated him to be the "carrier" when getting trays of milk from the cafeteria. All of these interventions supported Derek to participate while receiving discriminatory sensory input (i.e., input that does not activate the arousal systems and generate a "fight or flight" response).

The occupational therapist provided Derek's mother with information about interventions that worked for Derek in the classroom and how she could adapt these in the home environment.

Over a period of several months, Derek became more interactive with other students, as well as with his sister at home. The family found that Derek could interact with others via email, and he has two pen pals this way. During email interactions, Derek did not have to worry about extra sensory experiences interfering with his socialization; he frequently piled books on his lap during these sessions, an adaptation of the blanket from school.

CASE #6 – CAMERON (MIDDLE SCHOOL)

Pre-Assessment Process

Referral: Cameron's initial referral to special services occurred as a toddler, and he has been receiving related services since that time. He is currently making the transition to middle school—where he will be changing classes and teachers hourly. He will have to maneuver around a new building and will want to participate in school-related extracurricular activities.

This is not a new referral, but an ongoing case. Whenever a student with special needs transitions to a new environment, the demands and supports also change. In this case, the occupational and physical therapists are instrumental in assessing the environment demands of the new environment and recommending modifications.

History: Cameron is the oldest of four children. He was born 3 months prematurely and had anoxia at birth that resulted in spastic quadraplegia. His parents noted that at age 1, he was not sitting up. They took him to a neurologist who diagnosed Cameron with cerebral palsy. They enrolled Cameron in an early intervention program where he received occupational, physical, and speech-language therapy until he was 5 years old. Beginning in kindergarten, Cameron attended the local elementary school in regular education with paraprofessional support, as well as occupational and physical therapy and adaptive physical education as related services. Cameron uses a power wheelchair for mobility and a laptop computer for written assignments.

Pre-Assessment Hypothesis

The occupational therapist obtained a copy of this school district's ADA plan for accessibility for each of its buildings including the middle school. The occupational and physical therapist made a list of potential problem areas Cameron might encounter during this transition to a new building and new program. The therapist was particularly concerned about activities of daily living skills including toileting, eating, and dressing for physical education class. Other questions centered around how independent Cameron could be in this new environment and what task trade-offs would be necessary in order for him to be successful at the middle school level.

Assessment Plan

The preliminary plan was for the occupational and physical therapist to walk through the middle school building with the elementary school principal from Cameron's current school, the middle school principal, the building maintenance supervisor, Cameron and a friend of his choice, and Cameron's parents. The occupational and physical therapist had made a list of areas of the building or certain programs that might be particularly difficult for Cameron to access. They determined the accessibility of the cafeteria, restroom, locker room, library, track, office, locker area, and hall areas with doors.

The teams also decided to have a meeting with the sending and receiving staff members from the elementary and middle school so they could discuss curricular modifications that had been useful and would be possible in this new setting.

Findings and Interpretation

The middle school building is a one-story building with virtually no steps (one exception is one step up into some of the outside entrances). One entrance did not have a step, but Cameron was unable to enter the building independently as there were no automatic door openers on any of the outside entrances. Once inside the building, Cameron could easily access the office, the library, the commons areas, and the gymnasium. The boys restroom was not accessible, as the entrance into it was not wide enough for Cameron's wheelchair. The seventh grade wing of the building had double fire doors dividing it from the rest of the building that are required by fire code to be kept closed. Cameron was unable to open the heavy doors by pushing against them with his wheelchair.

Once inside this wing, Cameron could reach the padlock on the upper locker but he was unable to rotate the padlock in order to open it. The hallways in this wing are quite narrow with double lockers on both sides, resulting in a very crowded hall when students change classes. The students sit at large round tables in the language arts class that Cameron easily maneuvered up to and fit underneath. The algebra class had chairs with attached desks that were packed tightly into the classroom, making it impossible for Cameron to enter past the doorway. This was also the case in his other core classes.

The gymnasium was accessible to Cameron but due to the old style, there was no seating on the floor level. The bleachers started right outside the perimeter of the basketball court, making it difficult for Cameron to sit safely on the gym floor. There were no ramps or lifts up to the bleacher level. Cameron could also not access his physical education class when they went outside, as there was a step down onto the track. Cameron was interested in attending and announcing football games. The bleachers were not accessible to him.

This team conducted the assessment of the next environment for Cameron in the spring of the year prior to his entrance into middle school so the district would have adequate time to make modifications. The family, district administrators, and therapists sat down and made a specific plan for Cameron, including where classes would be scheduled (so time issues could be addressed as well).

This assessment time also enabled the members to discuss what situations might require extra staff support for Cameron to be successful in this educational environment. Cameron and his parents also met the middle school principal and became familiar with the building and programs.

Program Planning

The team used the information from the assessment of the middle school for Cameron's IEP meeting. The district agreed to make the building and programs accessible to Cameron. Cameron's parents were part of this team and helped in making decisions for how modifications could best be made for Cameron.

They made the following decisions and actions:

1. The outside entrance closest to the office had an automatic door opener installed that Cameron could operate. This was the one entrance that did not have an outside step up, and was the one the students used most frequently.

2. The restroom in the wing for Cameron's classes was large, so they installed a stall that met ADA standards without compromising other uses.

3. Automatic door openers for the double doors to the 7th grade wing were installed, and it was agreed to work on installing these in the other wings in subsequent years.

4. The family agreed to locate a digital lock for Cameron's locker.

5. The team discussed the narrow halls at great length. The teachers were clear that the "crowdedness" served a very important socialization function and so wanted to enable Cameron to participate in this activity, even though to adults it was chaotic. The team decided to develop a progress monitoring plan for this activity and see how Cameron managed without physical changes.

6. The counselors agreed to limit the number of children in classes with too many desks (and the *teachers* were happy), so that Cameron and other children could get around successfully; the administration hired an additional teacher for the 7th grade team to accommodate the shift in scheduling and used a room in the 8th grade wing for this activity.

7. The administration got an estimate for one new set of bleachers at one end of the gym and agreed to replace one section each year.

8. An architect and the occupational therapist collaborated to identify a strategy for getting to the field from the building for physical education class and other sports activities.

Intervention Planning

As you can see from this case, not all children require the same type of approach, and sometimes a more "institutional" approach is in everyone's best interest. Cameron already knew the cognitive, language, and other learning strategies for himself, and his condition is stable, but he needed the environment to be more user friendly to support him being there. This is a great role for occupational therapy in schools—to support these transitions.

Outcome

The district had to scramble to complete the plans by the start of school, and Cameron and his family visited the school several times during the summer so that Cameron could practice getting around. Their strategy was that if it was all very familiar to him, the disruptions would be less upsetting to Cameron's overall functioning. They also went to school during the various enrollment periods so there would be more traffic, and this additional challenge seemed to excite Cameron. The teachers and

Cameron collected data on his timeliness in the halls when changing classes, and found that he was late like many other children at first, but that he was able to socially broker his needs in the hall to get to his next class. This helped Cameron get immersed very quickly, and he was one of the first children everyone knew at school. The speech-language pathologist and occupational therapist came to school to program some "cool" phrases into his computer for those times when he could not produce language fast enough for the needs of the situation; everyone loved this.

CASE #7 – SARAH (HIGH SCHOOL)

Pre-Assessment Process

Referral: Sarah is a 16-year-old student who was a passenger in a vehicle involved in an accident in May of the previous school year. She sustained an injury to the left parietal region. Sarah has been an inpatient at an area rehabilitation hospital through the summer and is returning to school on a limited basis at the start of the school year.

This referral is being made to the high school's special education team in order for Sarah's current functioning level to be assessed and an appropriate program to be developed.

Students with Traumatic Brain Injury (TBI) may have emotional or affective difficulties, memory difficulties, attention problems, and perceptual and motor problems. Any of these may affect the student's ability to complete simple tasks, such as following directions and completing simple self-care tasks. Physical sequelae of TBI could include reduced stamina, seizures, headaches, and hearing and vision losses (Tyler, 1992). Cognitive problems of TBI could include memory, intellectual functioning, attention and concentration, language, and academic functioning.

A student's ability to adjust to TBI is often influenced by any affective problems, personality disturbances, behavior problems, pre-injury personality traits, the family's ability to cope, the sense of guilt over the injury circumstances, or denial of illness. In addition peers, teachers, and family must learn about the new characteristics and challenges before them; it is often helpful to offer them reading materials about TBI so that they can feel a sense of control over their own coping with the changes that will occur. Most states have a brain injury association that provides materials and support for families and service providers.

History: Sarah has been a regular education student who was just completing her sophomore year in high school. She was a member of the high school Color Guard and the spirit club. Sarah was a passenger in a car driven by another high school student when the driver lost control of the car on a gravel road and hit another vehicle head on. Neither girl was wearing her seat belt. Sarah was thrown from the car and sustained serious head injuries. The driver sustained internal injuries, was hospitalized and released after 1 week. Sarah is the only child in her two-parent family. Sarah's father is an accountant and her mother is a homemaker.

Both parents are quite involved with Sarah, although Sarah's mother is the primary care provider.

Pre-Assessment Hypothesis

A student who has sustained a serious head injury needs to have coordinated services between the medical and educational setting. Because Sarah has sustained a serious head injury with resulting difficulties in both cognitive and motor areas, the school-based therapist will want to observe Sarah in the rehab setting prior to school starting and gain as much information as possible from Sarah's medical team.

The referral and history suggests that Sarah will only be able to fully participate in the school environment with modifications and assistance. It will be important to conduct ongoing assessment of Sarah's abilities, as she is still in a recovery phase from her head injury.

Assessment Plan

The occupational and speech-language therapist will visit the rehab center where Sarah is receiving daily outpatient occupational, physical, and speech-language therapy. They will also visit with Sarah and her mom and observe therapy sessions with the various disciplines. In addition, the professionals decide to hold a joint team meeting in which Sarah's entire rehab team, as well as the team from the high school, meet to discuss Sarah's strengths and needs and plan for her transition back to high school.

The school's state Department of Education was operating a TBI state grant designed to assist school districts in understanding about TBIs of their students and assist teams in planning for these students. The team also consulted with these experts to obtain additional information and training for the school team.

Findings and Interpretations

The team used a combination of record review, observation, and interview prior to Sarah returning to school to collect data. The rehab team reported that Sarah has right hemiparesis with limitations in all movements of her right upper extremity. Sarah has limitations in all shoulder, elbow, wrist, and hand movements. She has right side neglect and does not use her arm or hand unless prompted. She also has limited sensory awareness of her right upper extremity. Sarah is able to get dressed and undressed, complete most of her own self-grooming with minimal assistance, and feed herself with utensils (although overall, she is slower than her peers). Sarah walks with a slight limp, but is functionally walking on different surfaces and up and down stairs. She has mild disorientation with directions and spatial relations. Sarah has gained good comprehension and expression skills.

Sarah's goals are to get back to school full-time, drive again, attend extracurricular activities, and spend time with her friends. This includes participating in Color Guard again. She would also like to be able to use her right arm and hand better so that she looks more "normal". When asked about post-high school goals, Sarah said she plans on attending a local community college or vocational school but does not know what she wants to study.

Considering what Sarah would like to accomplish is extremely important; Sarah is old enough to speak for herself and has the power to participate in or sabotage the team's plans. This is true with all children for whom therapists provide services, but because Sarah is an adolescent it is extremely important that she feels a part of the process. The therapist must consider this even more when designing a program for an adolescent who does not want to "stand out" (or in Sarah's words, "look like a freak"). The therapist must place as much emphasis on Sarah's mental health needs as on her physical needs.

Program Planning

The team planned a number of activities designed to enable Sarah to be as successful as possible in her school program. Several of these activities were:

1. Continuing contact with the rehab center where Sarah is receiving outpatient therapy. The school-based therapists and the hospital-based therapists arranged to talk weekly about Sarah's program. This allowed for the school-based therapist to convey information regarding Sarah's ability to function in the school environment to the hospital-based therapist. This arrangement also allowed for consistency across therapists and environments.

2. Sarah would continue to attend the medically-based rehab center therapy sessions 4 days each week.

3. The school team arranged Sarah's class schedule so that she attends afternoon classes and can attend her outpatient therapy sessions in the morning. This would allow Sarah to be at school over the lunch hour and for three classes in the afternoon, which would also allow her to attend after school extracurricular activities.

4. The collaborative teams set a goal to transition Sarah to school-based therapy over the next 6 months. The occupational therapist would continue to work on increasing functional capabilities of Sarah's right upper extremity, while at the same time working on modifications to support her participation.

5. The occupational therapist would teach Sarah precautions regarding lack of sensitivity of her right arm and hand.

6. Sarah will begin attending Color Guard practice and participating in practices to the extent she is able. With the consent of the sponsor and other Color Guard members, the therapist will attend these practices to observe, get ideas for how Sarah can practice, and make modifications so Sarah can participate in some routines.

7. Transition planning will begin with the development of Sarah's IEP.

8. The hospital-based therapist will explore driving options for Sarah and any modifications that she might need; the driver's education teacher at school will work with Sarah on driving simulations and knowledge and safety skill development.

Target Outcome 1

Sarah will execute a 3-minute Color Guard routine keeping in time with the other performers by May (36 weeks).

Intervention Approach

Provide environmental adaptations to accommodate Sarah's limitations.

Provide natural opportunities for Sarah to continue to use her right arm and hand (e.g., Color Guard).

Continue to teach Sarah one-handed techniques to complete activities of daily living.

Consult with high school faculty and staff, as well as with Sarah's peer group, regarding Sarah's return to school.

Intervention Procedures

Color Guard practices were a viable means of providing both therapeutic intervention for Sarah's arm and hand, developing better spatial relationships, and re-integrating Sarah into a small supportive peer group. Practices were held 3 days each week: 1 day during band class and 2 other days after school. Color Guard uses long plastic poles with flags on one end to develop routines to music. Sarah had been instrumental in starting Color Guard at the school and had co-developed many of the initial routines. The therapist looked at the movements necessary to hold and move the poles, and the speed and strength required. The therapist then modified some movements with the help of the rest of the Color Guard team so that Sarah could participate in at least one routine.

When occupational therapists are implementing best practices, they understand how to "see" the performance component needs in the person's chosen daily life activities. The therapist might have a difficult time convincing Sarah to complete her exercises for her arms, but Sarah is very interested in re-joining the Color Guard. The routines contain the same movements and endurance requirements that a more clinical therapy regime would contain. By using the high interest activity, both the therapist and Sarah have a better chance at a successful outcome (both for Color Guard participation and for rehabilitation).

Outcome

Sarah initially just attended and observed at the Color Guard practices with the therapist. The other girls consulted with Sarah on the routines they were developing and solicited any suggestions she could make. By the second week, Sarah was attempting to move the pole by holding it with her right hand and moving the pole with her left hand. This provided therapeutic activity for Sarah that was motivating for her. The team developed new "moves" which Sarah could also complete. By the first of November, Sarah partially participated in a Color Guard performance at the half time of a football game.

Sarah began attending school full-time the second semester, and outpatient rehabilitation by occupational therapy was reduced to once a week. A physical education class was included in her class schedule to allow for continuing therapeutic activity in her school day. The occupational therapist and the adaptive physical education teacher worked on an individual program for Sarah during this period.

Sarah was able to use her right arm and hand as a gross assist only and developed some of her own ways of completing tasks that she preferred. As a senior student, Sarah was able to participate in a job shadowing program through the high school to help introduce her to a variety of careers that she might consider.

CASE #8 – TAMMY (19 YEARS OLD)

Pre-Assessment Process

Referral: Tammy has been enrolled in special education programs throughout her entire school career. This referral is being made in order to gain supported employment opportunities through the State Division for Vocational Rehabilitation as part of her transition to post-high school employment. The primary concern expressed by Tammy, the parents, and school personnel was that Tammy lacked definite plans for the future. Without ongoing and timely intervention, it was likely that she would be spending unproductive time at home or in a sheltered workshop. These two options were unacceptable to Tammy and her family.

Supported employment is defined in federal statute as a highly individualized approach for assisting individuals with significant disabilities to obtain and maintain employment. Supported employment includes three essential components:

1. Paid work.
2. Employment in integrated community settings.
3. The availability of on-going support and training as needed to assure job retention or subsequent job placement.

Tammy's case illustrates her "transition" from student to a productive adult worker role. Her transition program began at age 14, when the transition coordinator employed by the special education cooperative along with Tammy's IEP team started planning for Tammy's post-secondary transition. The law regarding transition in IDEA 97 states:

Sec. 1414

(II) (vii)(I) beginning at age 14, and updated annually, a statement of the transition service needs of the child under the applicable components of the child's IEP that focuses on the child's courses of study (such as participation in advanced-placement courses or a vocational education program);

(II) beginning at age 16 (or younger, if determined appropriate by the IEP Team), a statement of needed transition services for the child, including, when appropriate, a statement of the interagency responsibilities or any needed linkages;

It is important that this transition be timely and smooth. Without a timely referral and attention to Tammy's transition needs, it is likely that a significant delay or gap in services would have occurred and possibly resulted in Tammy losing valuable skills and confidence.

History: Tammy was enrolled in special education services throughout her public school career due to her primary disability of moderate mental retardation. Her high school education included basic academics, some school and home based training in independent living activities, and vocational preparation activities that included community-based instruction. During her last year of high school, Tammy spent a half day every day in a work position at a local restaurant.

Tammy lived with her parents, who are very supportive and desire to see Tammy assume a worker role in the community. They also expressed anxiety about Tammy traveling independ-

ently in the community. Tammy's home was on the public bus route that provided access to needed transportation, although Tammy did not know how to use the bus system independently. Tammy's family assumed responsibility for food preparation, shopping, and house maintenance; Tammy assisted with house cleaning. Tammy had a history of some incoordination and judgement limitations when handling cleaning equipment and materials. This interfered with her ability to perform independently in this area. Tammy performs self-care activities independently, with occasional reminders from her mother. Tammy's recreational activities were almost always family-centered and family-initiated.

Pre-Assessment Hypothesis

The information gathered from Tammy and the referral sources indicated that employment was the primary concern. School personnel and Tammy's parents also felt that she would need significant help finding, learning about, and retaining a job, thus requiring the referral for supported employment services. Although Tammy could not identify specific job-related interests, she expresses a strong desire to work and earn money. Tammy's dependence on her parents for transportation, along with her difficulty with judgment and handling materials in a coordinated manner, required further investigation.

Assessment Plan

Two occupational therapists, a job developer, a job coach, Tammy, and her parents served as the supported employment service team. To gain needed information that would assist the team in placing Tammy in a paid community job, the team decided that some in-depth interviews with Tammy, her parents, and school personnel would be needed. The interviews would help the team identify Tammy's interests and abilities as they might apply to a job. The team decided that it would be important to assess not only job-related interests and abilities, but also her specific abilities at home, in the community, and recreationally. Needs or abilities in these areas can directly impact employment.

The Canadian Occupational Performance Measure (COPM) provides a structure for interviewing, and also provides an evidence-based method for making plans for Tammy (i.e., the COPM has been shown to reflect changes in a person's status and performance satisfaction) (Law, Polatajko, Pollack, McColl, Carswell, & Baptiste, 1994).

In addition to interviews, the team needed to gain information about what Tammy was able to do, how she learned, and how she operated in a variety of community environments. This would require a situational observation of Tammy's performance in a variety of relevant situations, such as on the city bus, at a downtown restaurant, crossing streets, and using city services. During this observation process, team members planned to identify Tammy's strengths and interests, while noting any supports that were required to ensure successful performance (e.g., inability to plan needed time to get to appointments) along with strategies to overcome these barriers.

Findings and Interpretations

The therapist interviewed Tammy and her parents using the COPM. They emphasized the worker role issues, since this was an overall priority for Tammy. Everyone agreed that "personal care" and "paid work" were priorities. Tammy wanted to have a job, and to be able to get to her job independently; her parents stated that she needed to be able to get ready for work by herself as well.

Tammy was highly skilled in many areas and able to learn new skills effectively (e.g., identifying the correct bus, placing an order in a restaurant, crossing streets safely) when given the opportunity to follow a model and to practice. Tammy learned quickly in the actual community environment that required a specific skill (e.g., a store, restaurant, city bus, bank).

She was unable to readily generalize across learning environments or situations. Tammy appeared to enjoy spending time in the community with people other than her family, however she lacked confidence to do this without some sort of support and assistance. In the self-care area, Tammy required cueing from her mother to shower and wash her hair on a regular basis. She also had some difficulty selecting matching clothes from her closet. Tammy's coordination was observed in a variety of functional contexts (carrying a food tray in a restaurant, walking over uneven surfaces, running to catch a bus, climbing the stairs of the bus, walking to her seat on a moving bus) and it was determined that her coordination was largely functional and safe. In situations where coordination and judgment were both needed (e.g., walking across a newly mopped floor), Tammy had more difficulty. With explicit instruction and demonstration, she was able to learn to walk around (compensation) the wet area even if this took her out of her way.

When a functional situational assessment process is used, it is important for the therapist to observe and record skills and needs within the context. It cannot be assumed, for example, that an individual's ability to safely cross a street with a crossing light means that he or she can also cross safely at an unmarked intersection. A functional assessment allows the team to focus on an individual's strengths (vs. weaknesses) in a variety of relevant situations. Family members generally understand and can actively contribute to such an assessment process that builds cooperation, a sense of shared planning, and problem-solving.

Based on extensive observations and interviews used to assess Tammy's work-related interests and needs, the team was able to identify the critical conditions that would need to be present in a job for Tammy. Tammy would require a job where supervision was always around, and a setting where co-workers would be able to redirect or instruct Tammy when she ran into difficulty. It was clear based on the assessment that Tammy would not do well working independently or working without frequent contact with others. Assessment of Tammy's ability to learn new tasks (e.g., riding the public bus) led the team to recommend that she have on-the-job "coaching" available in order to learn a job (i.e., explicit demonstration, practice, and feedback). The team felt that an employer would not be able to assume total responsibility for training Tammy given her unique learning needs.

The assessment process also allowed team members to identify Tammy's job-related interests. After spending time at a local restaurant, Tammy expressed that she would like to "help" with a salad bar and to "wash" tables. She also stated that she liked the uniforms worn by restaurant workers. Among other interests, it became clear that Tammy liked spectator sports, particularly professional football. The team was then able to incorporate her interests into a job search effort.

Program Planning

The supported employment service team focused primary attention on the performance area of work. Activities of daily living and leisure/recreation received a secondary focus, as the team felt that they would impact employment.

Community-based programs utilize a team-oriented effort to plan programs, and therefore resemble the individual within the environment. The contribution that the occupational therapist makes on the team is unique and vital, but is incorporated into natural life tasks along with the contributions of the other team members. Community-based programs demonstrate this important principle very well, and therefore provide a model for all program planning across the life span.

In Tammy's case, the team had to consider not only a work outcome, but how home life and recreation/leisure activities might impact work. The team members decided upon a five-step process that would lead to the development of an appropriate program plan for Tammy. These steps are to:

1. Identify Tammy's individual strengths, interests, and her desired outcome for the service provision process.

2. Identify a Frame of Reference.

3. Clarify community service provision outcomes (i.e., paid employment).

4. Develop goals that reflect anticipated outcomes.

5. Develop objectives to achieve goals.

Target Outcome 1

Tammy will maintain paid work for 6 months.

Intervention Approach

• Support to obtain employment.

• In-home coaching and consultation to design adaptations that provide cues for the "getting ready" routine.

• On-the-job training and support with needed modifications or adaptations.

• Job coaching for transport to and from job site.

Intervention Procedures (Examples)

The following intervention sequence will be implemented:

1. Analyze the work environment and specific job tasks to identify opportunities (e.g., a supportive co-worker, color coding on salad bar

ingredients) and barriers (e.g., typical business use of many written notices and written instructions for workers) for Tammy.

2. Observe Tammy doing the work activities, collect data on work task performance, and adapt environment or teaching methods to allow Tammy to succeed.

3. Meet with employer and co-workers to discuss job adaptations needed, and provide support and direction regarding interaction with Tammy.

4. Meet with parents and Tammy to design home routines and supports, so that they can reduce their involvement in her morning routine and enable Tammy to have her own consequences.

Outcome

Tammy receives supported employment services from the Community Developmental Disability Organization. This supported employment program designs and provides individualized community-based services that lead to paid employment.

Occupational therapists are critical members of the team and utilize their skills in functional assessment, environmental, and job analysis, as well as adaptation to maximize opportunities for employment success. Tammy's service environments are the environments she uses on a regular basis, and include her home, the city bus system, and her job. Utilization of natural community environments or assessment and training promotes meaningful learning and retention of skills and behaviors. Enabling Tammy to operate in a variety of natural environments allows the team to bypass her problems with generalization, while greatly increasing the efficiency of her intervention program.

Tammy, with the help of the supported employment service team, obtained a paid job at a local pizza restaurant. She required extensive on-the-job training by a job coach for the first few months of employment. Additionally, the job coach provided explicit training in the use of the public transportation system until Tammy was able to demonstrate independent and consistent use. Tammy's parents were very supportive in prompting Tammy to shower regularly and launder her uniform. They also prompted Tammy to get ready each morning and to catch the bus at the appropriate time. After several months of direct support by the occupational therapist and the job coach, Tammy demonstrated competence traveling and necessitated very occasional follow-up from the supported employment team. Her co-workers and employer assumed responsibility for daily support and training and reported tremendous satisfaction with Tammy's performance. The supported employment team gradually became consultants to the employer, but remained available on an as-needed basis.

CASE #10 – PROVIDING SERVICES TO WESTWOOD CHARTER SCHOOL

Charter schools have specific educational missions. The Westwood Charter School, which will serve as our example of population-based services, provides an alternative learning experience for educationally disadvantaged and high-risk students in grades 9 to 12 from a rural county. This school has the mission "to provide an authentic, nurturing, and academically challenging learning environment for high school students which is connected to the world outside of school, is meaningful for students, and promotes their positive sense of community and enthusiasm for learning." This school was developed in response to a longitudinal study of drop-out rates in participating LEAs that revealed 120 students in a 7-year period left high school prior to graduation. The previous year's students included six who were parents, two who were living on their own, six who were involved in the legal system, and five who were in custody of the welfare agency or were assigned to a social worker.

The principal of Westwood Charter School had formerly been an administrator and a teacher in the neighboring school district, and he had worked with occupational therapists on his teams before coming to Westwood. He discussed the member requirements of the professional teams for this new school with his board of directors, and they decided that an occupational therapist would be a useful addition.

Determining Needs

The occupational therapist's initial strategies included interviewing the administrative and teaching staff, reviewing the longitudinal study that led to the formation of Westwood Charter School, reviewing the records of the previous year's students, and discussing the mission and vision of Westwood Charter School with the staff.

During the interviews, the occupational therapist considered the information within the framework of the AOTA Uniform Terminology (i.e., listening for information about critical performance areas, performance components, and performance contexts). The Uniform Terminology framework provided an organizational structure for the planning process.

The occupational therapist determined that the students enrolled in Westwood Charter School were having life challenges that revealed the relationships among the performance areas, performance components, and performance contexts.

1. Some students were having difficulty with their worker and student roles (i.e., performance areas). Difficulties seemed to have related several factors:

    a. Some students have limited social awareness and skills (i.e., the performance components) for their worker and student roles.

    b. Some students were struggling to understand their particular work cultures (i.e., the performance context) and its demands.

c. Some students seemed to need skills training for the work tasks themselves (e.g., study skills for student role, task performance expertise for the work role).

d. Some students seemed to be unable to relate their own actions to the consequences in particular contexts, and therefore did not take responsibility for outcomes.

2. Some students were having difficulty establishing and maintaining social relationships (including family, peers) to support them in their roles as student, family member, and friend.

a. Some students seemed to lack awareness of social demands and cues.

b. Some students expressed lack of confidence in their ability to develop and maintain relationships.

c. Some students seemed to have difficulty creating a sense of autonomy (i.e., feeling effective as an individual who can take control of one's own life).

The occupational therapist checked back with the staff regarding these impressions about needs. The Westwood staff agreed that these were key issues to address in their curriculum and with individual students. They felt that these were the issues that interfered with the students' success and satisfaction with their lives, and that many of the negative situations that arose had their roots in these dilemmas.

Identifying Performance Factors

Once the occupational therapist had a clear overall understanding of the needs, she could use her unique occupational perspective to characterize the supports and barriers to performance within the Westwood Charter School system.

Supports for Performance Within the Westwood Charter School

A particularly strong support for the students' performance is the staff at Westwood Charter School (i.e., a performance context variable). They are very willing to receive and integrate new information and suggestions, and seem clear about the mission of their school to support the students to have a successful and satisfying life.

The curriculum is also a support for planning (this would be both a task variable and a contextual variable). Charter schools in general have great flexibility to be innovative and design non-traditional curriculums. The Westwood Charter School is structured around the development of individual learning plans that assist student performance and achievement in core academic areas, Internet and other learning technologies, and out-of-school/field-based learning experiences, including service-learning.

Academic goals of the Westwood Charter School are using six-trait writing to improve communication, demonstrating improvement in both narrative and expository reading comprehension, and demonstrating improvement in the area of mathematical problem-solving. Westwood Charter School also has non-academic goals for its students. These include promoting students' positive sense of community and promoting students' sense of resilience. These academic and non-academic goals set the stage for effective intervention planning on the areas of need.

The faculty have also designed a set of standards for enhancing students' overall critical thinking skills across the curriculum. Some of these standards include making informed decisions by examining options and anticipating consequences of actions, transferring learning from one context to another, working effectively in groups to accomplish a goal, identifying personal interests and goals and pursuing them, and recognizing the influence of diverse cultural perspectives on human thought and behavior. These goals and standards provide many opportunities for an occupational therapy perspective and intervention strategies.

Potential Barriers to Performance at Westwood Charter School

The Westwood students have multiple risk factors that create barriers to their success, including being teen parents, being removed from their biological family home, being involved with the legal system, failing in a traditional educational placement, and/or having learning and behavioral difficulties and attention problems. In addition, these students have a sense of failure and generally lack motivation and a sense of responsibility for their own actions. Reports from the admissions records indicate that many of their psychosocial issues have not been identified or explored.

The occupational therapist also noted that classroom arrangements feel and look chaotic. There are no "quiet" areas to reduce sensory stimuli to enhance student learning. Some students wear headphones to listen to music while working on the computers but often have the volume up so high that their music interferes with other students' learning. Lights are bright everywhere, both students and staff are talking most of the time, and the traffic flow between areas seems disruptive to other students' learning. The occupational therapist notes that she will explore environmental redesign to accommodate a wider range of sensory processing needs while working.

Designing the Intervention Program

The occupational therapist decided to organize the intervention plan using the Ecology of Human Performance framework because it provides both a method for characterizing the occupational therapy perspective on person/task/environment interaction as critical to performance, and a structure for organizing the intervention options for the staff.

Intervention Plan

The occupational therapist met with the school administrator to discuss general plans, then met with the whole staff to cover general information, and finally met with the respective teams to collaborate on specific ideas for effective interventions for each team's students. This strategy provided the occupational therapist with an opportunity to explain the overall occupational therapy perspective and then apply those concepts to specific problems. This strategy also set the stage for more effective use of her skills and expertise in the future.

During the meeting with the administrator, they discussed the possibility of resource allocation to enable the occupational therapist to provide peer coaching and supports for staff related to job exploration. Since the administrator was anxious for the community to view the school as a positive community resource, he decided that this might be a good use of resources initially and wanted to make sure that staff knew that he would support using money to include the occupational therapist in their implementation processes.

The staff meeting provided an opportunity for teaching and dialogue. The occupational therapist discussed her perspectives on supporting and designing successful performance options, and illustrated her perspective by using a case from their school (a student everyone was familiar with).

Characterizing the Occupational Therapy Perspective for Tom

Performance Areas:

1. Tom needs to develop effectiveness in his roles as worker and student (i.e., work and productive activities).

2. Tom needs to examine work options related to his own skills and interests (i.e., vocational exploration, work performance).

3. Tom needs to develop effectiveness in socialization options and performance (i.e., play/leisure activities).

Performance Components:

Tom needs psychosocial skills to support performance in work, student, and peer roles (i.e., psychological – values, interests, self-concept; social – roles, conduct, interpersonal skills, self-expression; self-management – coping, time management, self-control).

Performance Contexts:

1. Tom needs to understand the demands and supports available within particular life environments (e.g., temporal, social, cultural, and physical features)

They discussed how each of them viewed the student's strengths and needs, and the occupational therapist made comparisons and contrasts among perspectives. She demonstrated how her perspective provided unique and useful information for their thinking and problem-solving. This facilitated the follow-up meetings with teams and individualized planning, because it provided a framework for their thinking and questions related to particular students.

The occupational therapist provided guidance and expertise in several areas as described in the following examples.

1. Exploring employment options in the community through job shadowing and use of job coaches. The occupational therapist assisted with task analyzing the jobs and matching the tasks required with the students' abilities (i.e., application of Alter and Prevent interventions).

2. Assessing the educational environments to identify the sensory features that either increase or decrease the students' ability to complete work. The occupational therapist provided consultation to the classroom teachers and administrator regarding rearranging the physical environment to provide low lighting and sound absorbing partitions with large floor cushions and comfortable chairs in one area of the classroom (application of Adapt intervention).

3. Providing sensory processing information for students and staff so that each person could become more aware of their own sensory preferences and dislikes. The therapist used the Adult Sensory Profile; staff completed the tool, and they discussed their patterns in the group. Then staff administered the Adult Sensory Profile with their students as well (application of Establish/Restore intervention).

4. Designing community-based activities to increase the students' positive sense of community as well as positive feelings about themselves. The occupational therapist collaborated with Early Head Start (EHS) and Head Start to arrange volunteer experiences for students. The charter school students read to students at Head Start on a regular basis and assisted the EHS provider on home visits by playing with the siblings of the EHS child while the EHS provider visited with the parent(s). Additional activities included pairing up charter school students who have behavior and motivation difficulties with early elementary students with similar difficulties as learning buddies, as well as cooking a weekly meal for a community congregate meal site. This included planning the meal, purchasing the groceries, cooking and serving the meal, and cleaning up (application of Create, Prevent, and Alter interventions).

Planning a trip to visit the NICU to learn about the complications of pre-maturity as they relate to teenage pregnancies, lack of prenatal care, and the effects of drug and alcohol use on babies (Application of Establish/Restore, Adapt, and/or Prevent interventions).

Offering creative outlets to explore the students' self-concept and self-expression. The occupational therapist designed activities to encourage students to be more expressive about their feelings and themselves. An example of one activity was using mannequin heads that the students were able to complete with various materials to represent how they see themselves or how they think others see them. This activity was followed up with discussion and feedback (application of Establish/Restore, Adapt, Create, and Prevent interventions).

Conducting Program Evaluation

The staff used the program evaluation protocol for their whole school to evaluate the overall effectiveness of the occupational therapy services. This protocol includes methods for evaluating both the overall outcomes and the specific activities. The students and staff identified criteria for success of activities prior to beginning, and then were able to complete an evaluation of each suggested activity or modification using these criteria. An example of criteria for the first activity is:

Percentage of students who are successful part-time employees:
- *Have been employed consistently at the same job.*
- *Received acceptable performance evaluation from their employer.*
- *Interviewed with unsuccessful students to identify mismatch issues.*
- *Have job satisfaction (self-reported).*

The occupational therapist and school administrator met quarterly to review the occupational therapy utilization for the last quarter. They used several sources of information during these reviews, including billing records (which included time and types of activities), feedback forms from teams and other staff, satisfaction information from community partners, data from student performance, and records about the patterns and nature of usage (e.g., which teams used the occupational therapist in what ways during the quarter). They discussed more effective methods for using these services, and drafted a plan for the next quarter at each meeting.

The overall evaluation criteria for the Westwood Charter School included measures of academic progress as well as measures of non-academic performance, such as attendance records, parent satisfaction survey, student and teacher reflections, student drawings, School Climate Survey, Social Skills Rating System (SSRS), and The Adolescent Resiliency Attitudes Scale (ARAS). The administrator had an advisory team that reviewed these materials for presenting to the board. When occupational therapy services became part of their discussion, the occupational therapist would either attend the meetings or provide the needed information. Once a year, the occupational therapist provided an analysis of the overall contribution of her services to the schools' current outcomes, as well as suggestions for the future.

References for this Case Study:

Kansas Public Charter Schools Grant Application submitted by USD 341 Oskaloosa (1998-99)

Williams, Jennifer. (1999). Interview. [Personal communication regarding development of the intervention planning].

REFERENCES

Brogren, E. Hadders-Algra, M., & Forssberg, H. (1996). Postural control in children with spastic diplegia: Muscle activity during perturbations in sitting. *Developmental Medicine and Child Neurology, 38*(5), 379-388.

Cermak, S. (1993). Performance of normal Chinese adults and right CVA patients on the Random Chinese World Cancellation Test. *Clinical Neuropsychologist,1*(3), 239-249.

Crott, H. W., Giesel, M., & Hoffman, C. (1998). The process of inductive interference in groups: The use of hypothesis and target testing in sequential rule discovery tasks. *Journal of Personality and Social Psychology, 75*(4), 938-952.

Dunn, W. (1997). The impact of sensory processing abilities on the daily lives of young children and their families. *Infants and Young Children, 9*(4), 23-25.

Dunn, W. & Brown, T. (1997). Factor analysis on the sensory profile from a national sample of children without disabilities. *American Journal of Occupational Therapy, 51*(70), 490-495.

Erhardt, R. (1990). *Developmental visual dysfunction: Models for assessment and management.* San Antonio, TX: Therapy Skills Builders.

Evans-Morris, S. & Dunn-Klein, M. (1987). *Pre-feeding skills.* San Antonio, TX: Therapy Skill Builders.

Green, E. M., Mulcahy, C. M., & Pountey, T. E. (1995). An investigation into the development of early postural control. *Developmental Medicine and Child Neurology, 37*(5), 437-448.

Kandel, E., Schwartz, J., & Jessell, T. (2000). *Principles of neural science.* New York, NY: McGraw-Hill Companies.

Larnet, G. & Ekberg, O. (1995). Positioning improves the oral and pharyngeal swallowing function in children with cerebral palsy. *ACTA-PAEDIATRICA, 84*(6), 689-692.

Law, M., Polatajko, H., Pollack, N., McColl, M. A., Carswell, A., & Baptiste, S. (1994). Pilot testing of the COPM: Clinical and measurement issues. *Canadian Journal of Occupational Therapy, 61*(4), 191-197.

Myhr, U., Von-Wendt, L., Norrlin, S., & Radell, U. (1995). Five-year follow-up of functional sitting position in children with cerebral palsy. *Developmental Medicine and Child Neurology, 37*(7), 587-596.

Noronha, J., Bundy, A., & Groll, J. (1989). The effect of positioning on the hand function of body with cerebral palsy. *American Journal of Occupational Therapy, 43*(8), 507-512.

Royeen, C. B. & Lane, S. J. (1991). Tactile processing and sensory defensiveness. In A. Fisher, E. Murray, & A. Bundy (Eds.), *Sensory integration: Theory and practice* (pp. 108-133). Philadelphia, PA: FA Davis Company.

Salisbury, C., & Dunst, C. (1997). *Homes, school, and community partnerships: Building inclusive teams. Collaborative Teams for Students with Severe Disabilities* (pp. 57-82). Baltimore, MD: Paul H. Brookes Publishing Co.

Turnbull, A. P., Blue-Banning, M., Turbiville, V., & Park, J. (1999). From parent education to partnership education: A call for a transformed focus. *Topics in Early Childhood Special Education, 19*(3), 164-172.

Tyler, S. (1992). The development of ecosystemic approach as a humanistic education psychology. *Education Psychology, 12*(1), 15-24.

Vergara, E. (1993). *Foundations for practice in the neonatal intensive care unit and early intervention.* Rockville, MD: AOTA.

Williamson, G., & Szczepanski, M. (1999). Coping frame of reference. In P. Kramer & J. Hinojosa (Eds.), *Frames of reference for pediatric occupational therapy* (2nd ed.) (pp. 431-468). Baltimore, MD: Williams & Wilkins.

A Uniform Terminology for Occupational Therapy, Third Edition

American Occupational Therapy Association

This is an official document of the American Occupational Therapy Association. This document is intended to provide a generic outline of the domain of concern of occupational therapy and is designed to create common terminology for the profession and to capture the essence of occupational therapy succinctly for others.

It is recognized that the phenomena that constitute the profession's domain of concern can be categorized, and labeled, in a number of different ways. This document is not meant to limit those in the field, formulating theories or frames of reference, who may wish to combine or refine particular constructs. It is also not meant to limit those who would like to conceptualize the profession's domain of concern in a different manner.

INTRODUCTION

The first edition of Uniform Terminology was approved and published in 1979 (AOTA, 1979). In 1989, the *Uniform Terminology for Occupational Therapy—Second Edition* (AOTA, 1989) was approved and published. The second document presented an organized structure for understanding the areas of practice for the profession of occupational therapy. The document outlined two domains. *Performance Areas* (activities of daily living [ADL], work and productive activities, and play or leisure) include activities that the occupational therapy practitioner[1] emphasizes when determining functional abilities. *Performance Components* (sensorimotor, cognitive, psychosocial, and psychological aspects) are the elements of performance that occupational therapists assess and, when needed, in which they intervene for improved performance.

This third edition has been further expanded to reflect current practice and to incorporate contextual aspects of performance. *Performance Areas, Performance Components, and Performance Contexts* are the parameters of occupational therapy's domain of concern. *Performance areas* are broad categories of human activity that are typically part of daily life. They are activities of daily living, work and productive activities, and play or leisure activities. *Performance components* are fundamental human abilities that—to varying degrees and in differing combinations—are required for successful engagement in performance areas. These components are sensorimotor, cognitive, and psychosocial and psychological. *Performance contexts* are situations or factors that influence an individual's engagement in desired and/or required performance areas. Performance contexts consist of *temporal aspects* (chronological, developmental, life cycle, and disability status) and *environmental aspects* (physical, social, and cultural). There is an interactive relationship among performance areas, performance components, and performance contexts. Function in performance areas is the ultimate concern of occupational therapy, with performance components considered as they relate to participation in performance areas. Performance areas and performance components are always viewed within performance contexts. Performance contexts are taken into consideration when determining function and dysfunction relative to performance areas and performance components, and in planning intervention. For example, the occupational therapist does not evaluate strength (a performance component) in isolation. Strength is considered as it affects necessary or desired tasks (performance areas). If the individual is interested in homemaking, the occupational therapy practitioner would consider the interaction of strength with homemaking tasks. Strengthening could be addressed through kitchen activities, such as cooking and putting groceries away. In some cases, the practitioner would employ an adaptive approach and recommend that the family switch from heavy stoneware to lighter weight dishes, or use lighter weight pots on the stove to enable the individual to make dinner safely without becoming fatigued or compromising safety.

Occupational therapy assessment involves examining performance areas, performance components, and performance contexts. Intervention may be directed toward elements of performance areas (e.g., dressing, vocational exploration), performance components (e.g., endurance, problem solving), or the environmental aspects of performance contexts. In the last case, the physical and/or social environment may be altered or augmented to improve and/or maintain function. After identifying the performance areas the individual wishes or needs to address, the occupational therapist assesses the features of the environments in which the tasks will be performed. If an individual's job requires cooking in a restaurant as opposed to leisure cooking at home, the occupational therapy practitioner faces several challenges to enable the individual's success in different environments. Therefore, the third critical aspect of performance is the performance context, the features of the environment that affect the person's ability to engage in functional activities.

This document categorizes specific activities in each of the performance areas (ADL, work and productive activities, play or leisure). This categorization is based on what is considered "typical", and is not meant to imply that a particular individual characterizes personal activities in the same manner as someone else. Occupational therapy practitioners embrace individual differences, and so would document the unique pattern of the individual being served, rather than forcing the "typical" pattern on him or her and family. For example, because of experience or culture, a particular individual might think of home management as an ADL task rather than "work and productive activities" (current listing). Socialization might be considered part of play or leisure activity instead of its current listing as part of "activities of daily living", because of life experience or cultural heritage.

EXAMPLES OF USE IN PRACTICE

Uniform Terminology—Third Edition defines occupational therapy's domain of concern, which includes performance areas, performance components, and performance contexts. While this document may be used by occupational therapy practitioners in a number of different areas (e.g., practice, documentation, charge systems, education, program development, marketing, research, disability classifications, and regulations), it focuses on the use of Uniform Terminology in practice. This document is not intended to define specific occupational therapy interventions. Examples of how performance areas, performance components, and performance contexts translate into practice are provided below.

- An individual who is injured on the job may have the potential to return to work and productive activities, which is a performance area. In order to achieve the outcome of returning to work and productive activities, the individual may need to address specific performance components such as strength, endurance, soft tissue integrity, time management, and the physical features of performance contexts, like structures and objects in his or her environment. The occupational therapy practitioner, in collaboration with the individual and other members of the vocational team, uses planned interventions to achieve the desired outcome. These interventions may include activities such as an exercise program, body mechanics instruction, and job site modifications, all of which may be provided in a work-hardening program.

- An elderly individual recovering from a cerebral vascular accident may wish to live in a community setting, which combines the performance areas of ADL with work and productive activities. In order to achieve the outcome of community living, the individual may need to address specific performance components, such as muscle tone, gross motor coordination, postural control, and self-management. It is also necessary to consider the sociocultural and physical features of performance contexts, such as support available from other persons, and adaptations of structures and objects within the environment. The occupational therapy practitioner, in cooperation with the team, utilizes planned interventions to achieve the desired outcome. Interventions may include neuromuscular facilitation, practice of object manipulation, and instruction in the use of adaptive equipment and home safety equipment. The practitioner and individual also pursue the selection and training of a personal assistant to ensure the completion of ADL tasks. These interventions may be provided in a comprehensive inpatient rehabilitation unit.

- A child with learning disabilities is required to perform educational activities within a public school setting. Engaging in educational activities is considered the performance area of work and productive activities for this child. To achieve the educational outcome of efficient and effective completion of written classroom work, the child may need to address specific performance components. These include sensory processing, perceptual skills, postural control, motor skills, and the physical features of performance contexts, such as objects (e.g., desk, chair) in the environment. In cooperation with the team, occupational therapy interventions may include activities like adapting the student's seating in the classroom to improve postural control and stability, and practicing motor control and coordination. This program could be developed by an occupational therapist and supported by school district personnel.

- The parents of an infant with cerebral palsy may ask to facilitate the child's involvement in the performance areas of activities of daily living and play. Subsequent to assessment, the therapist identifies specific performance components, such as sensory awareness and neuromuscular control. The practitioner also addresses the physical and cultural features of performance contexts. In collaboration with the parents, occupational therapy interventions may include activities such as seating and positioning for play, neuromuscular facilitation techniques to enable eating, facilitating parent skills in caring for and playing with their infant, and modifying the play space for accessibility. These interventions may be provided in a home-based occupational therapy program.

- An adult with schizophrenia may need and want to live independently in the community, which represents the performance areas of activities of daily living, work and productive activities, and leisure activities. The specific performance categories may be medication routine, functional mobility, home management, vocational exploration, play or leisure performance, and social interaction. In order to achieve the outcome of living independently, the individual may need to address specific performance components such as topographical orientation, memory, categorization, problem solving, interests, social conduct, time management, and sociocultural features of performance contexts, such as social factors (e.g., influence of family and friends) and roles. The occupational therapy practitioner, in cooperation with the team, utilizes planned interventions to achieve the desired outcome. Interventions may include activities such as training in the use of public transportation, instruction in budgeting skills, selection of and participation in social activities, and instruction in social conduct. These interventions may be provided in a community-based mental health program.

- An individual with a history of substance abuse may need to reestablish family roles and responsibilities, which represent the performance areas of activities of daily living, work and productive activities, and leisure activities. In order to achieve the outcome of family participation, the individual may need to address the performance components of roles, values, social conduct, self-expression, coping skills, self-control, and the sociocultural features of performance contexts, such as custom, behavior, rules, and rituals. The occupational therapy practitioner, in cooperation with the team, utilizes planned intervention to achieve the desired outcomes. Interventions may include roles and values exercises, instruction in stress management techniques, identification of family roles and activities, and support to develop family leisure routines. These interventions may be provided in an inpatient acute care unit.

PERSON-ACTIVITY-ENVIRONMENT FIT

Person-activity-environment fit refers to the match among skills and abilities of the individual; the demands of the activity; and the characteristics of the physical, social, and cultural environments. It is the interaction among the performance areas, performance components, and performance contexts that is important and determines the success of the performance. When occupational therapy practitioners provide services, they attend to all of these aspects of performance and the interaction among them. They also attend to each individual's unique personal history. The personal history includes one's skills and abilities (performance components), the past performance of specific life tasks (performance areas), and experience within particular environments (performance contexts). In addition to personal history, anticipated life tasks and role demands influence performance.

When considering the person-activity-environment fit, variables such as novelty, importance, motivation, activity tolerance, and quality are salient. Situations range from those that are completely familiar, to those that are novel and have never been experienced. Both the novelty and familiarity within a situation contribute to the overall task performance. In each situation, there is an optimal level of novelty that engages the individual sufficiently and provides enough information to perform the task. When too little novelty is present, the individual may miss cues and opportunities to perform. When too much novelty is present, the individual may become confused and distracted, inhibiting effective task performance.

Humans determine that some stimuli and situations are more meaningful than others. Individuals perform tasks they deem important. It is critical to identify what the individual wants or needs to do when planning interventions.

The level of motivation an individual demonstrates to perform a particular task is determined by both internal and external factors. An individual's biobehavioral state (e.g., amount of rest, arousal, tension) contributes to the potential to be responsive. The features of the social and physical environments (e.g., persons in the room, noise level) provide information that is either adequate or inadequate to produce a motivated state.

Activity tolerance is the individual's ability to sustain a purposeful activity over time. Individuals must not only select, initiate, and terminate activities, but they must also attend to a task for the needed length of time to complete the task and accomplish their goals.

The quality of performance is measured by standards generated by both the individual and others in the social and cultural environments in which the performance occurs. Quality is a continuum of expectations set within particular activities and contexts.

I. Performance Areas	II. Performance Components	III. Performance Contexts

A. Activities of Daily Living
  1. Grooming
  2. Oral Hygiene
  3. Bathing/Showering
  4. Toilet Hygiene
  5. Personal Device Care
  6. Dressing
  7. Feeding and Eating
  8. Medication Routine
  9. Health Maintenance
  10. Socialization
  11. Functional Communication
  12. Functional Mobility
  13. Community Mobility
  14. Emergency Response
  15. Sexual Expression
B. Work and Productive Activities
  1. Home Management
    a. Clothing Care
    b. Cleaning
    c. Meal Preparation/Cleanup
    d. Shopping
    e. Money Management
    f. Household Maintenance
    g. Safety Procedures
  2. Care of Others
  3. Educational Activities
  4. Vocational Activities
    a. Vocational Exploration
    b. Job Acquisition
    c. Work or Job Performance
    d. Retirement Planning
    e. Volunteer Participation
C. Play or Leisure Activities
  1. Play or Leisure Exploration
  2. Play or Leisure Performance
	A. Sensorimotor Components
	  1. Sensory
	    a. Sensory Awareness
	    b. Sensory Processing
	      (1) Tactile
	      (2) Proprioceptive
	      (3) Vestibular
	      (4) Visual
	      (5) Auditory
	      (6) Gustatory
	      (7) Olfactory
	    c. Perceptual Processing
	      (1) Stereognosis
	      (2) Kinesthesia
	      (3) Pain Response
	      (4) Body Scheme
	      (5) Right-Left Discrimination
	      (6) Form Constancy
	      (7) Position in Space
	      (8) Visual-Closure
	      (9) Figure Ground
	      (10) Depth Perception
	      (11) Spatial Relations
	      (12) Topographical Orientation
	  2. Neuromusculoskeletal
	    a. Reflex
	    b. Range of Motion
	    c. Muscle Tone
	    d. Strength
	    e. Endurance
	    f. Postural Control
	    g. Postural Alignment
	    h. Soft Tissue Integrity
	  3. Motor
	    a. Gross Coordination
	    b. Crossing the Midline
	    c. Laterality
	    d. Bilateral Integration
	    e. Motor Control
	    f. Praxis
	    g. Fine Motor Coordination/Dexterity
	    h. Visual-Motor Integration
	    i. Oral-Motor Control
	B. Cognitive Integration and Components
	  1. Level of Arousal
	  2. Orientation
	  3. Recognition
	  4. Attention Span
	  5. Initiation of Activity
	  6. Termination of Activity
	  7. Memory
	  8. Sequencing
	  9. Categorization
	  10. Concept Formation
	  11. Spatial Operations
	  12. Problem Solving
	  13. Learning
	  14. Generalization
	C. Psychosocial Skills and Components
	  1. Psychological
	    a. Values
	    b. Interests
	    c. Self-Concept
	  2. Social
	    a. Role Performance
	    b. Social Conduct
	    c. Interpersonal Skills
	    d. Self-Expression
	  3. Self-Management
	    a. Coping Skills
	    b. Time Management
	    c. Self-Control
		A. Temporal Aspects
		  1. Chronological
		  2. Developmental
		  3. Life Cycle
		  4. Disability Status
		B. Environmental Aspects
		  1. Physical
		  2. Social
		  3. Cultural

UNIFORM TERMINOLOGY FOR OCCUPATIONAL THERAPY—THIRD EDITION

"Occupational Therapy" is the use of purposeful activity or interventions to promote health and achieve functional outcomes. "Achieving functional outcomes" means to develop, improve, or restore the highest possible level of independence of any individual who is limited by a physical injury or illness, a dysfunctional condition, a cognitive impairment, a psychosocial dysfunction, a mental illness, a developmental or learning disability, or an adverse environmental condition. Assessment means the use of skilled observation or evaluation by the administration and interpretation of standardized or nonstandardized tests and measurements to identify areas for occupational therapy services.

Occupational therapy services include, but are not limited to:

1. The assessment, treatment, and education of or consultation with the individual, family, or other persons
2. Interventions directed toward developing, improving, or restoring daily living skills; work readiness or work performance; play skills or leisure capacities; or enhancing educational performances skills
3. Providing for the development, improvement, or restoration of sensorimotor, oral-motor, perceptual or neuromuscular functioning; or emotional, motivational, cognitive, or psychosocial components of performance.

These services may require assessment of the need for and use of interventions such as the design, development, adaptation, application, or training in the use of assistive technology devices; the design, fabrication, or application of rehabilitative technology such as selected orthotic devices; training in the use of assistive technology, orthotic or prosthetic devices; the application of physical agent modalities as an adjunct to or in preparation for purposeful activity; the use of ergonomic principles; the adaptation of environments and processes to enhance functional performance; or the promotion of health and wellness (AOTA, 1993, p. 1117).

I. PERFORMANCE AREAS

Throughout this document, activities have been described as if individuals performed the tasks themselves. Occupational therapy also recognizes that individuals arrange for tasks to be done through others. The profession views independence as the ability to self-determine activity performance, regardless of who actually performs the activity.

A. *Activities of Daily Living*—Self-maintenance tasks.

1. *Grooming*—Obtaining and using supplies; removing body hair (use of razors, tweezers, lotions, etc.); applying and removing cosmetics; washing, drying, combing, styling, and brushing hair; caring for nails (hands and feet); caring for skin, ears, and eyes; and applying deodorant.
2. *Oral Hygiene*—Obtaining and using supplies; cleaning mouth; brushing and flossing teeth; or removing, cleaning, and reinserting dental orthotics and prosthetics.
3. *Bathing/Showering*—Obtaining and using supplies; soaping, rinsing, and drying all body parts; maintaining bathing position; transferring to and from bathing positions.
4. *Toilet Hygiene*—Obtaining and using supplies; clothing management; maintaining toileting position; transferring to and from toileting position; cleaning body; and caring for menstrual and continence needs (including catheters, colostomies, and suppository management).
5. *Personal Device Care*—Cleaning and maintaining personal care items, such as hearing aids, contact lenses, glasses, orthotics, prosthetics, adaptive equipment, and contraceptive and sexual devices.
6. *Dressing*—Selecting clothing and accessories appropriate for the time of day, weather, and occasion; obtaining clothing from storage area; dressing and undressing in a sequential fashion; fastening and adjusting clothing and shoes; and applying and removing personal devices, prostheses, or orthoses.

7. *Feeding and Eating*—Setting up food; selecting and using appropriate utensils and tableware; bringing food or drink to mouth; sucking, masticating, coughing, and swallowing; and management of alternative methods of nourishment.

8. *Medication Routine*—Obtaining medication, opening and closing containers, following prescribed schedules, taking correct quantities, reporting problems and adverse effects, and administering correct quantities using prescribed methods.

9. *Health Maintenance*—Developing and maintaining routines for illness prevention and wellness promotion, such as physical fitness, nutrition, and decreasing health risk behaviors.

10. *Socialization*—Accessing opportunities and interacting with other people in appropriate contextual and cultural ways to meet emotional and physical needs.

11. *Functional Communication*—Using equipment or systems to send and receive information, such as writing equipment, telephones, typewriters, communication boards, call lights, emergency systems, Braille writers, telecommunication devices for the deaf, and augmentative communication systems.

12. *Functional Mobility*—Moving from one position or place to another, such as in-bed mobility, wheelchair mobility, transfers (wheelchair, bed, car, tub/shower, toilet, chair, floor); performing functional ambulation and transporting objects.

13. *Community Mobility*—Moving self in the community and using public or private transportation, such as driving, or accessing buses, taxi cabs, or other public transportation systems.

14. *Emergency Response*—Recognizing sudden, unexpected hazardous situations, and initiating action to reduce the threat to health and safety.

15. *Sexual Expression*—Engaging in desired sexual activities.

B. *Work and Productive Activities*—Purposeful activities for self-development, social contribution, and livelihood.

1. *Home Management*—Obtaining and maintaining personal and household possessions and environment.
   a. *Clothing Care*—Obtaining and using supplies; sorting, laundering (hand, machine, and dry clean); folding; ironing; storing; and mending.
   b. *Cleaning*—Obtaining and using supplies; picking up; putting away; vacuuming; sweeping and mopping floors; dusting; polishing; scrubbing; washing windows; cleaning mirrors; making beds; and removing trash and recyclables.
   c. *Meal Preparation/Cleanup*—Planning nutritious meals; preparing and serving food; opening and closing containers, cabinets, and drawers; using kitchen utensils and appliances; cleaning up and storing food safely.
   d. *Shopping*—Preparing shopping lists (grocery and other); selecting and purchasing items; selecting method of payment; and completing money transactions.
   e. *Money Management*—Budgeting, paying bills, and using bank systems.
   f. *Household Maintenance*—Maintaining home, yard, garden appliances, vehicles, and household items.
   g. *Safety Procedures*—Knowing and performing preventive and emergency procedures to maintain a safe environment and prevent injuries.

2. *Care of Others*—Providing for children, spouse, parents, pets, or others, such as giving physical care, nurturing, communicating, and using age-appropriate activities.

3. *Educational Activities*—Participating in a learning environment through school, community, or work-sponsored activities, such as exploring educational interests, attending to instruction, managing assignments, and contributing to group experiences.

4. *Vocational Activities*—Participating in work-related activities.
   a. *Vocational Exploration*—Determining aptitudes, developing interests and skills, and selecting appropriate vocational pursuits.
   b. *Job Acquisition*—Identifying and selecting work opportunities, and completing application and interview processes.

c. *Work or Job Performance*—Performing job tasks in a timely and effective manner; incorporating necessary work behaviors.

d. *Retirement Planning*—Determining aptitudes, developing interests and skills, and identifying appropriate avocational pursuits.

e. *Volunteer Participation*—Performing unpaid activities for the benefit of selected individuals, groups, or causes.

C. *Play or Leisure Activities*—Intrinsically motivating activities for amusement, relaxation, spontaneous enjoyment, or self-expression.

1. *Play or Leisure Exploration*—Identifying interests, skills, opportunities, and appropriate play or leisure activities.

2. *Play or Leisure Performance*—Planning and participating in play or leisure activities; maintaining a balance of play or leisure activities with work and productive activities, and activities of daily living; obtaining, utilizing, and maintaining equipment and supplies.

II. PERFORMANCE COMPONENTS

A. *Sensorimotor Components*—The ability to receive input, process information, and produce output.

1. Sensory

   a. *Sensory Awareness*—Receiving and differentiating sensory stimuli.

   b. *Sensory Processing*—Interpreting sensory stimuli.

     (1) *Tactile*—Interpreting light touch, pressure, temperature, pain, and vibration through skin contact/receptors.

     (2) *Proprioceptive*—Interpreting stimuli originating in muscles, joints, and other internal tissues to give information about the position of one body part in relation to another.

     (3) *Vestibular*—Interpreting stimuli from the inner ear receptors regarding head position and movement.

     (4) *Visual*—Interpreting stimuli through the eyes, including peripheral vision and acuity, awareness of color and pattern.

     (5) *Auditory*—Interpreting and localizing sounds, and discriminating background sounds.

     (6) *Gustatory*—Interpreting tastes.

     (7) *Olfactory*—Interpreting odors.

   c. *Perceptual Processing*—Organizing sensory input into meaningful patterns.

     (1) *Stereognosis*—Identifying objects through proprioception, cognition, and the sense of touch.

     (2) *Kinesthesia*—Identifying the excursion and direction of joint movement.

     (3) *Pain Response*—Interpreting noxious stimuli.

     (4) *Body Scheme*—Acquiring an internal awareness of the body and the relationship of body parts to each other.

     (5) *Right-Left Discrimination*—Differentiating one side of the body from the other.

     (6) *Form Constancy*—Recognizing forms and objects as the same in various environments, positions, and sizes.

     (7) *Position in Space*—Determining the spatial relationship of figures and objects to self or other forms and objects.

     (8) *Visual-Closure*—Identifying forms or objects from incomplete presentations.

     (9) *Figure Ground*—Differentiating between foreground and background forms and objects.

     (10) *Depth Perception*—Determining the relative distance between objects, figures, or landmarks and the observer, and changes in planes of surfaces.

     (11) *Spatial Relations*—Determining the position of objects relative to each other.

     (12) *Topographical Orientation*—Determining the location of objects and settings and the route to the location.

2. Neuromusculoskeletal
   a. *Reflex*—Eliciting an involuntary muscle response by sensory input.
   b. *Range of Motion*—Moving body parts through an arc.
   c. *Muscle Tone*—Demonstrating a degree of tension or resistance in a muscle at rest and in response to stretch.
   d. *Strength*—Demonstrating a degree of muscle power when movement is resisted, as with objects or gravity.
   e. *Endurance*—Sustaining cardiac, pulmonary, and musculoskeletal exertion over time.
   f. *Postural Control*—Using righting and equilibrium adjustments to maintain balance during functional movements.
   g. *Postural Alignment*—Maintaining biomechanical integrity among body parts.
   h. *Soft Tissue Integrity*—Maintaining anatomical and physiological condition of interstitial tissue and skin.

3. Motor
   a. *Gross Coordination*—Using large muscle groups for controlled, goal-directed movements.
   b. *Crossing the Midline*—Moving limbs and eyes across the midsagittal plane of the body.
   c. *Laterality*—Using a preferred unilateral body part for activities requiring a high level of skill.
   d. *Bilateral Integration*—Coordinating both body sides during activity.
   e. *Motor Control*—Using the body in functional and versatile movement patterns.
   f. *Praxis*—Conceiving and planning a new motor act in response to an environmental demand.
   g. *Fine Coordination/Dexterity*—Using small muscle groups for controlled movements, particularly in object manipulation.
   h. *Visual-Motor Integration*—Coordinating the interaction of information from the eyes with body movement during activity.
   i. *Oral-Motor Control*—Coordinating oropharyngeal musculature for controlled movements.

B. *Cognitive Integration and Cognitive Components*—The ability to use higher brain functions.
   1. *Level of Arousal*—Demonstrating alertness and responsiveness to environmental stimuli.
   2. *Orientation*—Identifying person, place, time, and situation.
   3. *Recognition*—Identifying familiar faces, objects, and other previously presented materials.
   4. *Attention Span*—Focusing on a task over time.
   5. *Initiation of Activity*—Starting a physical or mental activity.
   6. *Termination of Activity*—Stopping an activity at an appropriate time.
   7. *Memory*—Recalling information after brief or long periods of time.
   8. *Sequencing*—Placing information, concepts, and actions in order.
   9. *Categorization*—Identifying similarities of and differences among pieces of environmental information.
   10. *Concept Formation*—Organizing a variety of information to form thoughts and ideas.
   11. *Spatial Operations*—Mentally manipulating the position of objects in various relationships.
   12. *Problem-Solving*—Recognizing a problem, defining a problem, identifying alternative plans, selecting a plan, organizing steps in a plan, implementing a plan, and evaluating the outcome.
   13. *Learning*—Acquiring new concepts and behaviors.
   14. *Generalization*—Applying previously learned concepts and behaviors to a variety of new situations.

C. *Psychosocial Skills and Psychological Components*—The ability to interact in society and to process emotions.
   1. Psychological
      a. *Values*—Identifying ideas or beliefs that are important to self and others.
      b. *Interests*—Identifying mental or physical activities that create pleasure and maintain attention.
      c. *Self-Concept*—Developing the value of the physical, emotional, and sexual self.
   2. Social
      a. *Role Performance*—Identifying, maintaining, and balancing functions one assumes or acquires in society (e.g., worker, student, parent, friend, religious participant).

b. *Social Conduct*—Interacting using manners, personal space, eye contact, gestures, active listening, and self-expression appropriate to one's environment.

c. *Interpersonal Skills*—Using verbal and nonverbal communication to interact in a variety of settings.

d. *Self-Expression*—Using a variety of styles and skills to express thoughts, feelings, and needs.

3. Self-Management

a. *Coping Skills*—Identifying and managing stress and related reactors.

b. *Time Management*—Planning and participating in a balance of self-care, work, leisure, and rest activities to promote satisfaction and health.

c. *Self-Control*—Modifying one's own behavior in response to environmental needs, demands, constraints, personal aspirations, and feedback from others.

III. PERFORMANCE CONTEXTS

Assessment of function in performance areas is greatly influenced by the contexts in which the individual must perform. Occupational therapy practitioners consider performance contexts when determining feasibility and appropriateness of interventions.

Occupational therapy practitioners may choose interventions based on an understanding of contexts, or may choose interventions directly aimed at altering the contexts to improve performance.

A. Temporal Aspects

1. *Chronological*—Individual's age.

2. *Developmental*—Stage or phase of maturation.

3. *Life Cycle*—Place in important life phases, such as career cycle, parenting cycle, or educational process.

4. *Disability Status*—Place in continuum of disability, such as acuteness of injury, chronicity of disability, or terminal nature of illness.

B. Environmental Aspects

1. *Physical*—Nonhuman aspects of contexts. Includes the accessibility to and performance within environments having natural terrain, plants, animals, buildings, furniture, objects, tools, or devices.

2. *Social*—Availability and expectations of significant individuals, such as spouse, friends, and caregivers. Also includes larger social groups which are influential in establishing norms, role expectations, and social routines.

3. *Cultural*—Customs, beliefs, activity patterns, behavior standards, and expectations accepted by the society of which the individual is a member. Includes political aspects, such as laws that affect access to resources and affirm personal rights. Also includes opportunities for education, employment, and economic support.

REFERENCES

American Occupational Therapy Association. (1979). *Occupational therapy output reporting system and uniform terminology for reporting occupational therapy services.* Rockville, MD: Author.

American Occupational Therapy Association. (1989). Uniform terminology for occupational therapy—Second edition. *American Journal of Occupational Therapy, 43,* 808-815.

American Occupational Therapy Association. (1993). Definition of occupational therapy practice for state regulation (Policy 5.3.1). *American Journal of Occupational Therapy, 47,* 1117-1121.

AUTHORS

The Terminology Task Force:
    Winifred Dunn, PhD, OTR, FAOTA Chairperson
    Mary Foto, OTR, FAOTA
    Jim Hinojosa, PhD, OTR, FAOTA Chairperson
    Barbara A. Boyt Schell, PhD, OTR/L, FAOTA
    Linda Kohlman Thomson, MOT, OTR, OT(C), FAOTA
    Sarah D. Hertfelder, MEd, MOT, OTR/L Staff Liaison for The Commission on Practice

Adopted by the Representative Assembly July 1994.

Note: This document replaces the following documents, all of which were rescinded by the 1994 Representative Assembly:
    Occupational Therapy Product Output Reporting System (1979)
    Uniform Terminology for Reporting Occupational Therapy Services—First Edition (1979)
    Uniform Occupational Therapy Evaluation Checklist (1981)
    Uniform Terminology for Occupational Therapy—Second Edition (1989)

UNIFORM TERMINOLOGY—THIRD EDITION: APPLICATION TO PRACTICE

Introduction

This document was developed to help occupational therapists apply *Uniform Terminology—Third Edition* to practice. The original grid format (Dunn, 1988) enabled occupational therapy practitioners to systematically identify deficit and strength areas of an individual and to select appropriate activities to address these areas in occupational therapy intervention (Dunn & McGourty, 1990). For the third edition, the profession is highlighting "Contexts" as another critical aspect of performance. A second grid provides therapy practitioners with a mechanism to consider the contextual features of performance in activities of daily living (ADL), work and productive activity, and play/leisure. "Performance Areas" and "Performance Components" (Figure A-1) focus on the individual. These features are embedded in the "Performance Contexts" (Figure A-2).

On the original grid (Dunn, 1988), the horizontal axis contains the Performance Areas of Activities of Daily Living, Work and Productive Activities, and Play or Leisure Activities (see Figure A-1). These Performance Areas are the functional outcomes occupational therapy addresses. The vertical axis contains the Performance Components, including Sensorimotor Components, Cognitive Components, and Psychosocial Components. The Performance Components are the skills and abilities that an individual uses to engage in the Performance Areas. During an occupational therapy assessment, the occupational therapy practitioner determines an individual's abilities and limitations in the Performance Components and how they affect the individual's functional outcomes in the Performance Areas.

Performance Components	Activities of Daily Living	Grooming	Oral Hygiene	Bathing/Showering	Toilet Hygiene	Personal Device Care	Dressing	Feeding and Eating	Medication Routine	Health Maintenance	Socialization	Functional Communication	Functional Mobility	Community Mobility	Emergency Response	Sexual Expression	Work and Productive Activities	Home Management	Care of Others	Educational Activities	Vocational Activities	Play or Leisure Activities	Play or Leisure Exploration	Play or Leisure Performance
A. *Sensorimotor Components*																								
1. Sensory																								
a. *Sensory Awareness*																								
b. *Sensory Processing*																								
(1) *Tactile*																								
(2) *Proprioceptive*																								
(3) *Vestibular*																								
(4) *Visual*																								
(5) *Auditory*																								
(6) *Gustatory*																								
(7) *Olfactory*																								
c. *Perceptual Processing*																								
(1) *Stereognosis*																								
(2) *Kinesthesia*																								
(3) *Pain Response*																								
(4) *Body Scheme*																								
(5) *Right-Left Discrimination*																								
(6) *Form Constancy*																								
(7) *Position in Space*																								
(8) *Visual-Closure*																								
(9) *Figure Ground*																								
(10) *Depth Perception*																								
(11) *Spatial Relations*																								
(12) *Topographical Orientation*																								
2. Neuromusculoskeletal																								
a. *Reflex*																								
b. *Range of Motion*																								
c. *Muscle Tone*																								
d. *Strength*																								
e. *Endurance*																								
f. *Postural Control*																								
g. *Postural Alignment*																								
h. *Soft Tissue Integrity*																								
3. Motor																								
a. *Gross Coordination*																								
b. *Crossing the Midline*																								
c. *Laterality*																								

Figure A-1. Uniform Terminology Grid (Performance Areas and Performance Components).

	Activities of Daily Living	Grooming	Oral Hygiene	Bathing/Showering	Toilet Hygiene	Personal Device Care	Dressing	Feeding and Eating	Medication Routine	Health Maintenance	Socialization	Functional Communication	Functional Mobility	Community Mobility	Emergency Response	Sexual Expression	Work and Productive Activities	Home Management	Care of Others	Educational Activities	Vocational Activities	Play or Leisure Activities	Play or Leisure Exploration	Play or Leisure Performance
d. Bilateral Integration																								
e. Motor Control																								
f. Praxis																								
g. Fine Coordination/ Dexterity																								
h. Visual-Motor Integration																								
i. Oral-Motor Control																								
B. Cognitive Integration and Cognitive Components																								
1. Level of Arousal																								
2. Orientation																								
3. Recognition																								
4. Attention Span																								
5. Initiation of Activity																								
6. Termination of Activity																								
7. Memory																								
8. Sequencing																								
9. Categorization																								
10. Concept Formation																								
11. Spatial Operations																								
12. Problem-Solving																								
13. Learning																								
14. Generalization																								
C. Psychosocial Skills and Psychological Components																								
1. Psychological																								
a. Values																								
b. Interests																								
c. Self-Concept																								
2. Social																								
a. Role Performance																								
b. Social Conduct																								
c. Interpersonal Skills																								
d. Self-Expression																								
3. Self-Management																								
a. Coping Skills																								
b. Time Management																								
c. Self-Control																								

Figure A-1 continued. Uniform Terminology Grid (Performance Areas and Performance Components).

Performance Contexts	Activities of Daily Living	Grooming	Oral Hygiene	Bathing/Showering	Toilet Hygiene	Personal Device Care	Dressing	Feeding and Eating	Medication Routine	Health Maintenance	Socialization	Functional Communication	Functional Mobility	Community Mobility	Emergency Response	Sexual Expression	Work and Productive Activities	Home Management	Care of Others	Educational Activities	Vocational Activities	Play or Leisure Activities	Play or Leisure Exploration	Play or Leisure Performance
A. Temporal Aspects 1. *Chronological*																								
2. *Developmental*																								
3. *Life Cycle*																								
4. *Disability Status* B. Environmental Aspects 1. *Physical*																								
2. *Social*																								
3. *Cultural*																								

Figure A-2. Uniform Terminology Grid (Performance Areas and Performance Contexts).

Special Note: The first application document (Dunn & McGourty, 1989) describes how to use the original *Uniform Terminology* grid with a variety of individuals. It is quite useful to introduce these concepts. However, the Third Edition of *Uniform Terminology* contains some changes in the Performance Areas and Performance Components lists. Be sure to check for the terminology currently approved in the Third Edition before applying this information in current practice environments.

With the addition of Performance Contexts into *Uniform Terminology*, occupational therapy practitioners must consider how to interface what the individual wants to do (i.e., performance area) with the contextual features that may support or block performance. Figure A-2 illustrates the interaction of Performance Areas and Performance Contexts as a model for therapists' planning.

The grid in Figure A-2 can be used to analyze the contexts of performance for a particular individual. For example, when working with a toddler with a developmental disability who needs to learn to eat, the occupational therapy practitioner would consider all the Performance Contexts features as they might impact on this toddler's ability to master eating. Unlike the grid in Figure A-1, in which the occupational therapy practitioner selects both Performance Areas (i.e., what the individual wants or needs to do) and the Performance Component (i.e., a person's strengths and needs), in this grid (Figure A-2) the occupational therapy practitioner only selects the Performance Area. After the Performance Area is identified through collaboration with the individual and significant others, the occupational therapy practitioner considers *all* Performance Contexts features as they might impact on performance of the selected task.

INTERVENTION PLANNING

Intervention planning occurs both within the general domain of concern of occupational therapy (i.e., Uniform Terminology) and by considering the profession's theoretical frames of reference that offer insights about how to approach the problem. In Figure A-1, the occupational therapy practitioner considers the Performance Areas that are of interest to the individual and the individual's strengths and concerns within the

Performance Components. The intervention strategies would emerge from the cells on the grid that are placed at the intersection of the Performance Areas and the targeted Performance Components (strength and/or concern). For example, if a child needed to improve sensory processing and fine coordination for oral hygiene and grooming, an occupational therapy practitioner might select a sensory integrative frame of reference to create intervention strategies, such as adding textures to handles and teaching the child sand and bean digging games. Dunn and McGourty (1989) discuss this in more detail.

When using Figure A-2, the occupational therapy practitioner considers the Performance Contexts features in relation to the desired Performance Area. The occupational therapy practitioner would analyze the individual's temporal, physical, social, and cultural contexts to determine the relevance of particular interventions. For example, if the child mentioned above was a member of a family in which having messy hands from sand play was unacceptable, the occupational therapy practitioner would consider alternate strategies that are more compatible with their lifestyle. For example, perhaps the family would be more interested in developing puppet play. This would still provide the child with opportunities to experience the textures of various puppets and the hand movements required to manipulate the puppets in play context, without adding the messiness of sand. When occupational therapy practitioners consider contexts, interventions become more relevant and applicable to individual's lives.

Case Example 1

Sophie, a 75-year-old lady who was widowed 3 years ago, is recovering from a cerebral vascular accident and has been transferred from an acute care unit to an inpatient medical rehabilitation unit. Prior to her admission, she was living in a small house in an isolated location and has no family living nearby. She was driving independently and frequently ran errands for her friends. She is adamant in her goal to return to her home after discharge. All of her friends are quite elderly and are not able to provide many resources for support.

Sophie and the team collaborated to identify her goals. Sophie decided that she wanted to be able to meet her daily needs with little or no assistance. Almost all of the Performance Areas are critical in order to achieve the outcome of community living in her own home. Being able to cook all of her meals, bathe independently, and have alternative transportation available is necessary. Because of their significant impact on the patient's function in the Performance Areas, some of the Performance Components that may need to be addressed are figure ground, muscle tone, postural control, fine coordination, memory, and self-management.

In the selection of occupational therapy interventions, it is critical to analyze the elements of Performance Contexts for the individual. The physical and social elements of her home environment do not support returning home without modifications to her home and additional social supports being established. Railings must be added to the front steps, provision of and instruction in the use of a tub seat, and instruction in the use of specialized transportation may need to occur. If this same individual had been living in an apartment in a retirement community prior to her CVA, the contexts of performance would support a return home with fewer environmental modifications being needed. Being independent in cooking might not be necessary due to meals being provided, and the bathroom might already be accessible and safe. If the individual had friends and family available, the social support network might already be established to assist with shopping and transportation needs. The occupational therapy interventions would be different due to the contexts in which the individual will be performing. Interventions must be selected with the impact of the Performance Contexts as an essential element.

Case Example 2

Malcolm is a 9-year-old boy who has a learning disability, which causes him to have a variety of problems in school. His teachers complain that he is difficult to manage in the classroom. Some of the Performance Components that may need to be addressed are his self-control such as interrupting, difficulty sitting during instruction, and difficulty with peer relations. Other children avoid him on the playground because he doesn't follow rules, doesn't play fair, and tends to anger quickly when confronted. The performance component impairment with concept formation is reflected in his sloppy and disorganized classroom assignments.

The critical elements of the Performance Contexts are the temporal aspect of age-appropriateness of his behavior and the social environmental aspect of his immature socialization. The significant cultural and temporal aspects of his family are that they place a high premium on athletic prowess.

The occupational therapy practitioner intervenes in several ways to address his behavior in the school environment. The occupational therapy practitioner focuses on structuring the classroom environment and facilitating consistent behavioral expectations for Malcolm by educational personnel. She also consults with the teachers to develop ways to structure activities that will support his ability to relate to other children in a positive way.

In contrast, another child with similar learning disabilities, but who is 12 years old and in the 7th grade might have different concerns. Elements of the Performance Contexts are the temporal aspect of the age-appropriateness of his behavior and the social environment context of school where "bullying" behavior is unacceptable and in which completing assignments is expected. In addressing the cultural Performance Contexts, the occupational therapy practitioner recognizes from meeting the parents that they have only average expectation for academic performance but value athletic accomplishments.

Since teachers at his school consider completion of home assignments to be part of average performance, the occupational therapy practitioner works with the child and parents on time management and reinforcement strategies to meet this expectation. After consultation with the coach, she works with the father to create activities to improve his athletic abilities. When occupational therapy practitioners consider family values as part of the contexts of performance, different intervention priorities may emerge.

AUTHORS

The Terminology Task Force:
   Winifred Dunn, PhD, OTR, FAOTA Chairperson
   Mary Foto, OTR, FAOTA
   Jim Hinojosa, PhD, OTR, FAOTA Chairperson
   Barbara A. Boyt Schell, PhD, OTR/L, FAOTA
   Linda Kohlman Thomson, MOT, OTR, OT(C), FAOTA
   Sarah D. Hertfelder, MEd, MOT, OTR/L Staff Liaison for the Commission on Practice 1994

Note: This document replaces the 1989 *Application of Uniform Terminology to Practice* that accompanied the *Uniform Terminology for Occupational Therapy—Second Edition.*

B.

Elements of Clinical Documentation (Revision)

American Occupational Therapy Association

These elements are provided to assist occupational therapy practitioners to document occupational therapy services. Occupational therapy practitioners determine the appropriate type of documentation and document the services provided within the time frames established by facilities, government agencies, and accreditation organizations. These elements do not address the specific content of documentation, which is unique to occupational therapy intervention for particular ages and types of impairments.

The purpose of documentation is to:
1. Provide a chronological record of the consumer's condition that details the complete course of therapeutic intervention.
2. Facilitate communication among professionals who contribute to the consumer's care.
3. Provide an objective basis to determine the appropriateness, effectiveness, and necessity of therapeutic intervention.
4. Reflects the practitioner's reasoning.

TYPES OF DOCUMENTATION

I. Evaluation Report
    A. Identification and Background Information
    B. Assessment Results
    C. Intervention or Treatment Plan
II. Contact, Treatment, or Visit Note
III. Progress Report
IV. Re-evaluation Report
V. Discharge or Discontinuation Report

I. Evaluation Report

Used to document the initial contact with the consumer, the data collected, the interpretation of the data, and the intervention plan. When an abbreviated evaluation process is used, such as screening, it is documented using only limited content areas applicable to the consumer and situation.
    A. Identification and Background Information (see Table B-1)
    B. Assessment Results (see Table B-2)
    C. Intervention or Treatment Plan (see Table B-3)

Table B-1.

Identification and Background Information

Content	Clarification
1. Name, age, sex, date of admission, treatment, diagnosis, and date of onset of current diagnosis.	Name may be omitted, depending on facility and department policies and procedures.
2. Referral source, services requested, and date of referral to occupational therapy.	Who requested occupational therapy services, what specific services were requested, and date services were requested.
3. Medical history and secondary problems or preexisting conditions, prior therapy.	Additional problems or conditions that may affect consumer function or outcomes.
4. Precautions and contraindications.	May be identified by referral source or occupational therapy practitioners.
5. Pertinent history that indicates prior levels of function and support systems.	Applicable developmental, educational, vocational, cultural, and socioeconomic history.
6. Present levels of function in performance areas determined by examination.[1]	Brief description of the consumer's level of performance in activities of daily living, work and productive activities, and play or leisure activities.
7. Performance contexts determined by examination.[1]	Description of those temporal aspects (chronological, developmental, life cycle, health status) and environmental (physical, social, cultural) features that affect the consumer's function in performance areas.
8. Consumer and family expectations.	Brief description of expected outcome of occupational therapy intervention.

[1]Refer to *Uniform Terminology for Occupational Therapy, Third Edition* (AOTA, 1994a), for specific performance areas, performance components, and performance contexts.

Table B-2.

Assessment Results

Content	Clarification
1. Tests and assessments administered and the results.	Name and type of assessment or test and the results; may include comparison with previous testing. State if standardized procedure not followed.
2. References to other pertinent reports and information.	Any additional sources of data or assessment results used.
3. Summary and analysis of evaluation findings.	State the type and severity of impairments identified and the functional limitations caused by the impairments in objective, functional, and measurable terms. Include the functional diagnosis.
4. Projected functional outcome(s).	Prognosis and anticipated level of performance (activities of daily living [ADL], work or productive activities, and play or leisure activities) the consumer will be able to achieve as a result of therapeutic intervention. May include a statement indicating the consumer does not have the potential to improve beyond current status.

Table B-3.

Intervention or Treatment Plan

Content	Clarification
1. Long-term functional goals	Functional limitations that must change in order to achieve the projected functional outcome.
	Degree the functional limitations will be decreased.
	Rationale for decreasing functional limitations.
	Functional change to occur by end of intervention.
	Consumer and/or family agreement with goals.
2. Short-term goals	Directly relate to long-term functional goals.
	Impairment that must change in order to achieve the projected functional outcome.
	Degree the impairment will be decreased.
	Functional ability that will result from a decrease in level of impairment.
	Change to occur in a brief period of time (e.g., 7, 14, or 30 days).
	Consumer and/or family agreement with goals.
3. Intervention or treatment procedures	Activities, techniques, and modalities selected to be used and how they relate to goals. May include family training and home programs.
	Identify assistive/adaptive equipment, orthotics, and/or prosthetics to meet consumer's environmental adaptation needs.
4. Type, amount, frequency, and duration of intervention or treatment	State skill and performance areas to be addressed and estimate the number, duration, and frequency of sessions to accomplish goals.
5. Recommendations	Need for occupational therapy services and necessary referrals to other professionals.

II. CONTACT, TREATMENT, OR VISIT NOTE

Used to document individual occupational therapy session or care coordination. May be very brief, such as in the use of a checklist, flow chart, or short narrative type notation (see Table B-4).

III. PROGRESS REPORT

Used periodically to document care coordination, interventions, progress toward functional goals, and to update goals and intervention or treatment plan (see Table B-5).

IV. RE-EVALUATION REPORT

Used to document sessions in which portions of the evaluation process are repeated or readministered. Usually occurs monthly or quarterly, depending on the setting (see Table B-6).

Table B-4.

Contact, Treatment, or Visit Note

Content	Clarification
1. Attendance and participation.	Therapy occurrence or reason for therapy not occurring as scheduled.
2. Activities, techniques, and modalities used	May be indicated by checklist or brief statement.
3. Assistive/adaptive equipment, prosthetics, and orthotics if issued or fabricated, and specific instructions for the application and/or use of the item.	State the device; note whether it was fabricated, sold, rented, or loaned; and state the effectiveness of the device.
4. Consumer's response to therapy.	Level of performance and anything unusual or significant that was a result of occupational therapy intervention.

Table B-5.

Progress Report

Content	Clarification
1. Activities, techniques, and modalities used.	Brief statement or intervention process.
2. Consumer's response to therapy, and the progress toward short- and long-term goal attainment and comparison with previous functional status.	State the consumer's physical and behavioral response to therapy, whether the goals are being achieved, if change has occurred, and how much change has occurred.
3. Goal continuance	Explanation for no or slow progress, reason for not meeting short-term goal(s), or need to continue current goal(s).
4. Goal modification when indicated by the response to therapy or by the establishment of new consumer needs.	State new goals and rationale for changes or additions.
5. Change in anticipated time to achieve goals.	If, for any reason, the therapy time frame is altered, include the reason for the change and the new anticipated time frame.
6. Assistive/adaptive equipment, prosthetics, and orthotics, if issued or fabricated, and specific instructions for the application and/or use of the item.	State the device; note whether it was fabricated, sold, rented, or loaned; and state the effectiveness of the device.
7. Consumer-related conferences and communication.	If occupational therapy practitioners participated in a conference or made a pertinent contact with a family member, agency, or health care professional, state this information with a brief summary of the conference or communication.
8. Home programs	Include a copy of the home program as established with the consumer. Include a statement regarding the consumer's ability to follow the program.
9. Consumer/caretaker instruction	What instruction was provided and in what format (i.e., verbal or written).
10. Plan	Specific procedures, communication, or consultations to be done in the future to address the goals.

Table B-6.

Re-Evaluation Report

Content	Clarification
1. Tests and assessments readministered and the results.	Name and type of test readministered. State if standardized procedure is not followed.
2. Comparative summary and analysis of previous evaluation findings.	Results analyzed and compared.with previous testing.
3. Reestablishment of projected functional outcome(s).	Anticipated level of performance (ADL, work or productive activities, and play or leisure activities) the consumer will be able to achieve as a result of therapeutic intervention. May include a statement of changes in previously established functional outcome(s) based on revised potential or goals of consumer.
4. Update of intervention or treatment plan	Revised or continued long-term functional goals; short-term goals; treatment procedures; and type, amount, and frequency of therapy.

Table B-7.

Discharge or Discontinuation Report

Content	Clarification
1. Therapy process	Summary of interventions used, consumer's responses, and number of sessions.
2. Goal attainment	Degree to which short- and long-term functional goals were achieved.
3. Functional outcome	Comparison of functional status prior to therapy and at discharge.
4. Home programs	Include the actual written home program that is to be followed after discharge.
5. Follow-up plans	State the schedule and specific plans.
6. Recommendations	State any recommendations pertaining to the consumer's future needs.
7. Referral(s) to other health care providers and community agencies	Indicate referral(s) or recommendations for referral(s) when additional or new services are needed.

V. DISCHARGE OR DISCONTINUATION REPORT

Used to document a summary of the course of therapy and any recommendations (see Table B-7).

FUNDAMENTAL ELEMENTS OF DOCUMENTATION

Each consumer of occupational therapy services must have a case record maintained as a permanent file. The record should be organized, legible, concise, clear, accurate, complete, current, and objective. Correct grammar and spelling should be used.

The following 10 elements should be present:

1. Consumer's full name and case number on each page of documentation.

2. Date stated as month, day, and year for each entry; time of intervention; and length of session.

3. Identification of type of documentation and department name.
4. Practitioner's signature with a minimum of first name or initial, last name, and professional designation.
5. Signature of the recorder directly at the end of the note without space left between the body of the note and the signature.
6. Countersignature by a registered occupational therapist (OTR) on documentation written by students and certified occupational therapy assistants (COTA) when required by law or the facility.
7. Compliance with confidentiality standards.
8. Acceptable terminology as defined by the facility.
9. Facility-approved abbreviations.
10. Errors corrected by drawing a single line through an error, and the correction initialed (liquid correction fluid and erasures are not acceptable), or facility requirements followed.

REFERENCES

American Occupational Therapy Association. (1994a). Uniform terminology for occupational therapy—Third edition. *American Journal of Occupational Therapy, 48*, 1047-1054.

American Occupational Therapy Association. (1994b). Uniform terminology—Third edition: Application to practice. American *Journal of Occupational Therapy, 48*, 1055-1059.

BIBLIOGRAPHY

Allen, C. K., Earhart, C. A., & Blue, T. (1992). *Occupational therapy treatment goals for the physically and cognitively disabled.* Bethesda, MD: American Occupational Therapy Association.

Allen, C., Foto, M., Moon-Sperling, T., & Wilson, D. (Eds.). (December 1989). A medical review approach to medicare outpatient documentation. *American Journal of Occupational Therapy, 43*, 793-800.

American Occupational Therapy Association. (1989). *Reports that work. AOTA self study series: Assessing function* (Chapter 9). Bethesda, MD: Author.

American Occupational Therapy Association. (1992). *Effective documentation for occupational therapy.* Bethesda, MD: Author.

American Occupational Therapy Association. (1994). Standards of practice for occupational therapy. *American Journal of Occupational Therapy, 48*, 1039-1043.

Hopkins, H. L., & Smith, H. D. (1993). *Willard and Spackman's occupational therapy* (8th ed.). Philadelphia, PA: Lippincott.

Stewart, D. L., & Abeln, S. H. (Eds.). (1993). *Documenting functional outcomes in physical therapy.* St. Louis, MO: Mosby.

Prepared by

Linda Kohlman Thomson, OT, OTR, OT(C), FAOTA
Mary Foto, OTR, FAOTA
for
Commission on Practice
Jim Hinojosa, PhD, OTR, FAOTA, Chair

Approved by the Representative Assembly April 1986
Revised 1994 and sent to the Representative Assembly FYI

This document replaces the 1986 *Guidelines for Occupational Therapy Documentation.* (*American Journal of Occupational Therapy, 40*, 830-832).

Note: If a document is revised, the previous version is superseded and, according to Parliamentary procedure, is automatically rescinded.

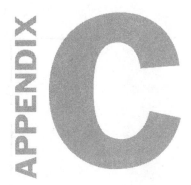

C. Examples of IEPs and IFSPs

The following pages include examples of IEPs and IFSPs.

NORTHEAST KANSAS EDUCATION SERVICE CENTER
Individualized Family Service Plan (IFSP)
For The Family of:

Child's Name:_____ SSN#_____DOB:_____
          (First, Middle Initial, Last)

Parent(s)
Name:_____

Complete
Address:_____

Setting where child spends
time:_____

Phone:
(home)_____(work)_____(other)_____

Parent's preferred language:_____

Date of consent for evaluation:_____

Primary Care Physician:_____ Phone:_____

Insurance
Name/Number_____

TYPE of PLAN *(please check)*

_____ Interim: Date:_____
_____ Initial: Date:_____
_____ Revised: Date(1)_____(2)_____(3)_____
_____ Transition: Date:_____

PROPOSED DATES OF: **ACTUAL DATES:**

Six month review:_____   _____
Annual review: _____   _____
Transition to Part B:_____   _____
Area's of Eligibility:_____   _____
Name of Family Service Coordinator:_____

Northeast Kansas Education Service Center
Individualized Family Service Plan (IFSP)
Family Concerns, Priorities, Resources

Date:_____

Child's Full
Name:_____DOB:_____

Family Concerns: (optional)   *Family Resources (Support) (optional)*

_____
_____
_____
_____
_____
_____
_____
_____

Setting where child spends most of his/her time: (Home, Daycare Center, Etc.)

_____
_____

Other services needed: Services that a child or family needs, but are neither required nor covered under Part C of IDEA. These are listed to provide a comprehensive picture of the child's total service needs. It is appropriate for the Family Service Coordinator to assist the family in securing these non-required but necessary services. (Includes immunizations, housing, respite, etc.)

_____

Other Services Needed: *Action Plan to Secure Service:*   *Person Responsible:*

_____   _____   _____

_____   _____   _____

_____   _____   _____

Northeast Kansas Education Service Center
Individualized Family Service Plan (IFSP)
CONSENT FOR SERVICES

Child's Full Name: _____ *DOB:* _____

I (we) agree to participate in the Northeast Kansas Education Service Center Infant Toddler program, and have had an explanation about parent rights, recordkeeping procedures, and policies. I (we) agree with the outcomes listed in this IFSP:

_____   _____
Name/Relationship   *Date*

_____   _____
Name/Relationship   *Date*

_____   _____
Name/Relationship   *Date*

ADDITIONAL TEAM MEMBERS

_____ *Signature/Title*   *Signature/Title*

_____   _____

_____   _____

_____   _____

IFSP REVIEW/CHANGE DOCUMENTATION: *Date:* _/_/_

Conference Summary:

_____

_____

_____

_____

_____

_____

Northeast Kansas Education Service Center
Individualized Family Services Plan (IFSP)

Review/Change Documenation Form

Child's Name: _____

IFSP REVIEW/CHANGE DOCUMENATION: **Date:** __/__/__

Conference Summary:

_____   _____
Family Service Coordinator   *Parent*

_____   _____
Other Team Member   *Other Party(s) present*

****

IFSP REVIEW/CHANGE DOCUMENTATION   **Date:** __/__/__

Conference Summary:

_____   _____
Family Service Coordinator   *Parent*

_____   _____
Other Team Member   *Other party(s) present*

Northeast Kansas Education Service Center
Annual Review Updated Assessment

Date:_____

Child's Full Name:_____DOB:_____

Cognitive (Thinking)
        Assessment: *Date:*   *By Whom:*

Summary:

Communication (Speech and Language)
        Assessment: *Date:*   *By Whom:*

Summary:

Social Emotional (Feelings)
        Assessment: *Date:*   *By Whom:*

Summary:

Adaptive (Self Help)
        Assessment: *Date:*   *By Whom:*

Summary:

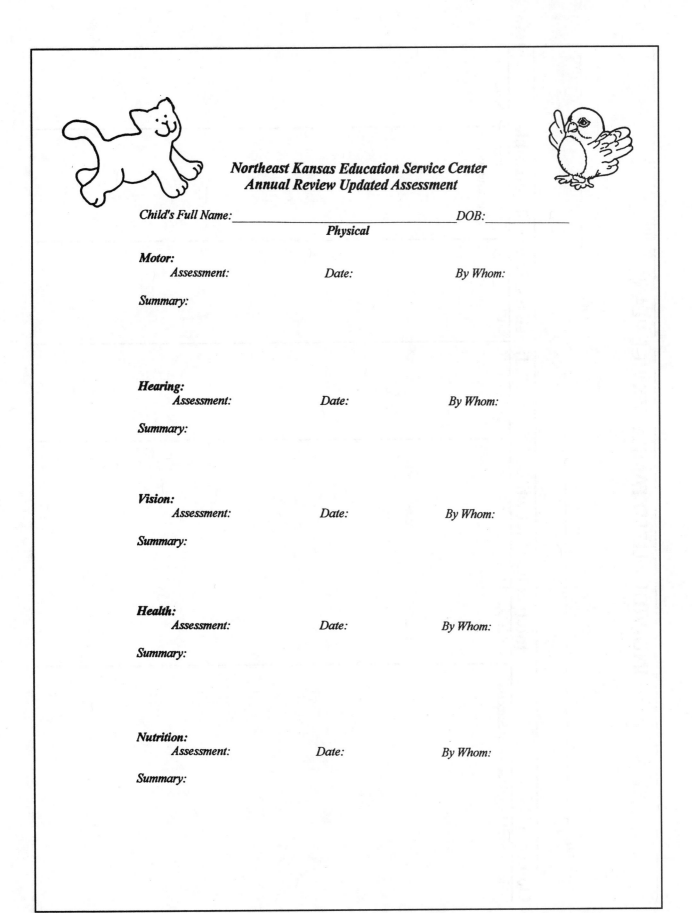

Northeast Kansas Education Service Center
Annual Review Updated Assessment

Child's Full Name:_____DOB:_____

Physical

Motor:
　　Assessment:　　　　　　Date:　　　　　　By Whom:

Summary:

Hearing:
　　Assessment:　　　　　　Date:　　　　　　By Whom:

Summary:

Vision:
　　Assessment:　　　　　　Date:　　　　　　By Whom:

Summary:

Health:
　　Assessment:　　　　　　Date:　　　　　　By Whom:

Summary:

Nutrition:
　　Assessment:　　　　　　Date:　　　　　　By Whom:

Summary:

INDIVIDUALIZED FAMILY SERVICE PLAN

Family: _____

Date: _____
Update: _____

Outcomes	Intervention/Activities	Timelines/Person Responsible			
Who, What Help, Degree of Success	Strategies/Materials	Initiation	Changed/ Achieved	Review Date Comments	Name

Child's Name_____

EARLY INTERVENTION PROGRAM SERVICES
(Eligible services under Part C)

Service:

Provider Name: Financial Responsibility:

Frequency: Projected Duration:

Location:

Basis: _____ Group _____ Individual

Initiation Date:

Service:

Provider Name: Financial Responsibility:

Frequency: Projected Duration:

Location:

Basis: _____ Group _____ Individual

Initiation Date:

Service:

Provider Name: Financial Responsibility:

Frequency: Projected Duration:

Location:

Basis: _____ Group _____ Individual

Initiation Date:

Service:

Provider Name: Financial Responsibility:

Frequency: Projected Duration:

Location:

Basis: _____ Group _____ Individual

Initiation Date:

INDIVIDUAL EDUCATION PLAN

Preferred First Name _____   Preferred Last _____

Legal First _____   Middle _____   Last _____

ID/SSN _____   Aux. ID _____   DOB _____   Ethnicity _____

Gender _____   Language of Student _____   Language of Home ____

Parent 1	Parent 2	Other
First Name _____	_____	_____
Last Name _____	_____	_____
Title _____	_____	_____
Rel to Child _____	_____	_____
Street _____	_____	_____
City _____	_____	_____
State _____	_____	_____
Zip _____	_____	_____
Home Phone _____	_____	_____
Work Phone #1 _____	_____	_____
Work Phone #2 _____	_____	_____
Co of Res. _____		

Enrollment Building_____   Attendance Building_____

Grade_____   Funding _____   Primary Exc _____   Secondary Exc _____

Procedural Dates

Pre-Assessment_____

Referral_____

Comp Eval Complete _____

Place Consent _____

Educational Status _____

IEP Meeting _____

Initiation _____

Vision Screen _____

Hearing Screen _____

Exit Status _____

Exit Date _____

HEALTH/PHYSICAL

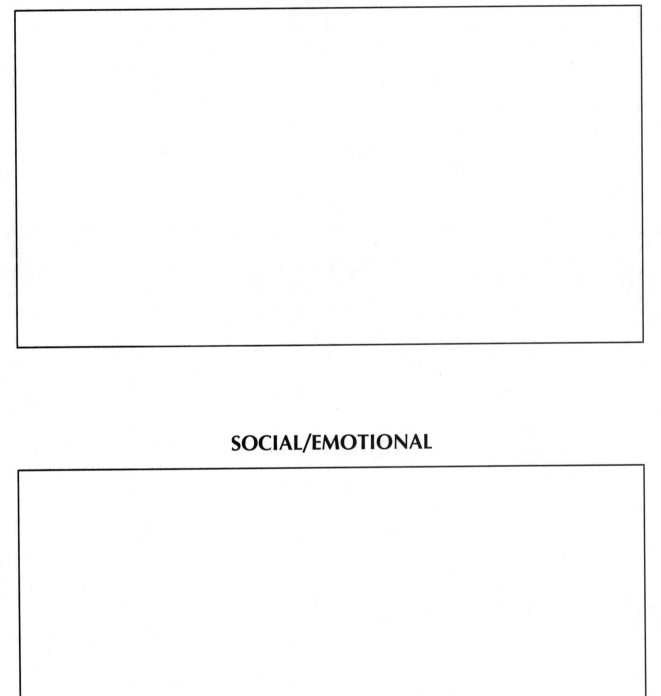

SOCIAL/EMOTIONAL

GENERAL INTELLIGENCE

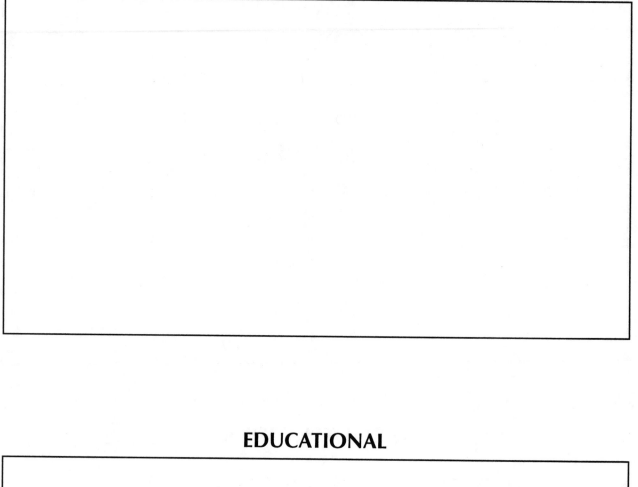

EDUCATIONAL

COMMUNICATION

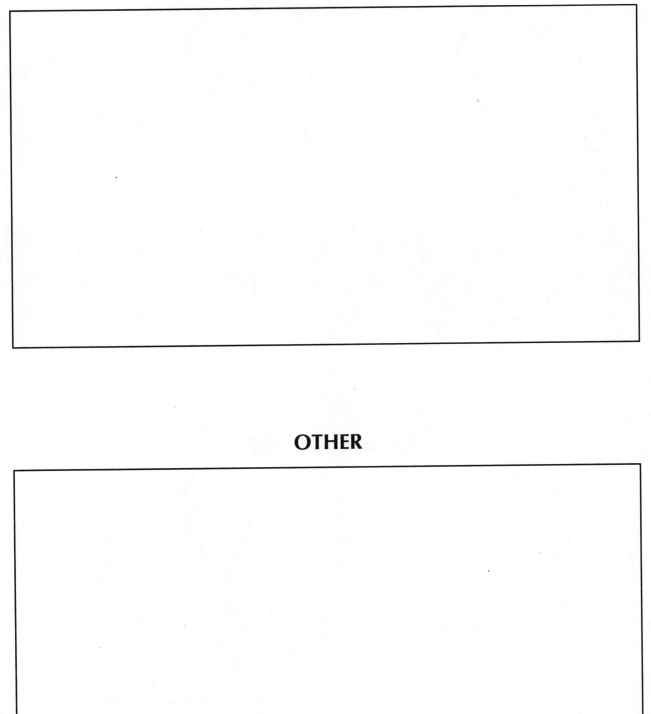

OTHER

INSTRUCTION

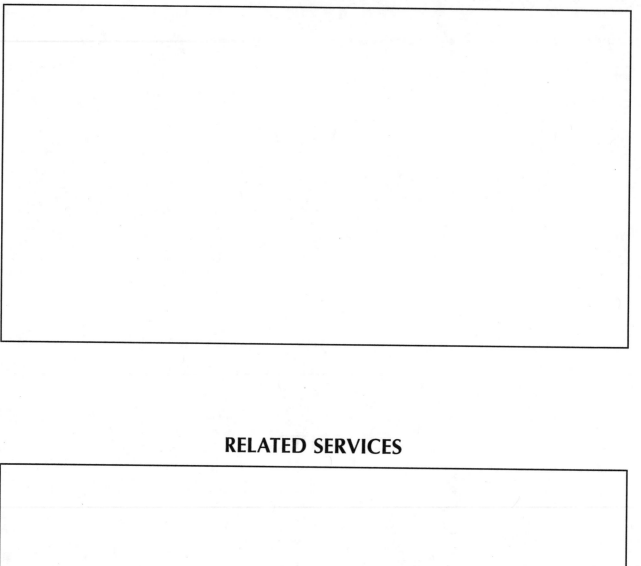

RELATED SERVICES

COMMUNITY EXPERIENCES

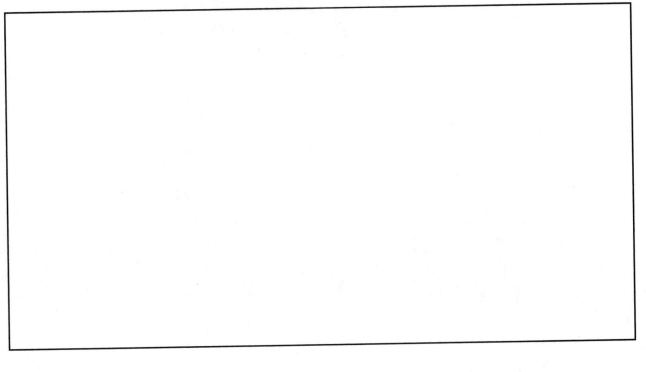

EMPLOYMENT AND OTHER POST-SCHOOL/
ADULT LIVING OUTCOMES

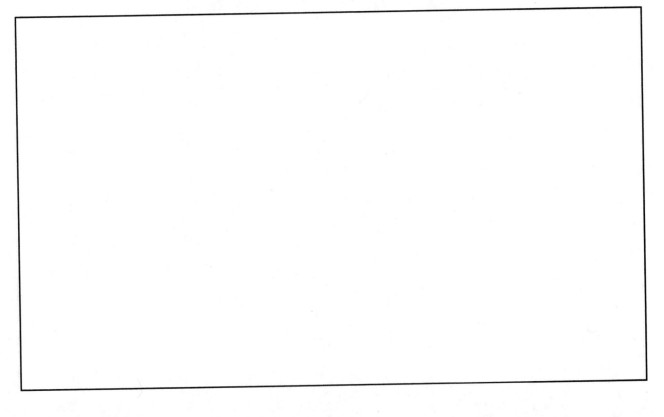

DAILY LIVING SKILLS

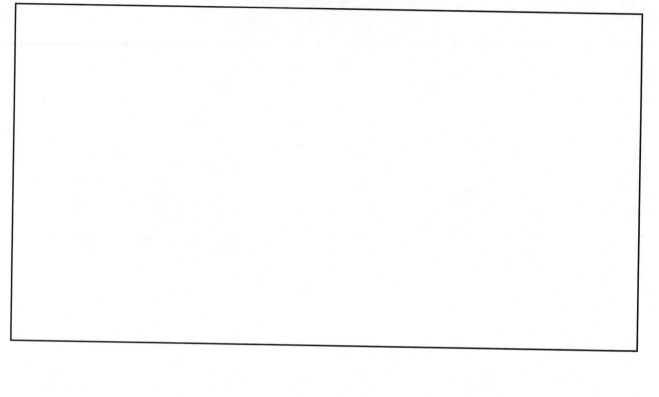

FUNCTIONAL VOCATIONAL EVALUATION

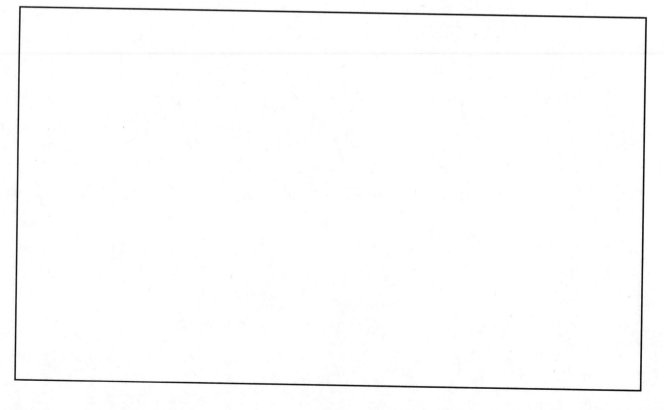

ACTION STATEMENTS

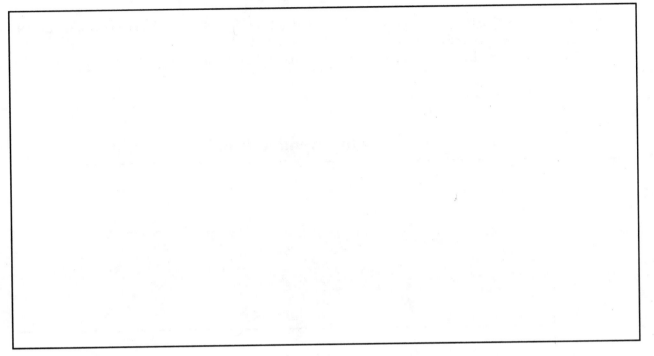

VOCATIONAL REHABILITATION

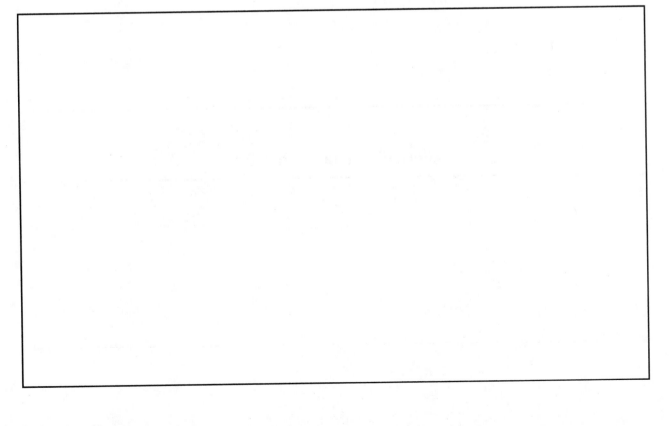

MISCELLANEOUS

Transportation Provided?   Yes - No   Extended School Previous Summer?   Yes - No
Has adaptive PE been considered?   Yes - No   Assistive Technology Plan?   Yes - No
Behavior Intervention Plan?   Yes - No   Alternative Graduation Plan?   Yes - No

Medical Diagnosis _____

Behavior Intervention Plan

Assistive Technology Plan

Alternative Graduation Plan

GOALS

1. _____

2. _____

3. _____

4. _____

5. _____

6. _____

7. _____

8. _____

9. _____

PARTICIPATION

Participation in General Education

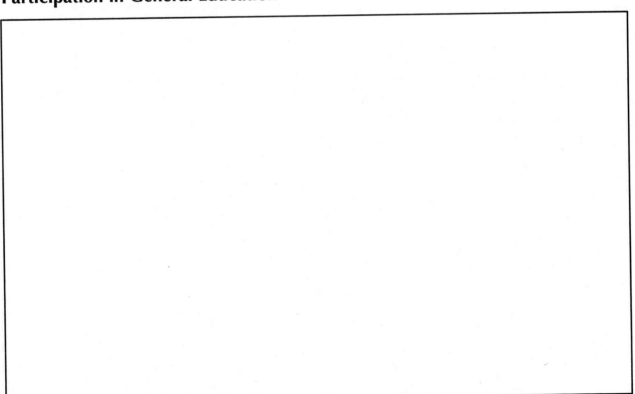

PARTICIPATION

Participation in Assessment

PARTICIPATION

Participation in Nonacademic Activities

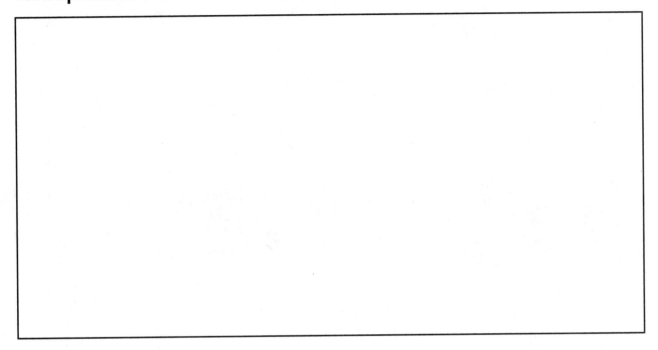

Participation in Extracurricular Activities

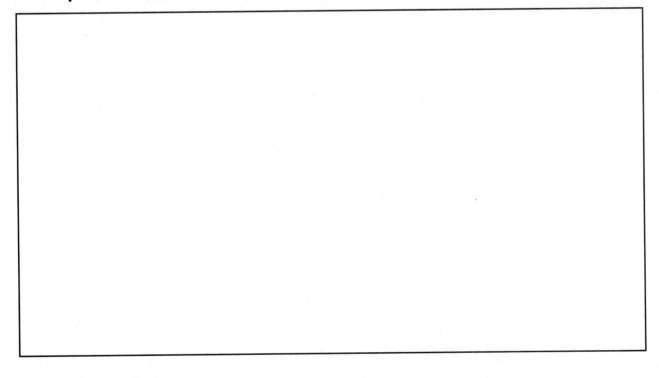

PARTICIPATION

Participation in Extended School Term

Special Considerations

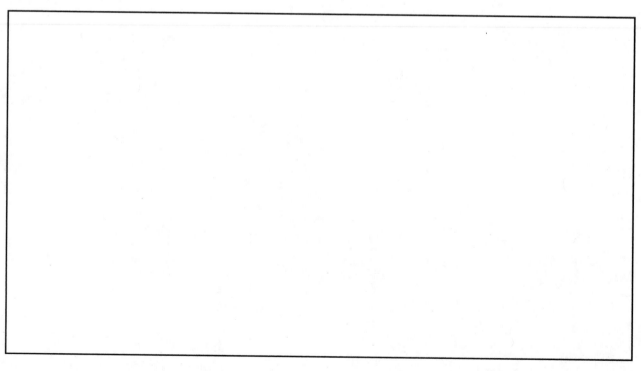

ANTICIPATED SERVICES TO BE PROVIDED

Line	Service	Setting	Provider (First, Mid, Last)	Min/ Day	Days/ Week	No. weeks	Start date	End date
1.								
2.								
3.								
4.								
5.								
6.								
7.								
8.								
9.								
10.								
11.								
12.								
13.								
14.								

ANTICIPATED SERVICES

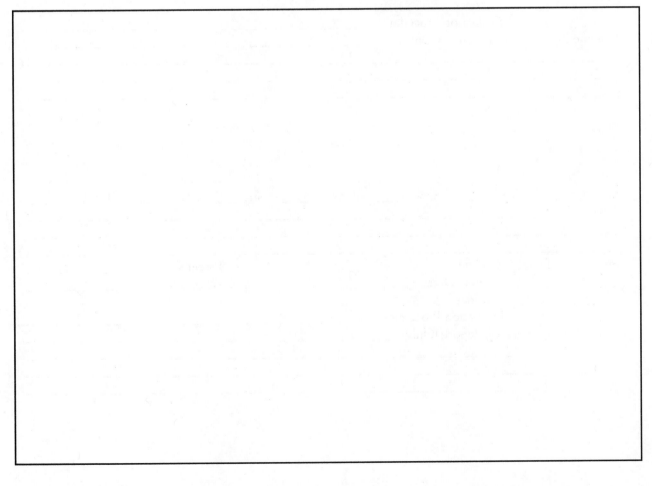

Line No. ____ Goal ____ Subj. ____ Bank _____ Str._____ Set ____ Objective ____

Text _____

_____

_____

Status   Date   Baseline   _____   Target Criteria _____

_____   _____   Baseline Date   _____   Target Date   _____

_____   _____   Provider   _____

_____   _____   Evaluation Procedure _____

Comments for Progress Reports Only _____

_____

_____

_____

_____

Line No. ____ Goal ____ Subj. ____ Bank _____ Str._____ Set ____ Objective ____

Text _____

_____

_____

Status   Date   Baseline   _____   Target Criteria _____

_____   _____   Baseline Date   _____   Target Date   _____

_____   _____   Provider   _____

_____   _____   Evaluation Procedure _____

Comments for Progress Reports Only _____

_____

_____

_____

_____

Line No. ____ Goal ____ Subj. ____ Bank _____ Str._____ Set ____ Objective ____

Text _____

_____

_____

Status   Date   Baseline   _____   Target Criteria _____

_____   _____   Baseline Date   _____   Target Date   _____

_____   _____   Provider   _____

_____   _____   Evaluation Procedure _____

Comments for Progress Reports Only _____

_____

_____

_____

_____

SIGNATURES

Name   Position   Date

_____   _____   _____

_____   _____   _____

_____   _____   _____

_____   _____   _____

_____   _____   _____

_____   _____   _____

_____   _____   _____

_____   _____   _____

_____   _____   _____

_____   _____   _____

_____   _____   _____

_____   _____   _____

*At age 18 all confidentiality and due process rights transfer from the parents to the student.

_____ The student has been informed regarding his/her rights.

_____ The parent(s) have been informed regarding the transfer of rights to the student.

Reports of the student's progress toward annual goals will be sent to the parents or the student, if age 18, according to the following schedule:

_____

_____

_____

_____

D. Reproducible Blank Forms from the Text

The following forms from the text have been included in this appendix for easy reproducibility:

- Legal Guardian's report of student's history form (Figure 5-4)
- Type 1 screening program tool (versions for children 3, 4, 5, and 6 years old) (Figure 5-9a through d)
- Intervention checklist for the classroom teacher (Figure 5-14)
- Occupational therapy referral form and behavior checklist (Figure 5-16)
- Common observations when sensory systems are poorly modulated (Figure 5-17)
- Relationship of frequently used standard scores to the bell curve (Figure 6-1)
- Sample ecological assessment for a preschooler at snack time (Figure 6-2)
- Best practice assessment planning guide (Figure 6-14)
- Data summary worksheet (Figure 7-1)
- Summary of task analysis worksheet (Figure 7-2)
- Context data worksheet (Figure 7-3)
- Worksheet to outline clinical reasoning data (Figure 7-4)
- Worksheet for outlining therapeutic interventions (Figure 7-5)
- Advanced worksheet for outlining therapeutic interventions (Figure 7-6)
- Sensory components of task performance (Figure 7-9)
- Sample Progress Monitoring Process (Table 8-1)
- Progress Monitoring Graph #1 (Figure 8-1)
- Progress Monitoring Graph #2 (Figure 8-2)

STUDENT HISTORY FORM (CONFIDENTIAL)

<u>General</u>

NAME _____ SEX_____ AGE ____
        (Last)   (First)   (Middle)

ADDRESS _____ CITY/STATE_____ ZIP _____

PHONE _____ DATE OF BIRTH_____

AGE AT TIME OF HISTORY _____ PLACE OF BIRTH _____

FATHER OR GUARDIAN'S NAME _____ AGE _____

OCCUPATION _____ HEALTH _____

MOTHER'S NAME _____ AGE _____

OCCUPATION _____ HEALTH _____

CHILD'S PHYSICIAN _____ PHONE _____

RELATIONSHIP OF INFORMANT TO CHILD _____

HOME SCHOOL _____ SUBDIVISION _____

<u>Family</u>

A. Are parents separated? _____ Divorced? _____

B. Has either parent remarried? _____ Which one? _____

C. With whom does the child live? _____

D. Check one: ( ) Natural Child ( ) Adopted Child ( ) Foster Child

E. Name of children in family (eldest to youngest – giving age): _____

F. Other living in the home: _____

<u>Developmental and Medical Background</u>

1. Prenatal: Was there any illness, infection, or unusual condition of mother during pregnancy?_____

2. Birth: Length of pregnancy? _____ Weight at birth? _____

Difficult or forced labor? _____ Instrument delivery? _____

Was there a delay in starting the baby to breathe? _____

Other comments: _____

Child's Health History: _____

3. A. Has the child ever had: Convulsions? _____ Seizures? _____

   Give details: (Identify illness being discussed with exact dates or ages when it occurred, etc.) _____

  B. Unexplained high fever: _____ How high? _____ Duration? _____

    When? _____ Circumstances: _____

  C. Is your child on medication or has he/she been on any in the past? _____

    Type? _____ Reason? _____ Date? _____

D. Present physical condition: Good _____ Fair _____ Poor _____

E. Please list any preschools and/or special programs your child has attended including therapy for speech,
   motor, etc.: _____

<u>Physical Factors</u>

A. At what age was he/she potty trained? _____

B. Does your child now have or has he/she ever had any of the following conditions?

  Difficulty: Talking? _____ Seeing? _____ Hearing? _____

  Falls or accidental injuries? _____ Does your child have trouble running or walking? _____

  How well does your child use: Scissors? Good _____ Fair _____ Poor _____

                          Pencils? Good _____ Fair _____ Poor _____

                          Crayons? Good _____ Fair _____ Poor _____

                          Right handed? _____ Left handed?_____

C. Has your child had any of the following?

  Serious accidents? _____ Date? _____

  Operations? _____ Date? _____

  Unusual illnesses? _____ Date? _____

  Unusual diseases? _____ Date? _____

D. To what things is the child allergic? _____

Legal Guardian's report of student's history form. (Reprinted with permission from Blue Valley
School District, Johnson County, KS.)

From Dunn, W. (2000). *Best Practice Occupational Therapy: In Community Service
with Children and Families.* Thorofare, NJ: SLACK Incorporated.

E. Has the child had any special problems in visual function? (Prolonged wandering of the eyes in infancy, crossed eyes, eyes turned out, drooped lids, failure to follow light or motions, reverses numbers or letters, i.e., sees "b" for "d" or "p" for "g", sees a "6" as a "9") _____

Has vision been tested? _____ Date or age tested? _____ Results: _____

F. Has the child ever had his ears examined by a physician? _____ At what age? _____

Results: _____

Has hearing been tested? _____ Was an audiometer used? _____ At what age? _____

Has your child ever had earaches/otitis media? _____ How often? _____

Have these been recurring? _____

G. Medical treatment being given out; for what conditions and by whom? _____

Family and Home Situation

A. What types of discipline do you use most often in guiding your child? Give examples: _____

_____

B. Are there any adults besides the parents who play an active part in guiding your child? If so, whom? ___

_____

C. Is he/she afraid of certain things, persons, animals, or situation? _____

Explain: _____

D. Has your child ever had temper tantrums? _____ At what age? _____

Explain: _____

E. What particular talents does your child have? _____

F. Are your child's sleeping habits regular? _____

G. Are your child's eating habits regular? _____

Does your child have strong likes or dislikes toward food textures? _____

Likes? _____ Dislikes? _____

H. How does your child respond to other siblings? _____

I. How do other siblings respond to this child? _____

J. Did your child seem to understand what was said to him/her before he/she learned to talk? _____

K. Were the child's wants anticipated before he attempted to speak? _____

L. Did your child use much gesture or sign language? _____

M. Did anyone "baby talk" to your child? _____

N. Is your child easily distracted or does he/she have trouble functioning if there is a lot of noise around?

_____

Legal Guardian's report of student's history form continued. (Reprinted with permission from Blue Valley School District, Johnson County, KS.)

From Dunn, W. (2000). *Best Practice Occupational Therapy: In Community Service with Children and Families.* Thorofare, NJ: SLACK Incorporated.

Developmental Skills Screening

Name: _____   Examiner: _____
Birthdate: _____   Date: _____

B = requires assistance of examiner   *A = accomplishes activity within normal time*

Age	Gross Motor	
3 years	1. Gets up from floor with partial trunk rotation	_____
	2. No longer walks with arms outstretched and shows uniformity of heel-toe gait	_____
	3. Balances on one foot for 1 second	_____
	4. Crawls through objects	_____
	5. Walks backwards	_____
	6. Catches large ball with arms fully extended	_____
	7. Throws small ball with torso participation	_____
	8. Alternates feet going upstairs holding rail	_____
	9. Jumps from bottom step with feet together	_____

Fine Motor
1. Inserts circle, square and triangle into formboard with rotations _____
2. Picks up cube without touching table _____
3. Builds 9-block tower _____
4. Imitates train of 3 or more blocks _____
5. Screws lid on jar _____
6. Demonstrates preferred hand using 3 fingers and thumb to grasp crayon _____
7. Copies circle _____
8. Copies horizontal line _____
9. Imitates cross _____
10. Uses scissors to snip at paper _____

Visual and/or Tactile
1. Hesitates at top of stairs when descending (depth perception) _____
2. Recognizes halves and fits together _____
3. Identifies familiar objects by touching and handling _____

Self-Help Skills
1. Undresses but needs help with fastenings _____
2. Puts on shoes and socks; may be incorrect _____
3. Unlaces shoes _____
4. Washes hands in appropriate sequence _____
5. Drinks from glass with one hand _____
6. Drinks through straw _____
7. No turning of spoon with minimum spilling _____
8. Pours from small container into glass with assistance _____
9. Uses fork to pierce food _____
10. Has BM and urinates in potty when reminders and assistance in wiping–boys may stand _____

Type 1 screening program tool. (Reprinted with permission from Blue Valley School District, Johnson County, KS.)

From Dunn, W. (2000). *Best Practice Occupational Therapy: In Community Service with Children and Families.* Thorofare, NJ: SLACK Incorporated.

Developmental Skills Screening

Name: _____   Examiner: _____
Birthdate: _____   Date: _____

B = requires assistance of examiner   *A = accomplishes activity within normal time*

Age	*Gross Motor*	
4 years	1. Walks with long swinging steps	_____
	2. Gets up from floor with no trunk rotation	_____
	3. Hops on toes with both feet	_____
	4. Balances on one foot for 2-5 seconds	_____
	5. Can touch end of nose with finger	_____
	6. Gallops	_____
	7. Walks on 3 ½" walking board stepping off 3 times	_____
	8. Catches large ball with hands moving in accordance with ball	_____
	9. Throws ball with elbow movement and no torso involvement	_____
	10. Holds rail to walk downstairs alternating feet	_____
	11. No evidence of ATNR	_____

Fine Motor
1. Adult grasp of pencil _____
2. Copies cross _____
3. Imitates square _____
4. Traces diamond _____
5. Cuts straight line _____
6. Draws man with 3 parts _____
7. Copies train of blocks _____
8. Copies bridge _____
9. Imitates gate _____

Visual and/or Tactile
1. Can identify closer of 2 objects _____
2. Matches identically shaped objects by size _____
3. Tactilly matches objects by size with vision occluded _____

Self-Help Skills
1. Undresses and unbuttons buttons _____
2. Puts coat on _____
3. Laces shoes _____
4. Identifies front and back _____
5. Uses fork appropriately _____
6. Pours from container without spilling _____
7. Blows nose _____
8. Goes to toilet on own – may need reminder to wipe _____
9. May call for mother at night for toileting _____

Type 1 screening program tool. (Reprinted with permission from Blue Valley School District, Johnson County, KS.)

From Dunn, W. (2000). *Best Practice Occupational Therapy: In Community Service with Children and Families.* Thorofare, NJ: SLACK Incorporated.

Developmental Skills Screening

Name: _____   Examiner: _____
Birthdate: _____   Date: _____

B = requires assistance of examiner   *A = accomplishes activity within normal time*

Age	Gross Motor	
5 years	1. Arms held near body with narrow stance in gait	_____
	2. Stands up without using hands for support	_____
	3. Can change from sitting, standing and squatting in serial manner	_____
	4. Makes 90 degrees pivot in standing	_____
	5. Distinguishes between own right and left	_____
	6. Walks full length of 3 ½" walking board	_____
	7. Sits up straight in chair	_____
	8. Skips on alternating feet	_____
	9. Bounces ball	_____
	10. May catch and kick ball simultaneously	_____
	11. Walks up and down stairs on alternating feet without rail	_____

Fine Motor
1. Copies square _____
2. Copies triangle _____
3. Draws man with 6 parts _____
4. Reach and placement of blocks show good accuracy _____
5. Copies gate of blocks _____
6. Cuts gate _____
7. Cuts curved line _____
8. Alternates supination and pronation irradically _____
9. Serial opposition with overflow and poor rhythm _____

Visual and/or Tactile
1. Differentiates square from rectangle _____
2. Localizes tactile stimuli to specific body part (arm, leg, etc.) _____
3. Mean of nystagmus to left – 8.9 seconds to right – 8.7 seconds _____

Self-Help Skills
1. Fastens buttons that are within sight _____
2. Washes and dries hands _____
3. May dress without prodding, but needs help with back fasteners _____
4. Brushes hair _____
5. Brushes teeth _____
6. Slow but independent feeding _____
7. Uses knife to spread _____
8. Needs reminders to wipe _____
9. No longer needs night toileting _____

Type 1 screening program tool. (Reprinted with permission from Blue Valley School District, Johnson County, KS.)

From Dunn, W. (2000). *Best Practice Occupational Therapy: In Community Service with Children and Families.* Thorofare, NJ: SLACK Incorporated.

Developmental Skills Screening

Name: _____   Examiner: _____
Birthdate: _____   Date: _____

B = requires assistance of examiner   *A = accomplishes activity within normal time*

Age
6 years

Gross Motor
1. Bows with feet together, legs and knees straight   _____
2. Balances on one foot with eyes open   _____
3. Walks on 1 ½" walking board with 2-3 falls   _____
4. Jumps over one foot obstacles   _____
5. Reaches for objects beyond arm's length with ease   _____
6. Kicks ball from running start   _____
7. Catches small ball and throws using optimal use of
   upper extremity   _____
8. Jumps from bottom step on toes   _____
9. Balances well on toes   _____
10. TLR prone and supine held for 20-30 seconds   _____
11. Body righting diminished   _____
12. Heel-toe walks forwards   _____

Fine Motor
1. Shows good thumb and index finger flexion in writing   _____
2. Draws square with sharp corners   _____
3. Copies diamond   _____

Visual and/or Tactile
1. Nystagmus mean to left – 10.5 seconds to right – 9.2 seconds   _____

Self-Help Skills
1. Dresses self; may need minimal assistance   _____
2. Ties shoe laces loosely   _____
3. Bathes self except for head and neck   _____
4. Uses fork to cut food to bite size   _____
5. Toilets self completely   _____

Type 1 screening program tool. (Reprinted with permission from Blue Valley School District, Johnson County, KS.)

From Dunn, W. (2000). *Best Practice Occupational Therapy: In Community Service with Children and Families.* Thorofare, NJ: SLACK Incorporated.

Student: _____ Teacher: _____ School: _____
Class/Subject:: _____ D.O.B.: _____ Date Completed: _____

Intervention Checklist
Classroom Teacher

What strategies have you tried to correct the problem? Please indicate those strategies you have applied to the problem and give an estimate of how long the strategy has been in effect in terms of days or weeks. Also comment on the success of these strategies in terms of "Yes" or "No":

	Specify:	Duration (Days/Weeks)	Success (Y-N)
Environmental Strategies			
1. Seating Change		_____	_____
2. Isolation (how often?)		_____	_____
3. Change to a different hour/same teacher		_____	_____
4. Change to a different teacher		_____	_____
5. Other		_____	_____
Organization Strategies			
1. Setting time limits for assignments/completion during class		_____	_____
2. Questioning at end of each sentence/paragraph to help focus on important information		_____	_____
3. Allowing additional time to complete task/take test		_____	_____
4. Highlighting main facts in the book		_____	_____
5. Organizing a notebook or providing folder to help organize work		_____	_____
6. Asking student to repeat directions given		_____	_____
7. Other		_____	_____
Motivational Strategies			
1. Checking papers by showing "C's" for correct		_____	_____
2. Sending home daily progress report		_____	_____
3. Immediate reinforcement of correct response		_____	_____
4. Keeping graphs and charts of student's progress		_____	_____
5. Conferencing with students parents		_____	_____
6. Conferencing with student's other teachers		_____	_____
7. Student reading lesson to aide, peer tutor or teacher		_____	_____
8. Home/school communication system for assignments		_____	_____
9. Using tapes of materials the rest of the class is reading		_____	_____
10. Student using tapes of materials at home or school		_____	_____
11. Classmate to take notes with carbon		_____	_____
12. Other		_____	_____
Presentation Strategies			
1. Giving assignments both orally and visually		_____	_____
2. Taping lessons so student can listen again		_____	_____
3. Allowing student to have sample or practice test		_____	_____
4. Providing legible material		_____	_____
5. Immediate correction of errors		_____	_____
6. Providing advance organizers		_____	_____
7. Providing tests in smaller blocks of questions/wider spaced		_____	_____
8. Providing tests in small segments/student hands in at end of each segment and gets next		_____	_____
9. Providing modified tests, fewer questions, simpler material		_____	_____
10. Giving tests orally		_____	_____
11. Other		_____	_____
Curriculum Strategies			
1. Providing opportunities for extra drill		_____	_____
2. Providing study guide (outline, etc., to follow)		_____	_____
3. Reducing quantity of material		_____	_____
4. Providing instructional materials geared to lower level of basic skills		_____	_____
5. Vocabulary flash cards		_____	_____
6. Vocabulary words in context		_____	_____
7. Special materials		_____	_____
8. Other		_____	_____

Are there any other strategies you have used that are not listed above? If "yes", please describe: (Duration and success):

Intervention checklist for the classroom teacher. (Reprinted with permission from Dunn, W. (1991) *Pediatric Occupational Therapy: Facilitating Effective Service Provision*. Thorofare, NJ: SLACK Incorporated.)

From Dunn, W. (2000). *Best Practice Occupational Therapy: In Community Service with Children and Families*. Thorofare, NJ: SLACK Incorporated.

Occupational Therapy Referral Form

_____ has been referred for an occupational therapy evaluation. To help with the evaluation, your input is very important. Please complete this questionnaire and return to the occupational therapist. The evaluation will be completed on _____. Thank you very much for your help!

Date of Referral: _____ Teacher: _____

Why do you feel this child should be evaluated by the occupational therapist? _____

Formal Evaluations:
1. I.Q./Name of Test: _____
   Data Given: _____
   Full Score: _____
      Verbal: _____
      Performance: _____
2. Academic Levels:
   Reading:_____ Date of Assessment: _____
   Spelling: _____ Date of Assessment: _____
   Math: _____ Date of Assessment:: _____
3. Other Pertinent Evaluations:
   Speech Evaluation Results:_____
   Special Evaluations (Given by Counselor or Special Teacher of LD resource teacher):_____
   VMI: _____
   Peabody Picture Vocabulary Test: _____
4. Health Evaluation:
   Medical Problems: _____
   Health Screening Results: _____
   Medications:_____

Checklist for Occupational Therapy

Please check the statements that are pertinent to this child.

Gross Motor
_____ Seems weaker than other children his/her age
_____ Does not have the endurance other children his/her age have for an activity
_____ Difficulty with hopping, jumping, skipping, or running as compared with others his/her age
_____ Appears stiff and awkward in his/her movements
_____ Clumsy, does not appear to know how body works, bumps into others or objects, never quite sits
             in chair correctly
_____ Does not seem to understand concepts such as right, left, front, or back as it relates to his/her body
_____ Shies away from playground equipment. May only play on one particular item
_____ Poor posture (always seems to be leaning against something, shoulders slump forward)

Fine Motor
_____ Difficulty with drawing, coloring, tracing
_____ Performs these activities quickly and result is usually sloppy
_____ Avoids fine motor activities
_____ Problem holding pencil, grasp may be very loose or very tight
_____ Printing is too dark, too light, too large, too small
_____ Does not seem to have a dominant hand

Academic
_____ Distractible
_____ Restless
_____ Slow worker
_____ Disorganized, messy desk
_____ Short attention span
_____ Hyperactive

Occupational therapy referral form and behavior checklist. (Reprinted with permission from Dunn, W. (1991) *Pediatric Occupational Therapy: Facilitating Effective Service Provision.* Thorofare, NJ: SLACK Incorporated.)

From Dunn, W. (2000). *Best Practice Occupational Therapy: In Community Service with Children and Families.* Thorofare, NJ: SLACK Incorporated.

Overreactive	Underreactive

Somatosensory (touch) system

Overreactive	Underreactive
____ defensive about others touching body	____ slow to respond
____ reacts emotionally or aggressively to touch	____ doesn't notice others
____ avoids selected textures in clothing selection	____ uses poor judgment regarding personal space
____ narrow range of clothing choices	____ mouths objects frequently
____ rigid rituals in personal hygiene	____ chews on pencils
____ extremely negative about dental work	____ doesn't seem to notice when someone brushes
____ picky eater, especially regarding textures	or touches arm or back
____ avoids haircuts, hair washing	____ allows drool to remain on face
____ withdraws from splashing water	____ leaves clothing twisted on body
____ pushes washcloth/towel away	
____ cries when hair is washed and dried	
____ pulls at hats and accessories	
____ gags easily with food textures/utensils in mouth	
____ avoids tasks that are wet/messy	
____ complains about tape or glue on skin	

Vestibular (movement) system

Overreactive	Underreactive
____ insecure about movement experiences	____ clumsy, lethargic
____ avoids or fears movement	____ slow to respond to movement demands
____ holds head upright, even when bending/leaning	____ poor endurance, tires easily
____ avoids new positions, especially of head	____ rocks in desk/chair
____ holds onto walls or banisters	____ craves movement
____ very clumsy on changeable surfaces, such as a field	
____ becomes disoriented after bending over sink, table	
____ becomes overly excited after a movement activity	
____ turns whole body to look at you (rather than just head)	

Proprioceptive (body position) system

Overreactive	Underreactive
____ tense muscles	____ weak grasp
____ rigidity, diminished fluidity of	____ poor endurance for tasks
____ locks joints to stabilize movement	____ tires easily, collapses
	____ hangs on objects for support
	____ can't lift heavy objects
	____ props to support self

Visual system

Overreactive	Underreactive
____ avoids bright lights, sunlight	____ doesn't notice when people come into the room
____ covers eyes in lighted room	____ difficulty finding objects in drawer, desk, on paper
____ watches everyone when they move around	____ trouble locating desired object on shelf, in drawer
____ covers part of the page when reading	

Auditory system

Overreactive	Underreactive
____ overreacts to unexpected sounds	____ doesn't respond to name being called
____ easily distracted in classroom	____ seems oblivious within an active environment
____ holds hands over ears	____ makes sounds constantly
____ can't work with background noise	
____ cries about sounds in environment (e.g., hair dryer)	

Common observations when sensory systems are poorly modulated. (Reprinted with permission from Dunn W. (1991) The sensorimotor systems: A framework for assessment and intervention. In F.P. Orelove & D. Sobsey (Eds.), *Educating children with multiple disabilities: A transdisciplinary approach* (2nd ed.) Baltimore,MD: Paul H. Brookes.)

From Dunn, W. (2000). *Best Practice Occupational Therapy: In Community Service with Children and Families.* Thorofare, NJ: SLACK Incorporated.

Relationship of frequently used standard scores to the bell curve. Shaded area denotes normal range. (Reprinted with permission from Sattler, J. M. (1988). *Assessment of Children* (3rd Edition). San Diego, CA: Jerome M. Sattler, Publisher, Inc.)

Percent of cases within sections of bell curve: 2% 13.5% 34% 34% 13.5% 2%

Standard deviations: -3.0 -2.0 -1.0 0.0 +1.0 +2.0 +3.0

Cumulative Percentages: 0.1% 2.0% 16% 50% 84% 98% 99.9%

Percentile Equivalents: 1 5 10 20 30 40 50 60 70 80 90 95 99

Z Scores: -3.0 -2.0 -1.0 0.0 +1.0 +2.0 +3.0

T Scores: 20 30 40 50 60 70 80

Stanines: 1 2 3 4 5 6 7 8 9

Percent in Stanines: 4% 7% 12% 17% 20% 17% 12% 7% 4%

IQ Composite Score (SB): 52 68 84 100 116 132 148

IQ Subtest Scores (SB): 26 34 42 50 58 66 74

IQ Composite Scores (Wechsler, KABC): 55 70 85 100 115 130 145

IQ Subtest Scores (Wechsler, KABC): 1 4 7 10 13 16 19

Bruininks-Oseretsky Composite Scores: 20 30 40 50 60 70 80

Bruininks-Oseretsky Subtest Scores: 0 5 10 15 20 25 30

Motor Free Visual Perception Test (Perceptual Quotient): 55 70 85 100 115 130 145

Test of Visual Perceptual Skills (Composite Scores): 55 70 85 100 115 130 145

TVPS Subtest Scores: 1 4 7 10 13 16 19

From Dunn, W. (2000). *Best Practice Occupational Therapy: In Community Service with Children and Families.* Thorofare, NJ: SLACK Incorporated.

Ecologically-Based Individualized Adaptation Inventory

Environment:

Activity:

Plan				Observation		
A Typical Toddler Inventory	An Inventory of the Patient	Skills Patient Can Probably Acquire	Skills Patient May Not Acquire	Adaptation Possibilities	Assessment	Daily Plan

Sample ecological assessment for a preschooler at snack time. (Reprinted with permission from *The Journal of the Association for the Severely Handicapped.*)

From Dunn, W. (2000). *Best Practice Occupational Therapy: In Community Service with Children and Families*. Thorofare, NJ: SLACK Incorporated.

Data collection strategy	Occupational performance: What they want and need to do	Context variable assessment	Person variables: Data during performance	Person variables: Formal assessment*
Records reviews				
Norm-referenced measurement				
Criterion-referenced measurement				
Informal measurement				
Skilled observation				
Interviews				
Ecological measures				

*Only included when necessary to verify or clarify; see text.

Best practice assessment planning guide.

From Dunn, W. (2000). *Best Practice Occupational Therapy: In Community Service with Children and Families.* Thorofare, NJ: SLACK Incorporated.

Person Variables	Activities of Daily Living	Work/Productive Activity	Play/Leisure Performance
Sensorimotor			
Cognitive			
Psychosocial			

Data summary worksheet. (Adapted from Dunn, W., Brown, C., McClain, L., & Westman, K. (1994). The ecology of human performance: A contextual perspective on human occupation. In C. Royeen (Ed.), *The practice of the future: Putting occupation back into therapy.* Washington, DC: AOTA.)

From Dunn, W. (2000). *Best Practice Occupational Therapy: In Community Service with Children and Families.* Thorofare, NJ: SLACK Incorporated.

Typical Performance Features of a Task	_____ 's Performance

Summary of task analysis worksheet. (Adapted from Dunn, W., Brown, C., McClain, L., & Westman, K. (1994). The ecology of human performance: A contextual perspective on human occupation. In C. Royeen (Ed.), *The practice of the future: Putting occupation back into therapy.* Washington, DC: AOTA.)

From Dunn, W. (2000). *Best Practice Occupational Therapy: In Community Service with Children and Families.* Thorofare, NJ: SLACK Incorporated.

	Code
Physical	
Social	
Cultural	
Temporal	
Code: s=supporting factor; b=barrier to performance; ?=could be either a support or barrier	

Context data worksheet. (Adapted from Dunn, W., Brown, C., McClain, L., & Westman, K. (1994). The ecology of human performance: A contextual perspective on human occupation. In C. Royeen (Ed.), *The practice of the future: Putting occupation back into therapy.* Washington, DC: AOTA.)

From Dunn, W. (2000). *Best Practice Occupational Therapy: In Community Service with Children and Families.* Thorofare, NJ: SLACK Incorporated.

Scientific Reasoning	Narrative Reasoning	Pragmatic Reasoning	Ethical Reasoning

Worksheet to outline clinical reasoning data. (Adapted from Dunn, W., Brown, C., McClain, L., & Westman, K. (1994). The ecology of human performance: A contextual perspective on human occupation. In C. Royeen (Ed.), *The practice of the future: Putting occupation back into therapy*. Washington, DC: AOTA.)

From Dunn, W. (2000). *Best Practice Occupational Therapy: In Community Service with Children and Families*. Thorofare, NJ: SLACK Incorporated.

Performance	Establish/Restore	Alter/Modify	Adapt	Prevent	Create

Worksheet for outlining therapeutic interventions. (Adapted from Dunn, W., Brown, C., McClain, L., & Westman, K. (1994). The ecology of human performance: A contextual perspective on human occupation. In C. Royeen (Ed.), *The practice of the future: Putting occupation back into therapy.* Washington, DC: AOTA.)

From Dunn, W. (2000). *Best Practice Occupational Therapy: In Community Service with Children and Families.* Thorofare, NJ: SLACK Incorporated.

Models of Service	Establish/Restore	Alter/Modify	Adapt	Prevent	Create
Direct					
Supervised Therapy					
Consult					

Advanced worksheet for outlining therapeutic interventions. (Adapted from Dunn, W., Brown, C., McClain, L., & Westman, K. (1994). The ecology of human performance: A contextual perspective on human occupation. In C. Royeen (Ed.), *The practice of the future: Putting occupation back into therapy.* Washington, DC: AOTA.)

From Dunn, W. (2000). *Best Practice Occupational Therapy: In Community Service with Children and Families.* Thorofare, NJ: SLACK Incorporated.

Routine/task _____ Sensory characteristics	What does the task routine hold? A | B | C	What does the particular environment hold?	What adaptations are likely to improve functional outcome?
Somato-sensory — light touch (tap, tickle)			
pain			
temperature (hot, cold)			
touch pressure (hug, pat, grasp)			
variable			
duration of stimulus (short, long)			
body surface contact (small, large)			
predictable			
unpredictable			
Vestibular — head position change			
speed change			
direction change			
rotary head movement			
linear head movement			
repetitive head movement (rhythmic)			
predictable			
unpredictable			
Proprio-ceptive — quick stretch stimulus			
sustained tension stimulus			
shifting muscle tension			
Visual — high intensity			
low intensity			
high contrast			
high similarity (low contrast)			
competitive			
variable			
predictable			
unpredictable			
Auditory — rhythmic			
variable			
constant			
competitive			
noncompetitive			
loud			
soil			
predictable			
unpredictable			
Olfactory/ Gustatory — mild			
strong			
predictable			
unpredictable			

Task: A = _____
Components: B = _____
             C = _____

Sensory components of task performance. (Reprinted with permission from Dunn, W. (1991). The sensorimotor systems: A framework for assessment and intervention. In F. P. Orelove & D. Sobsey (Eds.), *Educating children with multiple disabilities: A transdisciplinary approach* (2nd ed.). Baltimore: Paul H. Brookes.)

From Dunn, W. (2000). *Best Practice Occupational Therapy: In Community Service with Children and Families.* Thorofare, NJ: SLACK Incorporated.

Sample Progress Monitoring Process for _____

Outline of tasks	Patient's plan
Behavior	
Goal	
Hypothesis for observed behavior	
Intervention plan	
Measurement strategy	
Decision-making plan	

From Dunn, W. (2000). *Best Practice Occupational Therapy: In Community Service with Children and Families*. Thorofare, NJ: SLACK Incorporated.

Progress Monitoring Graph #1

Goal:

Sub-skill	Week																			
	1	2	3	4	5	6	7	8	9	10	11	12	13	14	15	16	17	18	19	20

6

5

4

3

2

1

0

KEY:
✓ = skill meets criteria   V = needed verbal prompt
O = not attempted/performed P = needed physical prompt

From Dunn, W. (2000). *Best Practice Occupational Therapy: In Community Service with Children and Families*. Thorofare, NJ: SLACK Incorporated.

Progress Monitoring Graph #2

Goal:

Minutes	Week																													
	1	2	3	4	5	6	7	8	9	10	11	12	13	14	15	16	17	18	19	20	21	22	23	24	25	26	27	28	29	30
10																														
9																														
8																														
7																														
6																														
5																														
4																														
3																														
2																														
1																														
0																														

Began Intervention   Changed Intervention

M
T
W
Th
F

From Dunn, W. (2000). *Best Practice Occupational Therapy: In Community Service with Children and Families.* Thorofare, NJ: SLACK Incorporated.

Public Law Number 105-17: Individuals with Disabilities Education Act (IDEA)

Miscellaneous Provisions

Publisher's Note: Please be aware of the varying effective dates for this legislation. Consult Miscellaneous Provisions – Effective Dates, to determine effective dates of legislation. Additionally, publisher has added notices indicating sections that are not immediately effective.

INDIVIDUALS WITH DISABILITIES EDUCATION ACT

20 U.S.C. Chapter 33

Part A–General Provisions

[Publisher's Note: Except as indicated, this Part is immediately effective]

Sec. 1400   Short title; table of contents; findings; purposes

(a) Short title

This Act may be cited as the "Individuals with Disabilities Education Act"

(b) [Omitted]

(c) Findings

The Congress finds the following:

(1) Disability is a natural part of the human experience and in no way diminishes the right of individuals to participate in or contribute to society. Improving educational results for children with disabilities is an essential element of our national policy of ensuring equality of opportunity, full participation, independent living, and economic self-sufficiency for individuals with disabilities.

(2) Before the date of the enactment of the Education for All Handicapped Children Act of 1975 (Public Law 94-142)—

(A) the special educational needs of children with disabilities were not being fully met;

(B) more than one-half of the children with disabilities in the United States did not receive appropriate educational services that would enable such children to have full equality of opportunity;

(C) 1,000,000 of the children with disabilities in the United States were excluded entirely from the public school system and did not go through the educational process with their peers;

(D) there were many children with disabilities throughout the United States participating in regular school programs whose disabilities prevented such children from having a successful educational experience because their disabilities were undetected; and

(E) because of the lack of adequate services within the public school system, families were often forced to find services outside the public school system, often at great distance from their residence and at their own expense.

(3) Since the enactment and implementation of the Education for All Handicapped Children Act of 1975, this Act has been successful in ensuring children with disabilities and the families of such children access to a free appropriate public education and in improving educational results for children with disabilities.

(4) However, the implementation of this Act has been impeded by low expectations, and an insufficient focus on apply-ing replicable research on proven methods of teaching and learning for children with disabilities.

(5) Over 20 years of research and experience has demonstrated that the education of children with disabilities can be made more effective by—

(A) having high expectations for such children and ensuring their access in the general curriculum to the maximum extent possible;

(B) strengthening the role of parents and ensuring that families of such children have meaningful opportunities to participate in the education of their children at school and at home;

(C) coordinating this Act with other local, educational service agency, State, and Federal school improvement efforts in order to ensure that such children benefit from such efforts and that special education can become a service for such children rather than a place where they are sent;

(D) providing appropriate special education and related services and aids and supports in the regular classroom to such children, whenever appropriate;

(E) supporting high-quality, intensive professional development for all personnel who work with such children in order to ensure that they have the skills and knowledge necessary to enable them—

(i) to meet developmental goals and, to the maximum extent possible, those challenging expectations that have been established for all children; and

(ii) to be prepared to lead productive, independent, adult lives, to the maximum extent possible;

(F) providing incentives for whole-school approaches and pre-referral intervention to reduce the need to label children as disabled in order to address their learning needs; and

(G) focusing resources on teaching and learning while reducing paperwork and requirements that do not assist in improving educational results.

(6) While States, local educational agencies, and educational service agencies are responsible for providing an education for all children with disabilities, it is in the national interest that the Federal Government have a role in assisting State and local efforts to educate children with disabilities in order to improve results for such children and to ensure equal protection of the law.

(7) (A) The Federal Government must be responsive to the governing needs of an increasingly more diverse society. A more equitable allocation of resources is essential for the Federal Government to meet its responsibility to provide an equal educational opportunity for all individuals.

(B) America's racial profile is rapidly changing. Between 1980 and 1990, the rate of increase in the population for white Americans was 6 percent, while the rate of increase for racial and ethnic minorities was much higher: 53 percent for Hispanics, 13.2 percent for African-Americans, and 107.8 percent for Asians.

(C) By the year 2000, this Nation will have 275,000,000 people, nearly one of every three of whom will be either African-American, Hispanic, Asian-American, or American Indian.

(D) Taken together as a group, minority children are comprising an ever larger percentage of public school students. Large-city school populations are overwhelmingly minority, for example: for fall 1993, the figure for Miami was 84 percent; Chicago, 89 percent; Philadelphia, 78 percent; Baltimore, 84 percent; Houston, 88 percent; and Los Angeles, 88 percent.

(E) Recruitment efforts within special education must focus on bringing larger numbers of minorities into the profession in order to provide appropriate practitioner knowledge, role models, and sufficient manpower to address the clearly changing demography of special education.

(F) The limited English proficient population is the fastest growing in our Nation, and the growth is occurring in many parts of our Nation. In the Nation's 2 largest school districts, limited English students make up almost half of all students initially entering school at the kindergarten level. Studies have documented apparent discrepancies in the levels of referral and placement of limited English proficient children in special education. The Department of Education has found that services provided to limited English proficient students often do not respond primarily to the pupil's academic needs. These trends pose special challenges for special education in the referral, assessment, and services for our Nation's students from non-English language backgrounds.

(8) (A) Greater efforts are needed to prevent the intensification of problems connected with mislabeling and high dropout rates among minority children with disabilities.

(B) More minority children continue to be served in special education than would be expected from the percentage of minority students in the general school population.

(C) Poor African-American children are 2.3 times more likely to be identified by their teacher as having mental retardation than their white counterpart.

(D) Although African-Americans represent 16 percent of elementary and secondary enrollments, they constitute 21 percent of total enrollments in special education.

(E) The drop-out rate is 68 percent higher for minorities than for whites.

(F) More than 50 percent of minority students in large cities drop out of school.

(9) (A) The opportunity for full participation in awards for grants and contracts; boards of organizations receiving funds under this Act; and peer review panels; and training of professionals in the area of special education by minority individuals, organizations, and historically black colleges and universities is essential if we are to obtain greater success in the education of minority children with disabilities.

(B) In 1993, of the 915,000 college and university professors, 4.9 percent were African-American and 2.4 percent were Hispanic. Of the 2,940,000 teachers, prekindergarten through high school, 6.8 percent were African-American and 4.1 percent were Hispanic.

(C) Students from minority groups comprise more than 50 percent of K-12 public school enrollment in seven States yet minority enrollment in teacher training programs is less than 15 percent in all but six States.

(D) As the number of African-American and Hispanic students in special education increases, the number of minority teachers and related service personnel produced in our colleges and universities continue to decrease.

(E) Ten years ago, 12 percent of the United States teaching force in public elementary and secondary schools were members of a minority group. Minorities comprised 21% of the national population at that time and were clearly underrepresented then among employed teachers. Today, the elementary and secondary teaching force is 13% minority, while 1/3 of the students in public schools are minority children.

(F) As recently as 1991, historically black colleges and universities enrolled 44 percent of the African-American teacher trainees in the Nation. However, in 1993, historically black colleges and universities received only 4 percent of the discretionary funds for special education and related services personnel training under this Act.

(G) While African-American students constitute 28 percent of total enrollment in special education, only 11.2 percent of individuals enrolled in preservice training programs for special education are African-American.

(H) In 1986-87, of the degrees conferred in education at the B.A., M.A., and Ph.D. levels, only 6, 8, and 8 percent, respectively, were awarded to African-American or Hispanic students.

(10) Minorities and underserved persons are socially disadvantaged because of the lack of opportunities in training and educational programs, undergirded by the practices in the private sector that impede their full participation in the mainstream of society.

(d) Purposes

The purposes of this title are—

(1)(A) to ensure that all children with disabilities have available to them a free appropriate public education that emphasizes special education and related services resigned to meet their unique needs and prepare them for employment and independent living;

(B) to ensure that the rights of children with disabilities and parents of such children are protected; and

(C) to assist States, localities, educational service agencies, and Federal agencies to provide for the education of all children with disabilities;

(2) to assist States in the implementation of a statewide, comprehensive, coordinated, multidisciplinary, interagency system of early intervention services for infants and toddlers with disabilities and their families;

(3) to ensure that educators and parents have the necessary tools to improve educational results for children with disabilities by supporting systemic-change activities; coordinated research and personnel preparation; coordinated technical assistance, dissemination, and support; and technology development and media services; and

(4) to assess, and ensure the effectiveness of, efforts to educate children with disabilities.

[Apr. 13, 1970, Pub. I. 91-230, Title VI, Part A, Sec. 601, as added, June 4, 1997, Pub. I. 105-17, Title I, Sec. 601, 111 Stat. 37.]

Sec. 1401   Definitions

Except as otherwise provided, as used in this Act:

(1) Assistive technology device

The term 'assistive technology device' means any item, piece of equipment, or product system, whether acquired commercially off the shelf, modified, or customized, that is used to increase, maintain, or improve functional capabilities of a child with a disability.

(2) Assistive technology service

The term 'assistive technology service' means any service that directly assists a child with a disability in the selection, acquisition, or use of an assistive technology device. Such term includes—

(A) the evaluation of the needs of such child, including a functional evaluation of the child in the child's customary environment;

(B) purchasing, leasing, or otherwise providing for the acquisition of assistive technology devices by such child;

(C) selecting, designing, fitting, customizing, adapting, applying, maintaining, repairing, or replacing of assistive technology devices;

(D) coordinating and using other therapies, interventions, or services with assistive technology devices, such as those associated with existing education and rehabilitation plans and programs;

(E) training or technical assistance for such child, or, where appropriate, the family of such child; and

(F) training or technical assistance for professionals (including individuals providing education and rehabilitation services), employers, or other individuals who provide services to, employ, or are otherwise substantially involved in the major life functions of such child.

(3) Child with a disability

(A) In general

The term 'child with a disability' means a child—

(i) with mental retardation, hearing impairments (including deafness), speech or language impairments, visual impairments (including blindness), serious emotional disturbance (hereinafter referred to as 'emotional disturbance'), orthopedic impairments, autism, traumatic brain injury, other health impairments, or specific learning disabilities; and

(ii) who, by reason thereof, needs special education and related services.

(B) Child aged 3 through 9

The term 'child with a disability' for a child aged 3 through 9 may, at the discretion of the State and the local educational agency, include a child—

(i) experiencing developmental delays, as defined by the State and as measured by appropriate diagnostic instruments and procedures, in one or more of the following areas: physical development, cognitive development, communication development, social or emotional development, or adaptive development; and

(ii) who, by reason thereof, needs special education and related services.

(4) Educational service agency

The term 'educational service agency'—

(A) means a regional public multiservice agency—

(i) authorized by State law to develop, manage, and provide services or programs to local educational agencies; and

(ii) recognized as an administrative agency for purposes of the provision of special education and related services provided within public elementary and secondary schools of the State; and

(B) includes any other public institution or agency having administrative control and direction over a public elementary or secondary school.

(5) Elementary school

The term 'elementary school' means a nonprofit institutional day or residential school that provides elementary education, as determined under State law.

(6) Equipment

The term 'equipment' includes—

(A) machinery, utilities, and built-in equipment and any necessary enclosures or structures to house such machinery, utilities, or equipment; and

(B) all other items necessary for the functioning of a particular facility as a facility for the provision of educational services, including items such as instructional equipment and necessary furniture; printed, published, and audio-visual instructional materials; telecommunications, sensory, and other technological aids and devices; and books, periodicals, documents, and other related materials.

(7) Excess costs

The term 'excess costs' means those costs that are in excess of the average annual per-student expenditure in a local educational agency during the preceding school year for an elementary or secondary school student, as may be appropriate, and which shall be computed after deducting—

(A) amounts received—

(i) under part B of this title;

(ii) under part A of title I of the Elementary and Secondary Education Act of 1965; or

(iii) under part A of title VII of that Act; and

(B) any State or local funds expended for programs that would qualify for assistance under any of those parts.

(8) Free appropriate public education

The term 'free appropriate public education' means special education and related services that—

(A) have been provided at public expense, under public supervision and direction, and without charge;

(B) meet the standards of the State educational agency;

(C) include an appropriate preschool, elementary, or secondary school education in the State involved; and

(D) are provided in conformity with the individualized education program required under Sec. 614(d).

(9) Indian

The term 'Indian' means an individual who is a member of an Indian tribe.

(10) Indian tribe

The term 'Indian tribe' means any Federal or State Indian tribe, band, rancheria, pueblo, colony, or community, including any Alaska Native village or regional village corporation (as defined in or established under the Alaska Native Claims Settlement Act).

(11) Individualized education program

The term 'individualized education program' or 'IEP' means a written statement for each child with a disability that is developed, reviewed, and revised in accordance with Sec. 1414(d).

(12) Individualized family service plan

The term 'individualized family service plan' has the meaning given such term in Sec. 1436.

(13) Infant or toddler with a disability

The term 'infant or toddler with a disability' has the meaning given such term in Sec. 1432.

(14) Institution of higher education

The term 'institution of higher education'—

(A) has the meaning given that term in Sec. 1201(a) of the Higher Education Act of 1965; and

(B) also includes any community college receiving funding from the Secretary of the Interior under the Tribally Controlled Community College Assistance Act of 1978.

(15) Local educational agency

(A) The term 'local educational agency' means a public board of education or other public authority legally constituted within a State for either administrative control or direction of, or to perform a service function for, public elementary or secondary schools in a city, county, township, school district, or other political subdivision of a State, or for such combination of school districts or counties as are recognized in a State as an administrative agency for its public elementary or secondary schools.

(B) The term includes—

(i) an educational service agency, as defined in paragraph (4); and

(ii) any other public institution or agency having administrative control and direction of a public elementary or secondary school.

(A) The term includes an elementary or secondary school funded by the Bureau of Indian Affairs, but only to the extent that such inclusion makes the school eligible for programs for which specific eligibility is not provided to the school in another provision of law and the school does not have a student population that is smaller than the student population of the local educational agency receiving assistance under this Act with the smallest student population, except that the school shall not be subject to the jurisdiction of any State educational agency other than the Bureau of Indian Affairs.

(16) Native language

The term 'native language', when used with reference to an individual of limited English proficiency, means the language normally used by the individual, or in the case of a child, the language normally used by the parents of the child.

(17) Nonprofit

The term 'nonprofit', as applied to a school, agency, organization, or institution, means a school, agency, organization, or institution owned and operated by one or more nonprofit corporations or associations no part of the net earnings of which inures, or may lawfully inure, to the benefit of any private shareholder or individual.

(18) Outlying area

The term 'outlying area' means the Untied States Virgin Islands, Guam, American Samoa, and the Commonwealth of the Northern Mariana Islands.

(19) Parent

The term 'parent'—

(A) includes a legal guardian; and

(B) except as used in Secs. 1415(b)(2) and 1439(a)(5), includes an individual assigned under either of those sections to be a surrogate parent.

(20) Parent organization

The term 'parent organization' has the meaning given that term in Sec. 1482(g).

(21) Parent training and information center

The term 'parent training and information center' means a center assisted under Sec. 1482 or 1483.

(22) Related services

The term 'related services' means transportation, and such developmental, corrective, and other supportive services (including speech-language pathology and audiology services, psychological services, physical and occupational therapy, recreation, including therapeutic recreation, social work services, counseling services, including rehabilitation counseling, orientation and mobility services, and medical services, except that such medical services shall be for diagnostic and evaluation purposes only) as may be required to assist a child with a disability to benefit from special education, and includes the early identification and assessment of disabling conditions in children.

(23) Secondary school

The term 'secondary school' means a nonprofit institutional day or residential school that provides secondary education, as determined under State law, except that it does not include any education beyond grade 12.

(24) Secretary

The term 'Secretary' means the Secretary of Education.

(25) Special education

The term 'special education' means specially designed instruction, at no cost to parents, to meet the unique needs of a child with a disability, including—

(A) instruction conducted in the classroom, in the home, in hospitals and institutions, and in other settings; and

(B) instruction in physical education.

(26) Specific learning disability

(A) In general

The term 'specific learning disability' means a disorder in one or more of the basic psychological processes involved in understanding or in using language, spoken or written, which disorder may manifest itself in imperfect ability to listen, think, speak, read, write, spell, or do mathematical calculations.

(B) Disorders included

Such term includes such conditions as perceptual disabilities, brain injury, minimal brain dysfunction, dyslexia, and developmental aphasia.

(C) Disorders not included

Such term does not include a learning problem that is primarily the result of visual, hearing, or motor disabilities, of mental retardation, of emotional disturbance, or of environmental, cultural, or economic disadvantage.

(27) State

The term 'State' means each of the 50 States, the District of Columbia, the Commonwealth of Puerto Rico, and each of the outlying areas.

(28) State educational agency

The term 'State educational agency' means the State board of education or other agency or officer primarily responsible for the State supervision of public elementary and secondary schools, or, if there is no such officer or agency, an officer or agency designated by the Governor or by State law.

(29) Supplementary aids and services

The term 'supplementary aids and services' means, aids, services, and other supports that are provided in regular education classes or other education-related settings to enable children with disabilities to be educated with nondisabled children to the maximum extent appropriate in accordance with Sec. 1412(a)(5).

(30) Transition services

The term 'transition services' means a coordinated set of activities for a student with a disability that—

(A) is designed within an outcome-oriented process, which promotes movement from school to post-school activities, including post-secondary education, vocational training, integrated employment (including supported employment), continuing and adult education, adult services, independent living, or community participation;

(B) is based upon the individual student's needs, taking into account the student's preferences and interests; and

(C) includes instruction, related services, community experiences, the development of employment and other post-school adult living objectives, and, when appropriate, acquisition of daily living skills and functional vocational evaluation.

[Apr. 13, 1970, Pub. I. 91-230, Title VI, Part A, Sec. 602, as added, June 4, 1997, Pub. I. 105-17, Title I, Sec. 602, III Stat. 42.)

Sec. 1402   Office of Special Education Programs

(a) Establishment

There shall be, within the Office of Special Education and Rehabilitative Services in the Department of Education, an Office of Special Education Programs, which shall be the principal agency in such Department for administering and carrying out this Act and other programs and activities concerning the education of children with disabilities.

(b) Director

The Office established under subsection (a) shall be headed by a Director who shall be selected by the Secretary and shall report directly to the Assistant Secretary for Special Education and Rehabilitative Services.

(c) Voluntary and uncompensated services

Not-with-standing Sec. 1342 of title 31, United States Code, the Secretary is authorized to accept voluntary and uncompensated services in furtherance of the purposes of this Act.

[Apr. 13, 1970, Pub. I, 91-230, Title VI, Part A, Sec. 603, as added, June 4, 1997, Pub. I. 105-17, Title I, Sec. 603, III Stat. 46.]

Sec. 1403   Abrogation of State sovereign immunity

(a) In general

A State shall not be immune under the eleventh amendment to the Constitution of the United States from suit in Federal court for a violation of this Act.

(b) Remedies

In a suit against a State for a violation of this Act, remedies (including remedies both at law and in equity) are available for such a violation to the same extent as those remedies are available for such a violation in the suit against any public entity other than a State.

(c) Effective date

Subsections (a) and (b) apply with respect to violations that occur in whole or part after the date of the enactment of the Education of the Handicapped Act Amendments of 1990.

[Apr. 13, 1970, Pub. I, 91-230, Title VI, Part A, Sec. 604, as added, June 4, 1997, Pub. I, 105-17, Title I, Sec. 604, III Stat. 47.]

Sec. 1404   Acquisition of equipment; construction or alteration of facilities

(a) In general

If the Secretary determines that a program authorized under this Act would be improved by permitting program funds to be used to acquire appropriate equipment, or to construct new facilities or alter existing facilities, the Secretary is authorized to allow the use of those funds for those purposes.

(b) Compliance with certain regulations

Any construction of new facilities or alteration of existing facilities under subsection (a) shall comply with the requirements of—

(1) appendix A of part 36 of title 28, Code of Federal Regulations (commonly known as the 'Americans with Disabilities Accessibility Guidelines for Buildings and Facilities'); or

(2) appendix A of part 101-19.6 of title 41, Code of Federal Regulations (commonly known as the 'Uniform Federal Accessibility Standards').

[Apr. 13, 1970, Pub. I, 91-230, Title VI, Part A, Sec. 605, as added, June 4, 1997, Pub. I, 105-17, Title I, Sec. 605, III Stat 47.]

Sec. 1405   Employment of individuals with disabilities

The Secretary shall ensure that each recipient of assistance under this Act makes positive efforts to employ and advance in employment qualified individuals with disabilities in programs assisted under this Act.

[Apr. 13, 1970, Pub. I, 91-230, Title VI, Part A, Sec. 606, as added, June 4, 1997, Pub. I, 105-17, Title I, Sec. 606, III Stat. 47.]

Sec. 1406   Requirements for prescribing regulations

(a) Public comment period

The Secretary shall provide a public comment period of at least 90 days on any regulation proposed under part B or part C of this Act on which an opportunity for public comment is otherwise required by law.

(b) Protections provided to children

The Secretary may not implement, or publish in final form, any regulation prescribed pursuant to this Act that would procedurally or substantively lessen the protections provided to children with disabilities under this Act, as embodied in regulations in effect on July 20, 1983 (particularly as such protections relate to parental consent to initial evaluation or initial placement in special education, least restrictive environment, related services, timelines, attendance of evaluation personnel at individualized education program meetings, or qualifications of personnel), except to the extent that such regulation reflects the clear and unequivocal intent of the Congress in legislation.

(c) Policy letters and statements

The Secretary may not, through policy letters or other statements, establish a rule that is required for compliance with, and eligibility under, this part without following the requirements of Sec. 553 of title 5, United States Code.

(d) Correspondence from Department of Education describing interpretations of this part

(1) In general

The Secretary shall, on a quarterly basis, publish in the Federal Register, and widely disseminate to interested entities through various additional forms of communication, a list of correspondence from the Department of Education received by individuals during the previous quarter that describes the interpretations of the Department of Education of this Act or the regulations implemented pursuant to this Act.

(2) Additional information

For each item of correspondence published in a list under paragraph (1), the Secretary shall identify the topic addressed by the correspondence and shall include such other summary information as the Secretary determines to be appropriate.

(e) Issues of national significance

If the Secretary receives a written request regarding a policy, question, or interpretation under part B of this Act, and determines that it raises an issue of general interest or applicability of national significance to the implementation of part B, the Secretary shall—

(1) include a statement to that effect in any written response;

(2) widely disseminate that response to State educational agencies, local educational agencies, parent and advocacy organizations, and other interested organizations, subject to applicable laws related to confidentiality of information; and

(3) not later than one year after the date on which the Secretary responds to the written request, issue written guidance on such policy, question, or interpretation through such means as the Secretary determines to be appropriate and consistent with law, such as a policy memorandum, notice of interpretation, or notice of proposed rulemaking.

(f) Explanation

Any written response by the Secretary under subsection (e) regarding a policy, question, or interpretation under part B of this Act shall include an explanation that the written response—

(1) is provided as informal guidance and is not legally binding; and

(2) represents the interpretation by the Department of Education of the applicable statutory or regulatory requirements in the context of the specific facts presented.

[Apr. 13, 1970, Pub. I, 91-230, Title VI, Part A, Sec. 607, as added, June 4, 1997, Pub. I, 105-17, Title I, Sec. 607, III Stat. 47.]

Part B—Assistance for Education of All Children with Disabilities

[Publisher's Note: Except as indicated, this Part is immediately effective]

Sec. 1411 Authorization; allotment; use of funds; authorization of appropriations

(a) Grants to States

(1) Purpose of grants

The Secretary shall make grants to States and the outlying areas, and provide funds to the Secretary of the Interior, to assist them to provide special education and related services to children with disabilities in accordance with this part.

(2) Maximum amounts

The maximum amount of the grant a State may receive under this section for any fiscal year is—

(A) the number of children with disabilities in the State who are receiving special education and related services—

(i) aged 3 through 5 if the State is eligible for a grant under Sec. 1419; and

(ii) aged 6 through 21; multiplied by

(B) 40% of the average per-pupil expenditure in public elementary and secondary schools in the United States.

(b) Outlying areas and freely associated states

(1) Funds reserved

From the amount appropriated for any fiscal year under subsection (j), the Secretary shall reserve not more than one percent, which shall be used—

(A) to provide assistance to the outlying areas in accordance with their respective populations of individuals aged 3 through 21; and

(B) for fiscal years 1998 through 2001, to carry out the competition described in paragraph (2), except that the amount reserved to carry out that competition shall not exceed the amount reserved for fiscal year 9196 for the competition under part B of this Act described under the heading "SPECIAL EDUCATION" in Public Law 104-134.

(2) Limitation for freely associated states

(A) Competitive grants

The Secretary shall use funds described in paragraph (1)(B) to award grants, on a competitive basis, to Guam, American Samoa, the Commonwealth of the Northern Mariana Islands, and the freely associated States to carry out the purposes of this part.

(B) Award basis

The Secretary shall award grants under subparagraph (A) on a competitive basis, pursuant to the recommendations of the Pacific Regional Educational Laboratory in Honolulu, Hawaii. Those recommendations shall be made by experts in the field of special education and related services.

(C) Assistance requirements

Any freely associated State that wishes to receive funds under this part shall include, in its application for assistance—

(i) information demonstrating that it will meet all conditions that apply to States under this part;

(ii) an assurance that, notwithstanding any other provision of this part, it will use those funds only for the direct provision of special education and related services to children with disabilities and to enhance its capacity to make a free appropriate public education available to all children with disabilities

(iii) the identity of the source and amount of funds, in addition to funds under this part, that it will make available to ensure that a free appropriate public education is available to all children with disabilities within its jurisdiction; and

(iv) such other information and assurances as the Secretary may require.

(D) Termination of eligibility

Notwithstanding any other provision of law, the freely associated States shall not receive any funds under this part for any program year that begins after September 30, 2001.

(E) Administrative costs

The Secretary may provide not more than five percent of the amount reserved for grants under this paragraph to pay the administrative costs of the Pacific Region Educational Laboratory under subparagraph (B).

(3) Limitation

An outlying area is not eligible for a competitive award under paragraph (2) unless it receives assistance under paragraph (1)(A).

(4) Special rule

The provisions of Public Law 95-134, permitting the consolidation of grants by the outlying areas, shall not apply to funds provided to those areas or to the freely associated States under this section.

(5) Eligibility for discretionary programs

The freely associated States shall be eligible to receive assistance under subpart 2 of part D of this Act until September 30, 2001.

(6) Definition

As used in this subsection, the 'term freely associated States' means the Republic of the Marshall Islands, the Federated States of Micronesia, and the Republic of Palau.

(c) Secretary of the Interior

From the amount appropriated for any fiscal year under subsection (j), the Secretary shall reserve 1.226 percent to provide assistance to the Secretary of the Interior in accordance with subsection (i).

(d) Allocations to States

(1) In general

After reserving funds for studies and evaluations under Sec. 1474(e), and for payments to the outlying areas and the Secretary of the Interior under subsections (b) and (c), the Secretary shall allocate the remaining amount among the States in accordance with paragraph (2) or subsection (e), as the case may be.

(2) Interim formula

Except as provided in subsection (e), the Secretary shall allocate the amount described in paragraph (1) among the States in accordance with Sec. 1411(a)(3), (4), and (5) and (b)(1), (2), and (3) of this Act, as in effect prior to the enactment of the Individuals with Disabilities Education Act Amendments of 1997, except that the determination of the number of children with disabilities receiving special education and related services under such Sec. 1411(a)(3) may, at the State's discretion, be calculated as of the last Friday in October or as of December 1 of the fiscal year for which the funds are appropriated.

(e) Permanent formula

(1) Establishment of base year

The Secretary shall allocate the amount described in subsection (d)(1) among the States in accordance with this subsection for each fiscal year beginning with the first fiscal year for which the amount appropriated under subsection (j) is more than $4,924,672,200.

(2) Use of base year

(A) Definition

As used in this subsection, the term 'base year' means the fiscal year preceding the first fiscal year in which this subsection applies.

(B) Special rule for use of base year amount

If a State received any funds under this section for the base year on the basis of children aged 3 through 5, but does not make a free appropriate public education available to all children with disabilities aged 3 through 5 in the State in any subsequent fiscal year, the Secretary shall compute the State's base year amount, solely for the purpose of calculating the State's allocation in that subsequent year under paragraph (3) or (4), by subtracting the amount allocated to the State for the base year on the basis of those children.

(3) Increase in funds

If the amount available for allocations to States under paragraph (1) is equal to or greater than the amount allocated to the States under this paragraph for the preceding fiscal year, those allocations shall be calculated as follows:

(A)(i) Except as provided in subparagraph (B), the Secretary shall

(I) allocate to each State the amount it received for the base year;

(II) allocate 85 percent of any remaining funds to States on the basis of their relative populations of children aged 3 through 21 who are of the same age as children with disabilities for whom the State ensures the availability of a free appropriate public education under this part; and

(III) allocate 15 percent of those remaining funds to States on the basis of their relative populations of children described in subclause (II) who are living in poverty.

(ii) For the purpose of making grants under this paragraph, the Secretary shall use the most recent population data, including data on children living in poverty, that are available and satisfactory to the Secretary.

(B) Notwithstanding subparagraph (A), allocations under this paragraph shall be subject to the following:

(i) No State's allocation shall be less than its allocation for the preceding fiscal year.

(ii) No State's allocation shall be less than the greatest of—

(I) the sum of—

(aa) the amount it received for the base year; and

(bb) one third of one percent of the amount by which the amount appropriated under subsection (j) exceeds the amount appropriated under this section for the base year;

(II) the sum of—

(aa) the amount it received for the preceding fiscal year; and

(bb) that amount multiplied by the percentage by which the increase in the funds appropriated from the preceding fiscal year exceeds 1.5 percent; or

(III) the sum of—

(aa) the amount it received for the preceding fiscal year; and

(bb) that amount multiplied by 90 percent of the percentage increase in the amount appropriated from the preceding fiscal year.

(iii) Notwithstanding clause (ii), no State's allocation under this paragraph shall exceed the sum of—

(I) the amount it received for the preceding fiscal year; and

(II) that amount multiplied by the sum of 1.5 percent and the percentage increase in the amount appropriated.

(C) If the amount available for allocations under this paragraph is insufficient to pay those allocations in full, those allocations shall be ratably reduced, subject to subparagraph (B)(i).

(4) Decrease in funds

If the amount available for allocations to States under paragraph (1) is less than the amount allocated to the States under this section for the preceding fiscal year, those allocations shall be calculated as follows:

(A) If the amount available for allocations is greater than the amount allocated to the States for the base year, each State shall be allocated the sum of—

(i) the amount it received for the base year; and

(ii) an amount that bears the same relation to any remaining funds as the increase the State received for the preceding fiscal year over the base year bears to the total of all such increases for all States.

(B)(i) If the amount available for allocations is equal to or less than the amount allocated to the States for the base year, each State shall be allocated the amount it received for the base year.

(ii) If the amount available is insufficient to make the allocations described in clause (i), those allocations shall be ratably reduced.

(f) State-level activities

(1) General

(A) Each State may retain not more than the amount described in subparagraph (B) for administration and other State-level activities in accordance with paragraphs (2) and (3).

(B) For each fiscal year, the Secretary shall determine and report to the State educational agency an amount that is 25 percent of the amount the State received under this section for fiscal year 1997, cumulatively adjusted by the Secretary for each succeeding fiscal year by the lesser of—

(i) the percentage increase, if any, from the preceding fiscal year in the State's allocation under this section; or

(ii) the rate of inflation, as measured by the percentage increase, if any, from the preceding fiscal year in the Consumer Price Index For All Urban Consumers, published by the Bureau of Labor Statistics of the Department of Labor.

(C) A State may use funds it retains under subparagraph (A) without regard to—

(i) the prohibition on commingling of funds in Sec.

1412(a)(18)(B); and

(ii) the prohibition on supplanting other funds in Sec. 1412(a)(18)(C).

(2) State administration

(A) For the purpose of administering this part, including Sec. 1419 (including the coordination of activities under this part with, and providing technical assistance to, other programs that provide services to children with disabilities)—

(i) each State may use not more than twenty percent of the maximum amount it may retain under paragraph (1)(A) for any fiscal year or $500,000 (adjusted by the cumulative rate of inflation since fiscal year 1998, as measured by the percentage increase, if any, in the Consumer Price Index For All Urban Consumers, published by the Bureau of Labor Statistics of the Department of Labor), whichever is greater; and

(ii) each outlying area may use up to five percent of the amount it receives under this section for any fiscal year or $35,000, whichever is greater.

(B) Funds described in subparagraph (A) may also be used for the administration of part C of this Act, if the State educational agency is the lead agency for the State under that part.

(3) Other state-level activities

Each State shall use any funds it retains under paragraph (1) and does not use for administration under paragraph (2) for any of the following:

(A) Support and direct services, including technical assistance and personnel development and training.

(B) Administrative costs of monitoring and complaint investigation, but only to the extent that those costs exceed the costs incurred for those activities during fiscal year 1985.

(C) To establish and implement the mediation process required by Sec. 1415(e), including providing for the costs of mediators and support personnel.

(D) To assist local educational agencies in meeting personnel shortages.

(E) To develop a State Improvement Plan under subpart 1 of part D.

(F) Activities at the State and local levels to meet the performance goals established by the State under Sec. 1412(a)(16) and to support implementation of the State Improvement Plan under subpart 1 of part D if the State receives funds under that subpart.

(G) To supplement other amounts used to develop and implement a Statewide coordinated services system designed to improve results for children and families, including children with disabilities and their families, but not to exceed one percent of the amount received by the State under this section. This system shall be coordinated with and, to the extent appropriate, build on the system of coordinated services developed by the State under part C of this Act.

(H) For subgrants to local educational agencies for the purposes described in paragraph (4)(A).

(4)(A) Subgrants to local educational agencies for capacity-building and improvement

In any fiscal year in which the percentage increase in the State's allocation under this section exceeds the rate of inflation (as measured by the percentage increase, if any, from the preceding fiscal year in the Consumer Price Index For All Urban Consumers, published by the Bureau of Labor Statistics of the Department of Labor), each State shall reserve, from its allocation under this section, the amount described in subparagraph (B) to make subgrants

to local educational agencies, unless that amount is less than $100,000, to assist them in providing direct services and in making systemic change to improve results for children with disabilities through one or more of the following:

(i) Direct services, including alternative programming for children who have been expelled from school, and services for children in correctional facilities, children enrolled in State-operated or State-supported schools, and children in charter schools.

(ii) Addressing needs or carrying out improvement strategies identified in the State's Improvement Plan under subpart 1 of part D.

(iii) Adopting promising practices, materials, and technology, based on knowledge derived from education research and other sources.

(iv) Establishing, expanding, or implementing interagency agreements and arrangements between local educational agencies and other agencies or organizations concerning the provision of services to children with disabilities and their families.

(v) Increasing cooperative problem-solving between parents and school personnel and promoting the use of alternative dispute resolution.

(B) Maximum subgrant

For each fiscal year, the amount referred to in subparagraph (A) is—

(i) the maximum amount the State was allowed to retain under paragraph (1)(A) for the prior fiscal year, or for fiscal year 1998, 25 percent of the State's allocation for fiscal year 1997 under this section; multiplied by

(ii) the difference between the percentage increase in the State's allocation under this section and the rate of inflation, as measured by the percentage increase, if any, from the preceding fiscal year in the Consumer Price Index For All Urban Consumers, published by the Bureau of Labor Statistics of the Department of Labor.

(5) Report on use of funds

As part of the information required to be submitted to the Secretary under Sec. 1412, each State shall annually describe—

(A) how amounts retained under paragraph (1) will be used to meet the requirements of this part;

(B) how those amounts will be allocated among the activities described in paragraphs (2) and (3) to meet State priorities based on input from local educational agencies; and

(C) the percentage of those amounts, if any, that will be distributed to local educational agencies by formula.

(g) Subgrants to local educational agencies

(1) Subgrants required

Each State that receives a grant under this section for any fiscal year shall distribute any funds it does not retain under subsection (f) (at least 75 percent of the grant funds) to local educational agencies in the State that have established their eligibility under Sec. 1413, and to State agencies that received funds under Sec. 1414A(a) of this Act for fiscal year 1997, as then in effect, and have established their eligibility under Sec. 1413, for use in accordance with this part.

(2) Allocations to local educational agencies

(A) Interim procedure

For each fiscal year for which funds are allocated to States under subsection (d)(2), each State shall allocate funds under paragraph (1) in accordance with Sec. 1411(d) of this Act, as in effect prior to the enactment of the Individuals with Disabilities Education Act Amendments of 1997.

(B) Permanent procedure

For each fiscal year for which funds are allocated to States under subsection (e), each State shall allocate funds under paragraph (1) as follows:

(i) Base payments

The State shall first award each agency described in paragraph (1) the amount that agency would have received under this section for the base year, as defined in subsection (e)(2)(A), if the State had distributed 75 percent of its grant for that year under Sec. 1411(d), as then in effect.

(ii) Allocation of remaining funds

After making allocations under clause (I), the State shall—

(I) allocate 85 percent of any remaining funds to those agencies on the basis of the relative numbers of children enrolled in public and private elementary and secondary schools within the agency's jurisdiction; and

(II) Allocate 15 percent of those remaining funds to those agencies in accordance with their relative numbers of children living in poverty, as determined by the State educational agency.

(3) Former chapter 1 state agencies

(A) To the extent necessary, the State—

(i) shall use funds that are available under subsection (f)(1)(A) to ensure that each State agency that received fiscal year 1994 funds under subpart 2 of part D of chapter 1 of title I of the Elementary and Secondary Education Act of 1965 receives, from the combination of funds under subsection (f)(1)(A) and funds provided under paragraph (1) of this subsection, an amount equal to—

(I) the number of children with disabilities, aged 6 through 21, to whom the agency was providing special education and related services on December 1 of the fiscal year for which the funds were appropriated, subject to the limitation in subparagraph (B); multiplied by

(II) the per-child amount provided under such subpart for fiscal year 1994; and

(ii) may use those funds to ensure that each local educational agency that received fiscal year 1994 funds under that subpart for children who had transferred from a State-operated or State-supported school or program assisted under that subpart receives, from the combination of funds available under subsection (f)(1)(A) and funds provided under paragraph (1) of this subsection, an amount for each such child, aged 3 through 21 to whom the agency was providing special education and related services on December 1 of the fiscal year for which the funds were appropriated, equal to the per-child amount the agency received under that subpart for fiscal year 1994.

(B) The number of children counted under subparagraph (A)(i)(I) shall not exceed the number of children aged 3 through 21 for whom the agency received fiscal year 1994 funds under subpart 2 of part D of chapter 1 of title I of the Elementary and Secondary Education Act of 1965.

(4) Reallocation of funds

If a State educational agency determines that a local educational agency is adequately providing a free appropriate public education to all children with disabilities residing in the area served by that agency with State and local funds, the State educational agency may reallocate any portion of the funds under this part that are not needed by that local agency to provide a free appropriate public education to other local educational agencies in the State that are not adequately providing special education and related services to all children with disabilities residing in the areas they serve.

(h) Definitions

For the purpose of this section—

(1) the term 'average per-pupil expenditure in public elementary and secondary schools in the United States' means—

(A) without regard to the source of funds—

(i) the aggregate current expenditures, during the second fiscal year preceding the fiscal year for which the determination is made (or, if satisfactory data for that year are not available, during the most recent preceding fiscal year for which satisfactory data are available) of all local educational agencies in the 50 States and the District of Columbia; plus

(ii) any direct expenditures by the State for the operation of those agencies; divided by

(B) the aggregate number of children in average daily attendance to whom those agencies provided free public education during that preceding year; and

(2) the term 'State' means each of the 50 States, the District of Columbia, and the Commonwealth of Puerto Rico.

(i) Use of amounts by Secretary of the Interior

(1) Provision of amounts for assistance

(A) In general

The Secretary of Education shall provide amounts to the Secretary of the Interior to meet the need for assistance for the education of children with disabilities on reservations aged 5 to 21, inclusive, enrolled in elementary and secondary schools for Indian children operated or funded by the Secretary of the Interior. The amount of such payment for any fiscal year shall be equal to 80 percent of the amount allotted under subsection (c) for that fiscal year.

(B) Calculation of number of children

In the case of Indian students aged 3 to 5, inclusive, who are enrolled in programs affiliated with the Bureau of Indian Affairs (hereafter in this subsection referred to as 'BIA') schools and that are required by the States in which such schools are located to attain or maintain State accreditation, and which schools have such accreditation prior to the date of enactment of the Individuals with Disabilities Education Act Amendments of 1991, the school shall be allowed to count those children for the purpose of distribution of the funds provided under this paragraph to the Secretary of the Interior. The Secretary of the Interior shall be responsible for meeting all of the requirements of this part for these children, in accordance with paragraph (2).

(C) Additional requirements

With respect to all other children aged 3 to 21, inclusive, on reservations, the State educational agency shall be responsible for ensuring that all of the requirements of this part are implemented.

(2) Submission of information

The Secretary of Education may provide the Secretary of the Interior amounts under paragraph (1) for a fiscal year only if the Secretary of the Interior submits to the Secretary of Education information that—

(A) demonstrates that the Department of the Interior meets the appropriate requirements, as determined by the Secretary of Education, of Secs. 1412 (including monitoring and evaluation activities) and 1413;

(B) includes a description of how the Secretary of the Interior will coordinate the provision of services under this part with local educational agencies, tribes and tribal organizations, and other private and Federal service providers;

(C) includes an assurance that there are public hearings, adequate notice of such hearings, and an opportunity for comment afforded to members of tribes, tribal governing bodies, and affected local school boards before the adoption of the policies, programs, and procedures described in subparagraph (A);

(D) includes an assurance that the Secretary of the Interior will provide such information as the Secretary of Education may require to comply with Sec. 1418;

(E) includes an assurance that the Secretary of the Interior and the Secretary of Health and Human Services have entered into a memorandum of agreement, to be provided to the Secretary of Education, for the coordination of services, resources, and personnel between their respective Federal, State, and local offices and with State and local educational agencies and other entities to facilitate the provision of services to Indian children with disabilities residing on or near reservations (such agreement shall provide for the apportionment of responsibilities and costs including, but not limited to, child find, evaluation, diagnosis, remediation or therapeutic measures, and (where appropriate) equipment and medical or personal supplies as needed for a child to remain in school or a program); and

(F) includes an assurance that the Department of the Interior will cooperate with the Department of Education in its exercise of monitoring and oversight of this application, and any agreements entered into between the Secretary of the Interior and other entities under this part, and will fulfill its duties under this part. Sec. 1416(a) shall apply to the information described in this paragraph.

(3) *Payments for education and services for Indian children with disabilities aged 3 through 5*

(A) *In general*

With funds appropriated under subsection (j), the Secretary of Education shall make payments to the Secretary of the Interior to be distributed to tribes or tribal organizations (as defined under Sec. 4 of the Indian Self-Determination and Education assistance Act) or consortia of the above to provide for the coordination of assistance for special education and related services for children with disabilities aged 3 through 5 on reservations served by elementary and secondary schools for Indian children operated or by the Department of the Interior. The amount of such payments under subparagraph (B) for any fiscal year shall be equal to 20 percent of the amount allotted under subsection (c).

(B) *Distribution of funds*

The Secretary of the Interior shall distribute the total amount of the payment under subparagraph (A) by allocating to each tribe or tribal organization an amount based on the number of children with disabilities ages 3 through 5 residing on reservations as reported annually, divided by the total of those children served by all tribes or tribal organizations.

(C) *Submission of information*

To receive a payment under this paragraph, the tribe or tribal organization shall submit such figures to the Secretary of the Interior as required to determine the amounts to be allocated under subparagraph (B). This information shall be compiled and submitted to the Secretary of Education.

(D) *Use of funds*

The funds received by a tribe or tribal organization shall be used to assist in child find, screening, and other procedures for the early identification of children aged 3 through 5, parent training, and the provision of direct services. These activities may be carried out directly or through contracts or cooperative agreements with the BIA, local educational agencies, and other public or private nonprofit organizations. The tribe or tribal organization is encour-

aged to involve Indian parents in the development and implementation of these activities. The above entities shall, as appropriate, make referrals to local, State, or Federal entities for the provision of services or further diagnosis.

(E) *Biennial report*

To be eligible to receive a grant pursuant to subparagraph (A), the tribe or tribal organization shall provide to the Secretary of the Interior a biennial report of activities undertaken under this paragraph, including the number of contracts and cooperative agreements entered into, the number of children contacted and receiving services for each year, and the estimated number of children needing services during the 2 years following the one in which the report is made. The Secretary of the Interior shall include a summary of this information on a biennial basis in the report to the Secretary of Education required under this subsection. The Secretary of Education may require any additional information from the Secretary of the Interior.

(F) *Prohibitions*

None of the funds allocated under this paragraph may be used by the Secretary of the Interior for administrative purposes, including child count and the provision of technical assistance.

(4) *Plan for coordination of services*

The Secretary of the Interior shall develop and implement a plan for the coordination of services for all Indian children with disabilities residing on reservations covered under this Act. Such plan shall provide for the coordination of services benefiting these children from whatever source, including tribes, the Indian Health Service, other BIA divisions, and other Federal agencies. In developing the plan, the Secretary of the Interior shall consult with all interested and involved parties. It shall be based on the needs of the children and the system best suited for meeting those needs, and may involve the establishment of cooperative agreements between the BIA, other Federal agencies, and other entities. The plan shall also be distributed upon request to States, State and local educational agencies, and other agencies providing services to infants, toddlers, and children with disabilities, to tribes, and to other interested parties.

(5) *Establishment of advisory board*

To meet the requirements of Sec. 1412(a)(21), the Secretary of the Interior shall establish, not later than 6 months after the date of the enactment of the Individuals with Disabilities Education Act Amendments of 1997, under the BIA, an advisory board composed of individuals involved in or concerned with the education and provision of services to Indian infants, toddlers, children, and youth with disabilities, including Indians with disabilities, Indian parents or guardians of such children, teachers, service providers, State and local educational officials, representatives of tribes or tribal organizations, representatives from State Interagency Coordinating Councils under Sec. 1441 in States having reservations, and other members representing the various divisions and entities of the BIA. The chairperson shall be selected by the Secretary of the Interior. The advisory board shall—

(A) assist in the coordination of services within the BIA and with other local, State, and Federal agencies in the provision of education for infants, toddlers, and children with disabilities;

(B) advise and assist the Secretary of the Interior in the performance of the Secretary's responsibilities described in this subsection;

(C) develop and recommend policies concerning effective inter- and intra-agency collaboration, including modifications to regulations, and the elimination of barriers to inter- and intra-agency programs and activities;

(D) provide assistance and disseminate information on best practices, effective program coordination strategies, and recommendations for improved education programming for Indian infants, toddlers, and children with disabilities; and

(E) provide assistance in the preparation of information required under paragraph (2)(D).

(6) Annual reports

(A) In general

The advisory board established under paragraph (5) shall prepare and submit to the Secretary of the Interior and to the Congress an annual report containing a description of the activities of the advisory board for the preceding year.

(B) Availability

The Secretary of the Interior shall make available to the Secretary of Education the report described in subparagraph (A).

(j) Authorization of appropriations

For the purpose of carrying out this part, other than Sec. 1419, there are authorized to be appropriated such sums as may be necessary.

[20 USC 1411 becomes effective beginning with funds appropriated for fiscal year 9198. Consult former IDEA until this date.]
[Apr. 13, 1970, Pub. I, 91-230, Title VI, Part B, Sec. 611, as added, June 4, 1997, Pub. I. 105-17, Title I, Sec. 611, III Stat. 49.]

Sec. 1412   State eligibility

(a) In general

A State is eligible for assistance under this part for a fiscal year if the State demonstrates to the satisfaction of the Secretary that the State has in effect policies and procedures to ensure that it meets each of the following conditions;

(1) Free appropriate public education

(A) In general

A free appropriate public education is available to all children with disabilities residing in the State between the ages of 3 and 21, inclusive, including children with disabilities who have been suspended or expelled from school.

(B) Limitation

The obligation to make a free appropriate public education available to all children with disabilities does not apply with respect to children:

(i) aged 3 through 5 and 18 through 21 in a State to the extent that is application to those children would be inconsistent with State law or practice, or the order of any court, respecting the provision of public education to children in those age ranges; and

(ii) aged 18 through 21 to the extent that State law does not require that special education and related services under this part be provided to children with disabilities who, in the educational placement prior to their incarceration in an adult correctional facility:

(I) were not actually identified as being a child with a disability under Sec. 1401(3) of this Act; or

(II) did not have an individualized education program under this part.

(2) Full educational opportunity goal

The State has established a goal of providing full educational opportunity to all children with disabilities and a detailed timetable for accomplishing that goal.

(3) Child find

(A) In general

All children with disabilities residing in the State, including children with disabilities attending private schools, regardless of the severity of their disabilities, and who are in need of special education and related services, are identified, located, and evaluated and a practical method is developed and implemented to determine which children with disabilities are currently receiving needed special education and related services.

(B) Construction

Nothing in this Act requires that children be classified by their disability so long as each child who has a disability listed in Sec. 1401 and who, by reason of that disability, needs special education and related services is regarded as a child with a disability under this part.

(4) Individualized education program

An individualized education program, or an individualized family service plan that meets the requirements of Sec. 1436(d), is developed, reviewed, and revised for each child with a disability in accordance with Sec. 1414(d).

[20 USC 1412(a)(4) becomes effective on July 1, 1998. Consult former IDEA until this date.]

(5) Least restrictive environment

(A) In general

To the maximum extent appropriate, children with disabilities, including children in public or private institutions or other care facilities, are educated with children who are not disabled, and special classes, separate schooling, or other removal of children with disabilities from the regular educational environment occurs only when the nature or severity of the disability of a child is such that education in regular classes with the use of supplementary aids and services cannot be achieved satisfactorily.

(B) Additional requirement

(i) In general

If the State uses a funding mechanism by which the State distributes State funds on the basis of the type of setting in which a child is served, the funding mechanism does not result in placements that violate the requirements of subparagraph (A).

(ii) Assurance

If the State does not have policies and procedures to ensure compliance with clause (i), the State shall provide the Secretary an assurance that it will revise the funding mechanism as soon as feasible to ensure that such mechanism does not result in such placements.

(6) Procedural safeguards

(A) In general

Children with disabilities and their parents are afforded the procedural safeguards required by Sec. 1415.

(B) Additional procedural safeguards

Procedures to ensure that testing and evaluation materials and procedures utilized for the purposes of evaluation and placement of children with disabilities will be selected and administered so as not to be racially or culturally discriminatory. Such materials or procedures shall be provided and administered in the child's native language or mode of communication, unless it clearly is not feasible to do so, and no single procedure shall be the sole criterion for determining an appropriate educational program for a child.

(7) Evaluation

Children with disabilities are evaluated in accordance with subsections (a) through (c) of Sec. 1414.

(8) Confidentiality

Agencies in the State comply with Sec. 1417(c) (relating to the confidentiality of records and information).

(9) Transition from part C to preschool programs

Children participating in early-intervention programs assisted under part C, and who will participate in preschool programs assisted under this part, experience a smooth and effective transition to those preschool programs in a manner consistent with Sec. 1437(a)(8). By the third birthday of such a child, an individualized education program or, if consistent with Secs. 1414(d)(2)(B) and 1436(d), an individualized family service plan, has been developed and is being implemented for the child. The local educational agency will participate in transition planning conferences arranged by the designated lead agency under Sec. 1437(a)(8).

(10) Children in private schools

(A) Children enrolled in private schools by their parents

(i) In general

To the extent consistent with the number and location of children with disabilities in the State who are enrolled by their parents in private elementary and secondary schools, provision is made for the participation of those children in the program assisted or carried out under this part by providing for such children special education and related services in accordance with the following requirements, unless the Secretary has arranged for services to those children under subsection(f):

(I) Amounts expended for the provision of those services by a local educational agency shall be equal to a proportionate amount of Federal funds made available under this part.

(II) Such services may be provided to children with disabilities on the premise of private, including parochial, schools, to the extent consistent with law.

(ii) Child-find requirement

The requirements of paragraph (3) of this subsection (relating to child find) shall apply with respect to children with disabilities in the State who are enrolled in private, including parochial, elementary and secondary schools.

(B) Children placed in, or referred to, private schools by public agencies

(i) In general

Children with disabilities in private schools and facilities are provided special education and related services, in accordance with an individualized education program, at no cost to their parents, if such children are placed in, or referred to, such schools or facilities by the State or appropriate local educational agency as the means of carrying out the requirements of this part or any other applicable law requiring the provision of special education and related services to all children with disabilities within such State.

(ii) Standards

In all cases described in clause (I), the State educational agency shall determine whether such schools and facilities meet standards that apply to State and local educational agencies and that children so served have all the rights they would have if served by such agencies.

(C) Payment for education of children enrolled in private schools without consent of or referral by the public agency

(i) In general

Subject to subparagraph (A), this part does not require a local educational agency to pay for the cost of education, including special education and related services, of a child with a disability at a private school or facility if that agency made a free appropriate public education available to the child and the parents elected to place the child in such private school or facility.

(ii) Reimbursement for private school placement

If the parents of a child with a disability, who previously received special education and related services under the authority of a public agency, enroll the child in a private elementary or secondary school without the consent of or referral by the public agency, a court or a hearing officer may require the agency to reimburse the parents for the cost of that enrollment if the court or hearing officer finds that the agency had not made a free appropriate public education available to the child in a timely manner prior to that enrollment.

(iii) Limitation on reimbursement

The cost of reimbursement described in clause (ii) may be reduced or denied—

(I) If—

(aa) at the most recent IEP meeting that the parents attended prior to removal of the child from the public school, the parents did not inform the IEP Team that they were rejecting the placement proposed by the public agency to provide a free appropriate public education to their child, including stating their concerns and their intent to enroll their child in a private school at public expense; or

(bb) 10 business days (including any holidays that occur on a business day) prior to the removal of the child from the public school, the parents did not give written notice to the public agency of the information described in division (aa);

(II) if, prior to the parents' removal of the child from the public school, the public agency informed the parents, through the notice requirements described in Sec. 1415(b)(7), of its intent to evaluate the child (including a statement of the purpose of the evaluation that was appropriate and reasonable), but the parents did not make the child available for such evaluation; or

(III) upon a judicial finding of reasonableness with respect to actions taken by the parents.

(iv) Exception

Notwithstanding the notice requirements in clause (iii)(I), the cost of reimbursement may not be reduced or denied for failure to provide such notice if—

(I) the parent is illiterate and cannot write in English;

(II) compliance with clause (iii)(I) would likely result in physical or serious emotional harm to the child;

(III) the school prevented the parent from providing such notice; or

(IV) the parents had not received notice, pursuant to Sec. 1415, of the notice requirement in clause (iii)(I).

(11) State educational agency responsible for general supervision

(A) In general

The State educational agency is responsible for ensuring that—

(i) the requirements of this part are met; and

(ii) all educational programs for children with disabilities in the State, including all such programs administered by any other State or local agency—

(I) are under the general supervision of individuals in the State who are responsible for educational programs for children with disabilities; and

(II) meet the educational standards of the State educational agency.

(B) Limitation

Subparagraph (A) shall not limit the responsibility of agencies in the State other than the State educational agency to provide, or pay for some or all of the costs of, a free appropriate public education for any child with a disability in the State.

(C) Exception

Notwithstanding subparagraphs (A) and (B), the Governor (or another individual pursuant to State law), consistent with State law, may assign to any public agency in the State the responsibility of ensuring that the requirements of this part are met with respect to children with disabilities who are convicted as adults under State law and incarcerated in adult prisons.

(12) Obligations related to and methods of ensuring services

(A) Establishing responsibility for services

The Chief Executive Officer or designee of the officer shall ensure that an interagency agreement or other mechanism for interagency coordination is in effect between each public agency described in subparagraph (B) and the State educational agency, in order to ensure that all services described in subparagraph (B)(i) that are needed to ensure a free appropriate public education are provided, including the provision of such services during the pendency of any dispute under clause (iii). Such agreement or mechanism shall include the following:

(i) Agency financial responsibility

An identification of, or a method for defining, the financial responsibility of each agency for providing services described in subparagraph (B)(i) to ensure a free appropriate public education to children with disabilities, provided that the financial responsibility of each public agency described in subparagraph (B),including the State Medicaid agency and other public insurers of children with disabilities, shall precede the financial responsibility of the local educational agency (or the State agency responsible for developing the child's IEP).

(ii) Conditions and terms of reimbursement

The conditions, terms, and procedures under which a local educational agency shall be reimbursed by other agencies.

(iii) Interagency disputes

Procedures for resolving interagency disputes (including procedures under which local educational agencies may initiate proceedings) under the agreement or other mechanism to secure reimbursement from other agencies or otherwise implement the provisions of the agreement or mechanism.

(iv) Coordination of services procedures

Policies and procedures for agencies to determine and identify the interagency coordination responsibilities of each agency to promote the coordination and timely and appropriate delivery of services described in subparagraph (B)(i).

(B) Obligation of public agency

(i) In general

If any public agency other than an educational agency is otherwise obligated under Federal or State law or assigned responsibility under State policy or pursuant to subparagraph (A), to provide or pay for any services that are also considered special education or related services (such as, but not limited to, services described in Secs. 1401(1) relating to assistive technology devices, 1401(2) relating to assistive technology services, 1401(22) relating to related services, 1401(29) relating to supplementary aids and services, and 1401(30) relating to transition services) that are necessary for ensuring a free appropriate public education to children with disabilities within the State, such public agency shall fulfill that obligation or responsibility, either directly or through contract or other arrangement.

(ii) Reimbursement for services by public agency

If a public agency other than an educational agency fails to provide or pay for the special education and related services described in clause (i), the local educational agency (or State agency responsible for developing the child's IEP) shall provide or pay for such services to the child. Such local educational agency or State agency may then claim reimbursement for the services from the public agency that failed to provide or pay for such services and such public agency shall reimburse the local educational agency or State agency pursuant to the terms of the interagency agreement or other mechanism described in subparagraph (A)(i) according to the procedures established in such agreement pursuant to subparagraph (A)(ii).

(C) Special rule

The requirements of subparagraph (A) may be met through—

(i) State statute or regulation;

(ii) Signed agreements between respective agency officials that clearly identify the responsibilities of each agency relating to the provision of services; or

(iii) Other appropriate written methods as determined by the Chief Executive Officer of the State or designee of the officer.

(13) Procedural requirements relating to local educational agency eligibility

The State educational agency will not make a final determination that a local educational agency is not eligible for assistance under this part without first affording that agency reasonable notice and an opportunity for a hearing.

(14) Comprehensive system of personnel development

The State has in effect, consistent with the purposes of this Act and with Sec. 1435(a)(8), a comprehensive system of personnel development that is designed to ensure an adequate supply of qualified special education, regular education, and related services personnel that meets the requirements for a State improvement plan relating to personnel development in subsections (b)(2)(B) and (c)(3)(D) of Sec. 1453.

[20 USC 1412(a)(14) becomes effective on July 1, 1998. Consult former IDEA until this date.]

(15) Personnel standards

(A) In general

The State educational agency has established and maintains standards to ensure that personnel necessary to carry out this part are appropriately and adequately prepared and trained.

(B) Standards described

Such standards shall—

(i) be consistent with any State-approved or State-recognized certification, licensing, registration, or other comparable requirements that apply to the professional discipline in which those personnel are providing special education or related services;

(ii) to the extent the standards described in subparagraph (A) are not based on the highest requirements in the State applicable to a specific profession or discipline, the State is taking steps to require retraining or hiring of personnel that meet appropriate professional requirements in the State; and

(iii) allow paraprofessionals and assistants who are appropriately trained and supervised, in accordance with State law, regulations, or written policy, in meeting the requirements of this part to be used to assist in the provision of special education and related services to children with disabilities under this part.

(C) Policy

In implementing this paragraph, a State may adopt a policy

that includes a requirement that local educational agencies in the State make an ongoing good-faith effort to recruit and hire appropriately and adequately trained personnel to provide special education and related services to children with disabilities, including, in a geographic area of the State where there is a shortage of such personnel, the most qualified individuals available who are making satisfactory progress toward completing applicable course work necessary to meet the standards described in subparagraph (B)(i), consistent with State law, and the steps described in subparagraph (B)(ii) within three years.

(16) Performance goals and indicators

The State—

(A) has established goals for the performance of children with disabilities in the State that—

(i) will promote the purposes of this Act, as stated in Sec. 1400(d); and

(ii) are consistent, to the maximum extent appropriate, with other goals and standards for children established by the State;

(B) has established performance indicators the State will use to assess progress toward achieving those goals that, at a minimum, address the performance of children with disabilities on assessments, drop-out rates, and graduation rates;

(C) will, every two years, report to the Secretary and the public on the progress of the State, and of children with disabilities in the State, toward meeting the goals established under subparagraph (A); and

(D) based on its assessment of that progress, will revise its State improvement plan under subpart 1 of part D as may be needed to improve its performance, if the State receives assistance under that subpart.

[20 USC 1412(a)(16) becomes effective on July 1, 1998. Consult former IDEA until this date.]

(17) Participation in assessments

(A) In general

Children with disabilities are included in general State and district-wide assessment programs, with appropriate accommodations, where necessary. As appropriate, the State or local educational agency—

(i) develops guidelines for the participation of children with disabilities in alternate assessments for those children who cannot participate in State and district-wide assessment programs; and

(ii) develops and, beginning not later than July 1, 2000, conducts those alternate assessments.

(B) Reports

The State educational agency makes available to the public, and reports to the public with the same frequency and in the same detail as it reports on the assessment of nondisabled children, the following:

(i) The number of children with disabilities participating in regular assessments.

(ii) The number of those children participating in alternate assessments.

(iii) (I) The performance of those children on regular assessments (beginning not later than July 1, 1998) and on alternate assessments (not later than July 1, 2000), if doing so would be statistically sound and would not result in the disclosure of performance results identifiable to individual children.

(II) Data relating to the performance of children described under subclause (I) shall be disaggregated—

(aa) for assessments conducted after July 1, 1998; and

(bb) for assessments conducted before July 1, 1998, if the State is required to disaggregate such data prior to July 1, 1998.

(18) Supplementation of State, local, and other Federal funds

(A) Expenditures

Funds paid to a State under this part will be expended in accordance with all the provisions of this part.

(B) Prohibition against commingling

Funds paid to a State under this part will not be commingled with State funds.

(C) Prohibition against supplantation and conditions for waiver by Secretary

Except as provided in Sec. 1413, funds paid to a State under this part will be used to supplement the level of Federal, State, and local funds (including funds that are not under the direct control of State or local educational agencies) expended for special education and related services provided to children with disabilities under this part and in no case to supplant such Federal, State, and local funds, except that, where the State provides clear and convincing evidence that all children with disabilities have available to them a free appropriate public education, the Secretary may waive, in whole or in part, the requirements of this subparagraph if the Secretary concurs with the evidence provided by the State.

(19) Maintenance of State financial support

(A) In general

The State does not reduce the amount of State financial support for special education and related services for children with disabilities, or otherwise made available because of the excess costs of educating those children, below the amount of that support for the preceding fiscal year.

(B) Reduction of funds for failure to maintain support

The Secretary shall reduce the allocation of funds under Sec. 1411 for any fiscal year following the fiscal year in which the State fails to comply with the requirement of subparagraph (A) by the same amount by which the State fails to meet the requirement.

(C) Waivers for exceptional or uncontrollable circumstances

The Secretary may waive the requirement of subparagraph (A) for a State, for one fiscal year at a time, if the Secretary determines that—

(i) granting a waiver would be equitable due to exceptional or uncontrollable circumstances such as a natural disaster or a precipitous and unforeseen decline in the financial resources of the State; or

(ii) the State meets the standard in paragraph (18)(C) of this section for a waiver of the requirement to supplement, and not to supplant, funds received under this part.

(D) Subsequent years

If, for any year, a State fails to meet the requirement of subparagraph (A), including any year for which the State is granted a waiver under subparagraph (C), the financial support required of the State in future years under subparagraph (A) shall be the amount that would have been required in the absence of that failure and not the reduced level of the State's support.

(E) Regulations

(i) The Secretary shall, by regulation, establish procedures (including objective criteria and consideration of the results of compliance reviews of the State conducted by the Secretary) for determining whether a grant to waiver under subparagraph (C)(ii).

(ii) The Secretary shall publish proposed regulations under clause (i) not later than 6 months after the date of the enactment of the Individuals with Disabilities Education Act Amendments of 1997, and shall issue final regulations under clause (i) not later than 1 year after such date of enactment.

(20) Public Participation

Prior to the adoption of any policies and procedures needed to comply with this section (including any amendments to such policies and procedures), the State ensures that there are public hearings, adequate notice of the hearings, and an opportunity for comment available to the general public, including individuals with disabilities and parents of children with disabilities.

(21) State advisory panel

(A) In general

The State has established and maintains an advisory panel for the purpose of providing policy guidance with respect to special education and related services for children with disabilities in the State.

(B) Membership

Such advisory panel shall consist of members appointed by the Governor, or any other official authorized under State law to make such appointments, that is representative of the State population and that is composed of individuals involved in, or concerned with, the education of children with disabilities, including—

(i) parents of children with disabilities;

(ii) individuals with disabilities;

(iii) teachers;

(iv) representatives of institutions of higher education that prepare special education and related services personnel;

(v) State and local education officials;

(vi) Administrators of programs for children with disabilities;

(vii) Representatives of other State agencies involved in the financing or delivery of related services to children with disabilities;

(viii) Representatives of private schools and public charter schools;

(ix) At least one representative of a vocational, community, or business organization concerned with the provision of transition services to children with disabilities; and

(x) Representatives from the State juvenile and adult corrections agencies.

(C) Special rule

A majority of the members of the panel shall be individuals with disabilities or parents of children with disabilities.

(D) Duties

The advisory panel shall—

(i) advise the State educational agency of unmet needs within the State in the education of children with disabilities;

(ii) comment publicly on any rules or regulations proposed by the State regarding the education of children with disabilities;

(iii) advise the State educational agency in developing evaluations and reporting on data to the Secretary under Sec. 1418;

(iv) advise the State educational agency in developing corrective action plans to address findings identified in Federal monitoring reports under this part; and

(v) advise the State educational agency in developing and implementing policies relating to the coordination of services for children with disabilities.

(22) Suspension and expulsion rates

(A) In general

The State educational agency examines data to determine if significant discrepancies are occurring in the rate of long-term suspensions and expulsions of children with disabilities—

(i) among local educational agencies in the State; or

(ii) compared to such rates for nondisabled children within such agencies.

(B) Review and revision of policies

If such discrepancies are occurring, the State educational agency reviews and, if appropriate, revises (or requires the affected State or local educational agency to revise) its policies, procedures, and practices relating to the development and implementation of IEPs, the use of behavioral interventions, and procedural safeguards, to ensure that such policies, procedures, and practices comply with this Act.

(b) State educational agency as provider of free appropriate public education or direct services

If the State educational agency provides free appropriate public education to children with disabilities, or provides direct services to such children, such agency—

(1) shall comply with any additional requirements of Sec. 1413(a), as if such agency were a local educational agency; and

(2) may use amounts that are otherwise available to such agency under this part to serve those children without regard to Sec. 1413(a)(2)(A)(i) (relating to excess costs).

(c) Exception for prior State plans

(1) In general

If a State has on file with the Secretary policies and procedures that demonstrate that such State meets any requirement of subsection (a), including any policies and procedures filed under this part as in effect before the effective date of the Individuals with Disabilities Education Act Amendments of 1997, the Secretary shall consider such State to have met such requirement for purposes of receiving a grant under this part.

(2) Modifications made by State

Subject to paragraph (3), an application submitted by a State in accordance with this section shall remain in effect until the State submits to the Secretary such modifications as the State deems necessary. This section shall apply to a modification to an application to the same extent and in the same manner as this section applies to the original plan.

(3) Modifications required by the Secretary

If, after the effective date of the Individuals with Disabilities Education Act Amendments of 1997, the provisions of this Act are amended (or the regulations developed to carry out this Act are amended), or there is a new interpretation of this Act by a Federal court or a State's highest court, or there is an official finding of noncompliance with Federal law or regulations, the Secretary may require a State to modify its application only to the extent necessary to ensure the State's compliance with this part.

(d) Approval by the Secretary

(1) In general

If the Secretary determines that a State is eligible to receive a grant under this part, the Secretary shall notify the State of that determination.

(2) Notice and hearing

The Secretary shall not make a final determination that a State is not eligible to receive a grant under this part until after providing the State—

(A) with reasonable notice; and

(B) with an opportunity for a hearing.

(e) Assistance under other Federal programs

Nothing in this title permits a State to reduce medical and other assistance available, or to alter eligibility, under titles V and

XIX of the Social Security Act with respect to the provision of a free appropriate public education for children with disabilities in the State.

(f) By-pass for children in private schools

(1) In general

If, on the date of enactment of the Education of the Handicapped Act Amendments of 1983, a State educational agency is prohibited by law from providing for the participation in special programs of children with disabilities enrolled in private elementary and secondary schools as required by subsection (a)(10)(A), the Secretary shall, notwithstanding such provision of law, arrange for the provision of services to such children through arrangements which shall be subject to the requirements of such subsection.

(2) Payments

(A) Determination of amounts

If the Secretary arranges for services pursuant to this subsection, the Secretary, after consultation with the appropriate public and private school officials, shall pay to the provider of such services for a fiscal year an amount per child that does not exceed the amount determined by dividing—

(i) the total amount received by the State under this part for such fiscal year; by

(ii) the number of children with disabilities served in the prior year, as reported to the Secretary by the State under Sec. 1418.

(B) Withholding of certain amounts

Pending final resolution of any investigation or complaint that could result in a determination under this subsection, the Secretary may withhold from the allocation of the affected State educational agency the amount the Secretary estimates would be necessary to pay the cost of services described in subparagraph (A).

(C) Period of payments

The period under which payments are made under subparagraph (A) shall continue until the Secretary determines that there will no longer be any failure or inability on the part of the State educational agency to meet the requirements of subsection (a)(10)(A).

(3) Notice and hearing

(A) In general

The Secretary shall not take any final action under this subsection until the State educational agency affected by such action has had an opportunity, for at least 45 days after receiving written notice thereof, to submit written objections and to appear before the Secretary or the Secretary's designee to show cause why such action should not be taken.

(B) Review of action

If a State educational agency is dissatisfied with the Secretary's final action after a proceeding under subparagraph (A), such agency may, not later than 60 days after notice of such action, file with the United States court of appeals for the circuit in which such State is located a petition for review of that action. A copy of the petition shall be forthwith transmitted by the clerk of the court to the Secretary. The Secretary thereupon shall file in the court the record of the proceedings on which the Secretary based the Secretary's action, as provided in Sec. 2112 of title 28, United States Code.

(C) Review of findings of fact

The findings of fact by the Secretary, if supported by substantial evidence, shall be conclusive, but the court, for good cause shown, may remand the case to the Secretary to take further evidence, and the Secretary may thereupon make new or modified findings of fact and may modify the Secretary's previous action, and shall file in the court the record of the further proceedings. Such new or modified findings of fact shall likewise be conclusive if supported by substantial evidence.

(D) Jurisdiction of court of appeals; review by United States Supreme Court

Upon the filing of a petition under subparagraph (B), the United States court of appeals shall have jurisdiction to affirm the action of the Secretary or to set it aside, in whole or in part. The judgement of the court shall be subject to review by the Supreme Court of the United States upon certiorari or certification as provided in Sec. 1254 of title 28, United States Code.

[Apr. 13, 1970, Pub. I, 91-230, Title VI, Part B, Sec. 612, as added, June 4, 1997, Pub. I, 105-17, Title I, Sec. 612, III Stat. 60.]

Sec. 1413 Local educational agency eligibility

(a) In general

A local educational agency is eligible for assistance under this part or a fiscal year if such agency demonstrates to the satisfaction of the State educational agency that it meets each of the following conditions:

(1) Consistency with State policies

The local educational agency, in providing for the education of children with disabilities within its jurisdiction, has in effect policies, procedures, and programs that are consistent with the State policies and procedures established under Sec. 1412.

(2) Use of amounts

(A) In general

Amounts provided to the local educational agency under this part shall be expended in accordance with the applicable provisions of this part and—

(i) shall be used only to pay the excess costs of providing special education related services to children with disabilities;

(ii) shall be used to supplement State, local, and other Federal funds and not to supplant such funds; and

(iii) shall not be used, except as provided in subparagraphs (B) and (C), to reduce the level of expenditures for the education of children with disabilities made by the local educational agency from local funds below the level of those expenditures for the preceding fiscal year.

(B) Exception

Notwithstanding the restriction in subparagraph (A)(iii), a local educational agency may reduce the level of expenditures where such reduction is attributable to—

(i) the voluntary departure, by retirement or otherwise, or departure for just cause, of special education personnel;

(ii) a decrease in the enrollment of children with disabilities;

(iii) the termination of the obligation of the agency, consistent with this part, to provide a program of special education to a particular child with a disability that is an exceptionally costly program, as determined by the State educational agency, because the child—

(I) has left the jurisdiction of the agency;

(II) has reached the age at which the obligation of the agency to provide a free appropriate public education to the child has terminated; or

(III) no longer needs such program of special education; or

(iv) the termination of costly expenditures for long-term purchases, such as the acquisition of equipment or the construction of school facilities.

(C) Treatment of Federal funds in certain fiscal years

(i) Notwithstanding clauses (ii) and (iii) of subparagraph (A), for any fiscal year for which amounts appropriated to carry out Sec. 1411 exceeds $4,100,000,000, a local educational agency may treat as local funds, for the purpose of such clauses, up to 20 percent of the amount of funds it receives under this part that exceeds the amount it received under this part for the previous fiscal year.

(ii) Notwithstanding clause (i), if a State educational agency determines that a local educational agency is not meeting the requirements of this part, the State educational agency may prohibit the local educational agency from treating funds received under this part as local funds under clause (i) for any fiscal year, only if it is authorized to do so by the State constitution or a State statute.

(D) Schoolwide programs under title I of the ESEA

Notwithstanding subparagraph (A) or any other provision of this part, a local educational agency may use funds received under this part for any fiscal year to carry out a schoolwide program under Sec. 1114 of the Elementary and Secondary Education Act of 1965, except that the amount so used in any such program shall not exceed—

(i) the number of children with disabilities participating in the schoolwide program; multiplied by

(ii)(I) the amount received by the local educational agency under this part for that fiscal year; divided by

(II) the number of children with disabilities in the jurisdiction of that agency.

(3) Personnel development

The local educational agency—

(A) shall ensure that all personnel necessary to carry out this part are appropriately and adequately prepared, consistent with the requirements of Sec. 1453(c)(3)(D); and

(B) to the extent such agency determines appropriate, shall contribute to and use the comprehensive system of personnel development of the State established under Sec. 1412(a)(14).

(4) Permissive use of funds

Notwithstanding paragraph (2)(A) or Sec. 1412(a)(18)(B) (relating to commingled funds), funds provided to the local educational agency under this part may be used for the following activities:

(A) Services and aids that also benefit nondisabled children

For the costs of special education and related services and supplementary aids and services provided in a regular class or other education-related setting to a child with a disability in accordance with the individualized education program of the child, even if one or more nondisabled children benefit from such services.

(B) Integrated and coordinated services system

To develop and implement a fully integrated and coordinated services system in accordance with subsection (f).

(5) Treatment of charter schools and their students

In carrying out this part with respect to charter schools that are public schools of the local educational agency, the local educational agency—

(A) serves children with disabilities attending those schools in the same manner as it serves children with disabilities in its other schools; and

(B) provides funds under this part to those schools in the same manner as it provides those funds to its other schools.

(6) Information for State educational agency

The local educational agency shall provide the State educational agency with information necessary to enable the State educational agency to carry out its duties under this part, including, with respect to paragraphs (16) and (17) of Sec. 1412(a), information relating to the performance of children with disabilities participating in programs carried out under this part.

(7) Public information

The local educational agency shall make available to parents of children with disabilities and to the general public all documents relating to the eligibility of such agency under this part.

(b) Exception for prior local plans

(1) In general

If a local educational agency or State agency has on file with the State educational agency policies and procedures that demonstrate that such local educational agency, or such State agency, as the case may be, meets any requirement of subsection (a), including any policies and procedures filed under this part as in effect before the effective date of the Individuals with Disabilities Education Act Amendments of 1997, the State educational agency shall consider such local educational agency or State agency, as the case may be, to have met such requirement for purposes of receiving assistance under this part.

(2) Modification made by local educational agency

Subject to paragraph (3), an application submitted by a local educational agency in accordance with this section shall remain in effect until it submits to the State educational agency such modifications as the local educational agency deems necessary.

(3) Modifications required by State educational agency

If, after the effective date of the Individuals with Disabilities Education Act Amendments of 1997, the provisions of this Act are amended (or the regulations developed to carry out this Act are amended), or there is a new interpretation of this Act by Federal or State courts, or there is an official finding of noncompliance with Federal or State law or regulations, the State educational agency may require a local educational agency to modify its application only to the extent necessary to ensure the local educational agency's compliance with this part or State law.

(c) Notification of local educational agency or State agency in case of ineligibility

If the State educational agency determines that a local educational agency or State agency is not eligible under this section, the State educational agency shall notify the local educational agency or State agency, as the case may be, of that determination and shall provide such local educational agency or State agency with reasonable notice and an opportunity for a hearing.

(d) Local educational agency compliance

(1) In general

If the State educational agency, after reasonable notice and an opportunity for a hearing, finds that a local educational agency or State agency that has been determined to be eligible under this section is failing to comply with any requirement described in subsection (a), the State educational agency shall reduce or shall not provide any further payments to the local educational agency or State agency until the State educational agency is satisfied that the local educational agency or State agency, as the case may be, is complying with that requirement.

(2) Additional requirements

Any State agency or local educational agency in receipt of a notice described in paragraph (1) shall, by means of public notice, take such measures as may be necessary to bring the pendency of an action pursuant to this subsection to the attention of the public within the jurisdiction of such agency.

(3) Consideration

In carrying out its responsibilities under paragraph (1), the State educational agency shall consider any decision made in a hearing held under Sec. 1415 that is adverse to the local educational agency or State agency involved in that decision.

(e) Joint establishment of eligibility

(1) Joint establishment

(A) In general

A State educational agency may require a local educational agency to establish its eligibility jointly with another local educational agency if the State educational agency determines that the local educational agency would be ineligible under this section because the local educational agency would not be able to establish and maintain programs of sufficient size and scope to effectively meet the needs of children with disabilities.

(B) Charter school exception

A State educational agency may not require a charter school that is a local educational agency to jointly establish its eligibility under subparagraph (A) unless it is explicitly permitted to do so under the State's charter school statute.

(2) Amount of payments

If a State educational agency requires the joint establishment of eligibility under paragraph (1), the total amount of funds made available to the affected local educational agencies shall be equal to the sum of the payments that each such local educational agency would have received under Sec. 1411(g) if such agencies were eligible for such payments.

(3) Requirements

Local educational agencies that establish joint eligibility under this subsection shall—

(A) adopt policies and procedures that are consistent with the State's policies and procedures under Sec. 1412(a); and

(B) be jointly responsible for implementing programs that receive assistance under this part.

(4) Requirements for educational service agencies

(A) In general

If an educational service agency is required by State law to carry out programs under this part, the joint responsibilities given to local educational agencies under this subsection shall—

(i) not apply to the administration and disbursement of any payments received by that educational service agency; and

(ii) be carried out only by that educational service agency.

(B) Additional requirement

Notwithstanding any other provision of this subsection, an educational service agency shall provide for the education of children with disabilities in the least restrictive environment, as required by Sec. 1412(a)(5).

(f) Coordinated services system

(1) In general

A local educational agency may not use more than 5 percent of the amount such agency receives under this part for any fiscal year, in combination with other amounts (which shall include amounts other than education funds), to develop and implement a coordinated services system designed to improve results for children and families, including children with disabilities and their families.

(2) Activities

In implementing a coordinated services system under this subsection, a local educational agency may carry out activities that include—

(A) improving the effectiveness and efficiency of service delivery, including developing strategies that promote accountability for results;

(B) service coordination and case management that facilitates the linkage of individualized education programs under this part and individualized family service plans under part C with individualized service plans under multiple Federal and State programs, such as title 1 of the Rehabilitation Act of 1973 (vocational rehabilitation), title XIX of the Social Security Act (Medicaid), and title XVI of the Social Security Act (supplemental security income);

(C) developing and implementing interagency financing strategies for the provision of education, health, mental health, and social services, including transition services and related services under this Act; and

(D) interagency personnel development for individuals working on coordinated services.

(3) Coordination with certain projects under Elementary and Secondary Education Act of 1965

If a local educational agency is carrying out a coordinated services project under title XI of the Elementary and Secondary Education Act of 1965 and a coordinated services project under this part in the same schools, such agency shall use amounts under this subsection in accordance with the requirements of that title.

(g) School-based improvement plan

(1) In general

Each local educational agency may, in accordance with paragraph (2), use funds made available under this part to permit a public school within the jurisdiction of the local educational agency to design, implement, and evaluate a school-based improvement plan that is consistent with the purposes described in Sec. 1451(b) and that is designed to improve educational and transitional results for all children with disabilities and, as appropriate, for other children consistent with subparagraphs (A) and (B) of subsection (a)(4) in that public school.

(2) Authority

(A) In general

A State educational agency may grant authority to a local educational agency to permit a public school described in paragraph (1) (through a school-based standing panel established under paragraph (4)(B)) to design, implement, and evaluate a school-based improvement plan described in paragraph (1) for a period not to exceed 3 years.

(B) Responsibility of local educational agency

If a State educational agency grants the authority described in subparagraph (A), a local educational agency that is granted such authority shall have the sole responsibility of oversight of all activities relating to the design, implementation, and evaluation of any school-based improvement plan that a public school is permitted to design under this subsection.

(3) Plan requirements

A school-based improvement plan described in paragraph (1) shall—

(A) be designed to be consistent with the purposes described in Sec. 1451(b) and to improve educational and transitional results for all children with disabilities and, as appropriate, for other children consistent with subparagraphs (A) and (B) of subsection (a)(4), who attend the school for which the plan is designed and implemented;

(B) be designed, evaluated, and, as appropriate, implemented by a school-based standing panel established in accordance with paragraph (4)(B);

(C) include goals and measurable indicators to assess the progress of the public school in meeting such goals; and

(D) ensure that all children with disabilities receive the services described in the individualized education programs of such children.

(4) Responsibilities of the local educational agency

A local educational agency that is granted authority under paragraph (2) to permit a public school to design, implement, and evaluate a school-based improvement plan shall—

(A) select each school under the jurisdiction of such agency that is eligible to design, implement, and evaluate such a plan;

(B) require each school selected under subparagraph (A), in accordance with criteria established by such local educational agency under subparagraph (C), to establish a school-based standing panel to carry out the duties described in paragraph (3)(B);

(C) establish—

(i) criteria that shall be used by such local educational agency in the selection of an eligible school under subparagraph (A);

(ii) criteria that shall be used by a public school selected under subparagraph (A) in the establishment of a school-based standing panel to carry out the duties described in paragraph (3)(B) and that shall ensure that the membership of such panel reflects the diversity of the community in which the public school is located and includes, at a minimum—

(I) parents of children with disabilities who attend such public school, including parents of children with disabilities from unserved and underserved populations, as appropriate;

(II) special education and general education teachers of such public school;

(III) special education and general education administrators, or the designee of such administrators, of such public school; and

(IV) related services providers who are responsible for providing services to the children with disabilities who attend such public school; and

(iii) criteria that shall be used by such local educational agency with respect to the distribution of funds under this part to carry out this subsection;

(D) disseminate the criteria established under subparagraph (C) to local school district personnel and local parent organizations within the jurisdiction of such local educational agency;

(E) require a public school that desires to design, implement, and evaluate a school-based improvement plan to submit an application at such time, in such manner, and accompanied by such information as such local educational agency shall reasonably require; and

(F) establish procedures for approval by such local educational agency of a school-based improvement plan designed under this subsection.

(5) Limitation

A school-based improvement plan described in paragraph (1) may be submitted to a local educational agency for approval only if a consensus with respect to any matter relating to the design, implementation, or evaluation of the goals of such plan is reached by the school-based standing panel that designed such plan.

(6) Additional requirements

(A) Parental involvements

In carrying out the requirements of this subsection, a local educational agency shall ensure that the parents of children with disabilities are involved in the design, evaluation, and, where appropriate, implementation of school-based improvement plans in accordance with this subsection.

(B) Plan approval

A local educational agency may approve a school-based improvement plan of a public school within the jurisdiction of such agency for a period of 3 years, if—

(i) the approval is consistent with the policies, procedures, and practices established by such local educational agency and in accordance with this subsection; and

(ii) a majority of parents of children who are members of the school-based standing panel, and a majority of other members of the school-based standing panel, that designed such plan agree in writing to such plan.

(7) Extension of plan

If a public school within the jurisdiction of a local educational agency meets the applicable requirements and criteria described in paragraphs (3) and (4) at the expiration of the 3-year approval period described in paragraph (6)(B), such agency may approve a school-based improvement plan of such school for an additional 3-year period.

(h) Direct services by the State educational agency

(1) In general

A State educational agency shall use the payments that would otherwise have been available to a local educational agency or to a State agency to provide special education and related services directly to children with disabilities residing in the area served by that local agency, or for whom that State agency is responsible, if the State educational agency determines that the local education agency or State agency, as the case may be—

(A) has not provided the information needed to establish the eligibility of such agency under this section;

(B) is unable to establish and maintain programs of free appropriate public education that meet the requirements of subsection (a);

(C) is unable or unwilling to be consolidated with one or more local educational agencies in order to establish and maintain such programs; or

(D) has one or more children with disabilities who can best be served by a regional or State program or service-delivery system designed to meet the needs of such children.

(2) Manner and location of education and services

The State educational agency may provide special education and related services under paragraph (1) in such manner and at such locations (including regional or State centers) as the State agency considers appropriate. Such education and services shall be provided in accordance with this part.

(i) State agency eligibility

Any State agency that desires to receive a subgrant for any fiscal year under Sec. 1411(g) shall demonstrate to the satisfaction of the State educational agency that—

(1) all children with disabilities who are participating in programs and projects funded under this part receive a free appropriate public education, and that those children and their parents are provided all the rights and procedural safeguards described in this part; and

(2) the agency meets such other conditions of this section as the Secretary determines to be appropriate.

(j) Disciplinary information

The State may require that a local educational agency include in the records of a child with a disability a statement of any current or previous disciplinary action that has been taken against the child and transmit such statement to the same extent that such disciplinary information is included in, and transmitted with, the student records of nondisabled children. The statement may include a description of any behavior engaged in by the child that required disciplinary action, a description of the disciplinary action taken, and any other information that is relevant to the safety of the child and other individuals involved with the child. If the State adopts such a policy, and the child transfers from one school to another, the transmission of any of the child's records must include both the child's current individualized education program and any such statement of current or previous disciplinary action that has been taken against the child.

[Apr. 13, 1970, Pub. I, 91-230, Title VI, Part B, Sec. 613, as added, June 4, 1997, Pub. I, 105-17, Title I, Sec. 613, III Stat. 73.]

Sec. 1414 Evaluations, eligibility determinations, individualized education programs, and educational placements

(a) Evaluations and reevaluations

(1) Initial evaluations

(A) In general

A State educational agency, other State agency, or local educational agency shall conduct a full and individual initial evaluation, in accordance with this paragraph and subsection (b), before the initial provision of special education and related services to a child with a disability under this part.

(B) Procedures

Such initial evaluation shall consist of procedures—

(i) to determine whether a child is a child with a disability (as defined in Sec. 1401(3)); and

(ii) to determine the educational needs of such child.

(C) Parental consent

(i) In general

The agency proposing to conduct an initial evaluation to determine if the child qualifies as a child with a disability as defined in Sec. 1401(3)(A) or 1401(3)(B) shall obtain an informed consent from the parent of such child before the evaluation is conducted. Parental consent for evaluation shall not be construed as consent for placement for receipt of special education and related services.

(ii) Refusal

If the parents of such child refuse consent for the evaluation, the agency may continue to pursue an evaluation by utilizing the mediation and due process procedures under Sec. 1415, except to the extent inconsistent with State law relating to parental consent.

(2) Reevaluations

A local educational agency shall ensure that a reevaluation of each child with a disability is conducted—

(A) if conditions warrant a reevaluation or if the child's parent or teacher requests a reevaluation, but at least once every 3 years; and

(B) in accordance with subsections (b) and (c).

(b) Evaluation procedures

(1) Notice

The local educational agency shall provide notice to the parents of a child with a disability, in accordance with subsections (b)(3), (b)(4), and (c) of Sec. 1415, that describes any evaluation procedures such agency proposes to conduct.

(2) Conduct of evaluation

In conducting the evaluation, the local educational agency shall—

(A) use a variety of assessment tools and strategies to gather relevant functional and developmental information, including information provided by the parent, that may assist in determining whether the child is a child with a disability and the content of the child's individualized education program, including information related to enabling the child to be involved in and progress in the general curriculum or, for preschool children, to participate in appropriate activities;

(B) not use any single procedure as the sole criterion for determining whether a child is a child with a disability or determining an appropriate educational program for the child; and

(C) use technically sound instruments that may assess the relative contribution of cognitive and behavioral factors, in addition to physical or developmental factors.

(3) Additional requirements

Each local educational agency shall ensure that—

(A) tests and other evaluation materials used to assess a child under this section—

(i) are selected and administered so as not to be discriminatory on a racial or cultural basis; and

(ii) are provided and administered in the child's native language or other mode of communication, unless it is clearly not feasible to do so; and

(B) any standardized tests that are given to the child—

(i) have been validated for the specific purpose for which they are used;

(ii) are administered by trained and knowledgeable personnel; and

(iii) are administered in accordance with any instructions provided by the producer of such tests;

(C) the child is assessed in all areas of suspected disability; and

(D) assessment tools and strategies that provide relevant information that directly assists persons in determining the educational needs of the child are provided.

(4) Determination of eligibility

Upon completion of administration of tests and other evaluation materials—

(A) the determination of whether the child is a child with a disability as defined in Sec. 1401(3) shall be made by a team of qualified professionals and the parent of the child in accordance with paragraph (5); and

(B) a copy of the evaluation report and the documentation of determination of eligibility will be given to the parent.

(5) Special rule for eligibility determination

In making a determination of eligibility under paragraph (4)(A), a child shall not be determined to be a child with a disability if the determinant factor for such determination is lack of instruction in reading or math or limited English proficiency.

(c) Additional requirements for evaluation and reevaluations

(1) Review of existing evaluation data

As part of an initial evaluation (if appropriate) and as part of any reevaluation under this section, the IEP Team described in subsection (d)(1)(B) and other qualified professionals, as appropriate, shall—

(A) review existing evaluation data on the child, including evaluations and information provided by the parents of the child, current classroom-based assessments and observations, and teacher and related services providers observation; and

(B) on the basis of that review, and input from the child's parents, identify what additional data, if any, are needed to determine—

(i) whether the child has a particular category of disability, as described in Sec. 1401(3), or, in case of a reevaluation of a child, whether the child continues to have such a disability;

(ii) the present levels of performance and educational needs of the child;

(iii) whether the child needs special education and related services, or in the case of a reevaluation of a child, whether the child continues to need special education and related services; and

(iv) whether any additions or modifications to the special education and related services are needed to enable the child to meet the measurable annual goals set out in the individualized education program of the child and to participate, as appropriate, in the general curriculum.

(2) Source of data

The local educational agency shall administer such tests and other evaluation materials as may be needed to produce the data identified by the IEP Team under paragraph (1)(B).

(3) Parental consent

Each local educational agency shall obtain informed parental consent, in accordance with subsection (a)(1)(C), prior to conducting any reevaluation of a child with a disability, except that such informed parent consent need not be obtained if the local educational agency can demonstrate that it had taken reasonable measures to obtain such consent and the child's parent has failed to respond.

(4) Requirements if additional data are not needed

If the IEP Team and other qualified professionals, as appropriate, determine that no additional data are needed to determine whether the child continues to be a child with a disability, the local educational agency—

(A) shall notify the child's parents of—

(i) that determination and the reasons for it; and

(ii) the right of such parents to request an assessment to determine whether the child continues to be a child with a disability; and

(B) shall not be required to conduct such an assessment unless requested to by the child's parents.

(5) Evaluations before change in eligibility

A local educational agency shall evaluate a child with a disability in accordance with this section before determining that the child is no longer a child with a disability.

(d) Individualized education programs

(1) Definitions

As used in this title:

(A) Individualized education program

The term 'individualized education program' or 'IEP' means a written statement for each child with a disability that is developed, reviewed, and revised in accordance with this section and that includes—

(i) a statement of the child's present levels of educational performance, including—

(I) how the child's disability affects the child's involvement and progress in the general curriculum; or

(II) for preschool children, as appropriate, how the disability affects the child's participation in appropriate activities;

(ii) a statement of measurable annual goals, including benchmarks or short-term objectives, related to—

(I) meeting the child's needs that result from the child's disability to enable the child to be involved in and progress in the general curriculum; and

(II) meeting each of the child's other educational needs that result from the child's disability;

(iii) a statement of the special education and related services and supplementary aids and services to be provided to the child, or on behalf of the child, and a statement of the program modifications or supports for school personnel that will be provided for the child—

(I) to advance appropriately toward attaining the annual goals;

(II) to be involved and progress in the general curriculum in accordance with clause (I) and to participate in extracurricular and other nonacademic activities; and

(III) to be educated and participate with other children with disabilities and nondisabled children in the activities described in this paragraph;

(iv) an explanation of the extent, if any, to which the child will not participate with nondisabled children in the regular class and in the activities described in clause (iii);

(v)(I) a statement of any individual modifications in the administration of State or districtwide assessments of such student achievement that are needed in order for the child to participate in such assessment; and

(II) if the IEP Team determines that the child will not participate in a particular State or districtwide assessment of student achievement (or part of such an assessment), a statement of—

(aa) why that assessment is not appropriate for the child; and

(bb) how the child will be assessed;

(vi) the projected date for the beginning of the services and modifications described in clause (iii), and the anticipated frequency, location, and duration of those services and modifications;

(vii)(I) beginning at age 14, and updated annually, a statement of the transition service needs of the child under the applicable components of the child's IEP that focuses on the child's courses of study (such as participation in advanced-placement courses or a vocational educational program);

(II) beginning at age 16 (or younger, if determined appropriate by the IEP Team), a statement of needed transition services for the child, including, when appropriate, a statement of the interagency responsibilities or any needed linkages; and

(III) beginning at least one year before the child reaches the age of majority under State law, a statement that the child has been informed of his or her rights under this title, if any, that will transfer to the child on reaching the age of majority under Sec. 1415(m); and

(viii) a statement of—

(I) how the child's progress toward the annual goals described in clause (ii) will be measured; and

(II) how the child's parents will be regularly informed (such as periodic report cards), at least as often as parents are informed of their nondisabled children's progress, of—

(aa) their child's progress toward the annual goals described in clause (ii); and (bb) the extent to which that progress is sufficient to enable the child to achieve the goals by the end of the year.

(B) Individualized education program team

The term 'individualized education program team' or 'IEP Team' means a group of individuals composed of—

(i) the parents of a child with a disability;

(ii) at least one regular education teacher of such child (if the child is, or may be, participating in the regular education environment);

(iii) at least one special education teacher, or where appropriate, at least one special education provider of such child;

(iv) a representative of the local educational agency who—

(I) is qualified to provide, or supervise the provision of, specially designed instruction to meet the unique needs of children with disabilities;

(II) is knowledgeable about the general curriculum; and

(III) is knowledgeable about the availability of resources of the local educational agency;

(v) an individual who can interpret the instructional implications of evaluation results, who may be a member of the team described in clauses (ii) through (vi);

(vi) at the discretion of the parent or the agency, other individuals who have knowledge or special expertise regarding the child, including related services personnel as appropriate; and

(vii) whenever appropriate, the child with a disability.

(2) Requirement that program be in effect

(A) In general

At the beginning of each school year, each local educational agency, State educational agency, or other State agency, as the case may be, shall have in effect, for each child with a disability in its jurisdiction, an individualized education program, as defined in paragraph (1)(A).

(B) Program for child aged 3 through 5

In the case of a child with a disability aged 3 through 5 (or, at the discretion of the State educational agency, a 2 year-old child with a disability who will turn age 3 during the school year), an individualized family service plan that contains the material described in Sec. 1436, and that is developed in accordance with this section, may serve as the IEP of the child if using that plan as the IEP is—

(i) consistent with State policy; and

(ii) agreed to by the agency and the child's parents.

(3) Development of IEP

(A) In general

In developing each child's IEP, the IEP Team, subject to subparagraph (C), shall consider—

(i) the strengths of the child and the concerns of the parents for enhancing the education of their child; and

(ii) the results of the initial evaluation or most recent evaluation of the child.

(B) Consideration of special factors

The IEP Team shall—

(i) in the case of a child whose behavior impedes his or her learning or that of others, consider, when appropriate, strategies, including positive behavioral interventions, strategies, and supports to address that behavior;

(ii) in the case of a child with limited English proficiency, consider the language needs of the child as such needs relate to the child's IEP;

(iii) in the case of a child who is blind or visually impaired, provide for instruction in Braille and the use of Braille unless the IEP Team determines, after an evaluation of the child's reading and writing skills, needs, and appropriate reading and writing media (including an evaluation of the child's future needs for instruction in Braille or the use of Braille), that instruction in Braille or the use of Braille is not appropriate for the child;

(iv) consider the communication needs of the child, and in the case of a child who is deaf or hard of hearing, consider the child's language and communication needs, opportunities for direct communications with peers and professional personnel in the child's language and communication mode, academic level, and full range of needs, including opportunities for direct instruction in the child's language and communication mode; and

(v) consider whether the child requires assistive technology devices and services.

(C) Requirement with respect to regular education teacher

The regular education teacher of the child, as a member of the IEP Team, shall, to the extent appropriate, participate in the development of the IEP of the child, including the determination of appropriate positive behavioral interventions and strategies and the determination of supplementary aids and services, program modifications, and support for school personnel consistent with paragraph (1)(A)(iii).

(4) Review and revision of IEP

(A) In general

The local educational agency shall ensure that, subject to subparagraph (B), the IEP Team—

(i) reviews the child's IEP periodically, but not less than annually to determine whether the annual goals for the child are being achieved; and

(ii) revises the IEP as appropriate to address—

(I) any lack of expected progress toward the annual goals and in the general curriculum, where appropriate;

(II) the results of any reevaluation conducted under this section;

(III) information about the child provided to, or by, the parents, as described in subsection (c)(1)(B);

(IV) the child's anticipated needs; or

(V) other matters.

(B) Requirement with respect to regular education teacher

The regular education teacher of the child, as a member of the IEP Team, shall, to the extent appropriate, participate in the review and revision of the IEP of the child.

(5) Failure to meet transition objectives

If a participating agency, other than the local educational agency, fails to provide the transition services described in the IEP in accordance with paragraph (1)(A)(vii), the local educational agency shall reconvene the IEP Team to identify alternative strategies to meet the transition objectives for the child set out in that program.

(6) Children with disabilities in adult prisons

(A) In general

The following requirements do not apply to children with disabilities who are convicted as adults under State law and incarcerated in adult prisons:

(i) The requirements contained in Sec. 1412(a)(17) and paragraph (1)(A)(v) of this subsection (relating to participation of children with disabilities in general assessments).

(ii) The requirements of subclauses (I) and (II) of paragraph (1)(A)(vii) of this subsection (relating to transition planning and transition services), do not apply with respect to such children whose eligibility under this part will end, because of their age, before they will be released from prison.

(B) Additional requirement

If a child with a disability is convicted as an adult under State law and incarcerated in an adult prison, the child's IEP Team may modify the child's IEP or placement notwithstanding the requirements of Secs. 1412(a)(5)(A) and 1414(d)(1)(A) if the State has demonstrated a bona fide security or compelling penological interest that cannot otherwise be accommodated.

[20 USC 1414(d), except for paragraph 6 concerning children with disabilities in adult prisons, becomes effective on July 1, 1998. Paragraph 6 is effective immediately. Consult former IDEA until this date.]

(e) Construction

Nothing in this section shall be construed to require the IEP Team to include information under one component of a child's IEP that is already contained under another component of such IEP.

(f) Educational placements

Each local educational agency or State educational agency shall ensure that the parents of each child with a disability are members of any group that makes decisions on the educational placement of their child.

[Apr. 13, 1970, Pub. I, 91-230, Title VI, Part B, Sec. 614, as added, June 4, 1997, Pub. I, 105-17, Title I, Sec. 614, III Stat. 81.]

Sec. 1415   Procedural safeguards

(a) Establishment of procedures

Any State educational agency, State agency, or local educational agency that receives assistance under this part shall establish and maintain procedures in accordance with this section to ensure that children with disabilities and their parents are guaranteed procedural safeguards with respect to the provision of free appropriate public education by such agencies.

(b) Types of procedures

The procedures required by this section shall include—

(1) an opportunity for the parents of a child with a disability to examine all records relating to such child and to participate in meetings with respect to the identification, evaluation, and educational placement of the child, and the provision of a free appropriate public education to such child, and to obtain an independent educational evaluation of the child;

(2) procedures to protect the rights of the child whenever the parents of the child are not known, the agency cannot, after reasonable efforts, locate the parents, or the child is a ward of the State, including the assignment of an individual (who shall not be an employee of the State educational agency, the local educational agency, or any other agency that is involved in the education or care of the child) to act as a surrogate for the parents;

(3) written prior notice to the parents of the child whenever such agency—

(A) proposes to initiate or change; or

(B) refuses to initiate or change;

the identification, evaluation, or educational placement of the child, in accordance with subsection (c), or the provision of a free appropriate public education to the child;

(4) procedures designed to ensure that the notice required by paragraph (3) is in the native language of the parents, unless it clearly is not feasible to do so;

(5) an opportunity for mediation in accordance with subsection (e);

(6) an opportunity to present complaints with respect to any matter relating to the identification, evaluation, or educational placement of the child, or the provision of a free appropriate public education to such child;

(7) procedures that require the parent of a child with a disability, or the attorney representing the child, to provide notice (which shall remain confidential)—

(A) to the State educational agency or local educational agency, as the case may be, in the complaint filed under paragraph (6); and

(B) that shall include—

(i) the name of the child, the address of the residence of the child, and the name of the school the child is attending;

(ii) a description of the nature of the problem of the child relating to such proposed initiation or change, including facts relating to such problem; and

(iii) a proposed resolution of the problem to the extent known and available to the parents at the time; and

(8) procedures that require the State educational agency to develop a model form to assist parents in filing a complaint in accordance with paragraph (7).

(c) Content of prior written notice

The notice required by subsection (b)(3) shall include—

(1) a description of the action proposed or refused by the agency;

(2) an explanation of why the agency proposes or refuses to take the action;

(3) a description of any other options that the agency considered and the reasons why those options were rejected;

(4) a description of each evaluation procedure, test, record, or report the agency used as a basis for the proposed or refused action;

(5) a description of any other factors that are relevant to the agency's proposal or refusal;

(6) a statement that the parents of a child with a disability have protection under the procedural safeguards of this part and, if this notice is not an initial referral for evaluation, the means by which a copy of a description of the procedural safeguards can be obtained; and

(7) sources for parents to contact to obtain assistance in understanding the provisions of this part.

(d) Procedural safeguards notice

(1) In general

A copy of the procedural safeguards available to the parents of a child with a disability shall be given to the parents, at a minimum—

(A) upon initial referral for evaluation;

(B) upon each notification of an individualized education program meeting and upon reevaluation of the child; and

(C) upon registration of a complaint under subsection (b)(6).

(2) Contents

The procedural safeguards notice shall include a full explanation of the procedural safeguards, written in the native language of the parents, unless it clearly is not feasible to do so, and written in an easily understandable manner, available under this section and under regulations promulgated by the Secretary relating to—

(A) independent educational evaluation;

(B) prior written notice;

(C) parental consent;

(D) access to educational records;

(E) opportunity to present complaints;

(F) the child's placement during pendency of due process proceedings;

(G) procedures for students who are subject to placement in an interim alternative educational setting;

(H) requirements for unilateral placement by parents of children in private schools at public expense;

(I) mediation;

(J) due process hearings, including requirements for disclosure of evaluation results and recommendations;

(K) State-level appeals (if applicable in that State);

(L) civil actions; and

(M) attorneys' fees

(e) Mediation

(1) In general

Any State educational agency or local educational agency that receives assistance under this part shall ensure that procedures are established and implemented to allow parties to disputes involving any matter described in subsection (b)(6) to resolve such disputes through a mediation process which, at a minimum, shall be available whenever a hearing is requested under subsection (f) or (k).

(2) Requirements

Such procedures shall meet the following requirements:

(A) The procedures shall ensure that the mediation process—

(i) is voluntary on the part of the parties;

(ii) is not used to deny or delay a parent's right to a due process hearing under subsection (f), or to deny any other rights afforded under this part; and

(iii) is conducted by a qualified and impartial mediator who is trained in effective mediation techniques.

(B) A local educational agency or a State agency may establish procedures to require parents who choose not to use the mediation process to meet, at a time and location convenient to the parents, with a disinterested party who is under contract with—

(i) a parent training and information center or community parent resource center in the State established under Sec. 1482 or 1483; or

(ii) an appropriate alternative dispute resolution entity; to encourage the use, and explain the benefits, of the mediation process to the parents.

(C) The State shall maintain a list of individuals who are qualified mediators and knowledgeable in laws and regulations relating to the provision of special education and related services.

(D) The State shall bear the cost of the mediation process, including the costs of meetings described in subparagraph (B).

(E) Each session in the mediation process shall be scheduled in a timely manner and shall be held in a location that is convenient to the parties to the dispute.

(F) An agreement reached by the parties to the dispute in the mediation process shall be set forth in a written mediation agreement.

(G) Discussions that occur during the mediation process shall be confidential and may not be used as evidence in any subsequent due process hearings or civil proceedings and the parties to the mediation process may be required to sign a confidentiality pledge prior to the commencement of such process.

(f) Impartial due process hearing

(1) In general

Whenever a complaint has been received under subsection (b)(6) or (k) of this section, the parents involved in such complaint shall have an opportunity for an impartial due process hearing, which shall be conducted by the State educational agency or by the local educational agency, as determined by State law or by the State educational agency.

(2) Disclosure of evaluations and recommendations

(A) In general

At least 5 business days prior to a hearing conducted pursuant to paragraph (1), each party shall disclose to all other parties all evaluations completed by that date and recommendations based on the offering party's evaluations that the party intends to use at the hearing.

(B) Failure to disclose

A hearing officer may bar any party that fails to comply with subparagraph (A) from introducing the relevant evaluation or recommendation at the hearing without the consent of the other party.

(3) Limitation on conduct of hearing

A hearing conducted pursuant to paragraph (1) may not be conducted by an employee of the State educational agency or the local educational agency involved in the education or care of the child.

(g) Appeal

If the hearing required by subsection (f) is conducted by a local educational agency, any party aggrieved by the findings and decision rendered in such a hearing may appeal such findings and decision to the State educational agency. Such agency shall conduct an impartial review of such decision. The officer conducting such review shall make an independent decision upon completion of such review.

(h) Safeguards

Any party to a hearing conducted pursuant to subsection (f) or (k), or an appeal conducted pursuant to subsection (g), shall be accorded—

(1) the right to be accompanied and advised by counsel and by individuals with special knowledge or training with respect to the problems of children with disabilities;

(2) the right to present evidence and confront, cross-examine, and compel the attendance of witnesses;

(3) the right to a written, or, at the option of the parents, electronic verbatim record of such hearing; and

(4) the right to written, or, at the option of the parents, electronic findings of fact and decisions (which findings and decisions shall be made available to the public consistent with the requirements of Sec. 1417(c) (relating to the confidentiality of data, information, and records) and shall also be transmitted to the advisory panel established pursuant to Sec. 1412(a)(21)).

(i) Administrative procedures

(1) In general

(A) Decision made in hearing

A decision made in a hearing conducted pursuant to subsection (f) or (k) shall be final, except that any party involved in such hearing may appeal such decision under the provisions of subsection (g) and paragraph (2) of this subsection.

(B) Decision made at appeal

A decision made under subsection (g) shall be final, except that any party may bring an action under paragraph (2) of this subsection.

(2) Right to bring civil action

(A) In general

Any party aggrieved by the findings and decision made under subsection (f) or (k) who does not have the right to an appeal under subsection (g), and any party aggrieved by the finding and decision under this subsection, shall have the right to bring a civil action with respect to the complaint presented pursuant to this section, which action may be brought in any State court of competent jurisdiction or in a district court of the United States without regard to amount in controversy.

(B) Additional requirements

In any action brought under this paragraph, the court—

(i) shall receive the records of the administrative proceedings;

(ii) shall hear additional evidence at the request of a party; and

(iii) basing its decision on the preponderance of the evidence, shall grant such relief as the court determines is appropriate.

(3) Jurisdiction of district courts; attorneys' fees

(A) In general

The district courts of the United States shall have jurisdiction of actions brought under this section without regard to the amount in controversy.

(B) Award of attorneys' fees

In any action or proceeding brought under this section, the court, in its discretion, may award reasonable attorneys' fees as part of the costs to the parents of a child with a disability who is the prevailing party.

(C) Determination of amount of attorneys' fees

Fees awarded under this paragraph shall be based on rates prevailing in the community in which the action or proceeding arose for the kind and quality of services furnished. No bonus or multiplier may be used in calculating the fees awarded under this subsection.

(D) Prohibition of attorneys' fees and related costs for certain services

(i) Attorneys' fees may not be awarded and related costs may not be reimbursed in any action or proceeding under this section for services performed subsequent to the time of a written offer of settlement to a parent if—

(I) the offer is made within the time prescribed by Rule 68 of the Federal Rules of Civil Procedure or, in the case of an administrative proceeding, at any time more than ten days before the proceeding begins;

(II) the offer is not accepted within 10 days; and

(III) the court or administrative hearing officer finds that the relief finally obtained by the parents is not more favorable to the parents than the offer of settlement.

(ii) Attorneys' fees may not be awarded relating to any meeting of the IEP Team unless such meeting is convened as a result of an administrative proceeding or judicial action, or, at the discretion of the State, for a mediation described in subsection (e) that this is conducted prior to the filing of a complaint under subsection (b)(6) or (k) of this section.

(E) Exception to prohibition on attorneys' fees and related costs

Notwithstanding subparagraph (D), an award of attorneys' fees and related costs may be made to a parent who is the prevailing party and who was substantially justified in rejecting the settlement offer.

(F) Reduction in amount of attorneys' fees

Except as provided in subparagraph (G), whenever the court finds that—

(i) the parent, during the course of the action or proceeding, unreasonably protracted the final resolution of the controversy;

(ii) the amount of the attorneys' fees otherwise authorized to be awarded unreasonably exceeds the hourly rate prevailing in the community for similar services by attorneys of reasonably comparable skill, reputation, and experience;

(iii) the time spent and legal services furnished were excessive considering the nature of the action or proceeding; or

(iv) the attorney representing the parent did not provide to the school district the appropriate information in the due process complaint in accordance with subsection (b)(7);

the court shall reduce, accordingly, the amount of the attorneys' fees awarded under this section.

(G) Exception to reduction in amount of attorneys' fees

The provisions of subparagraph (F) shall not apply in any action or proceeding if the court finds that the State or local educational agency unreasonably protracted the final resolution of the action or proceeding or there was a violation of this section.

(j) Maintenance of current educational placement

Except as provided in subsection (k)(7), during the pendency of any proceedings conducted pursuant to this section, unless the State or local educational agency and the parents otherwise agree, the child shall remain in the then-current educational placement of such child, or, if applying for initial admission to a public school, shall, with the consent of the parents, be placed in the public school program until all such proceedings have been completed.

(k) Placement in alternative educational setting

(1) Authority of school personnel

(A) School personnel under this section may order a change in the placement of a child with a disability—

(i) to an appropriate interim alternative educational setting, another setting, or suspension, for not more than 10 school days (to the extent such alternatives would be applied to children without disabilities); and

(ii) to an appropriate interim alternative educational setting for the same amount of time that a child without a disability would be subject to discipline, but for not more than 45 days if-

(I) the child carries a weapon to school or to a school function under the jurisdiction of a State or a local educational agency; or

(II) the child knowingly possesses or uses illegal drugs or sells or solicits the sale of a controlled substance while at school or a school function under the jurisdiction of a State or local educational agency.

(B) Either before or not later than 10 days after taking a disciplinary action described in subparagraph (A)—

(i) if the local educational agency did not conduct a functional behavioral assessment and implement a behavioral intervention plan for such child before the behavior that resulted in the suspension described in subparagraph (A), the agency shall convene an IEP meeting to develop an assessment plan to address that behavior; or

(ii) if the child already has a behavioral intervention plan, the IEP Team shall review the plan and modify it, as necessary, to address the behavior.

(2) Authority of hearing officer

A hearing officer under this section may order a change in the placement of a child with a disability to an appropriate interim alternative educational setting for not more than 45 days if the hearing officer—

(A) determines that the public agency has demonstrated by substantial evidence that maintaining the current placement of such child is substantially likely to result in injury to the child or to others;

(B) considers the appropriateness of the child's current placement;

(C) considers whether the public agency has made reasonable efforts to minimize the risk of harm in the child's current placement, including the use of supplementary aids and services; and

(D) determines that the interim alternative educational setting meets the requirements of paragraph (3)(B).

(3) Determination of setting

(A) In general

The alternative educational setting described in paragraph (1)(A)(ii) shall be determined by the IEP Team.

(B) Additional requirements

Any interim alternative educational setting in which a child is placed under paragraph (1) or (2) shall—

(i) be selected so as to enable the child to continue to participate in the general curriculum, although in another setting, and to continue to receive those services and modifications, including those described in the child's current IEP, that will enable the child to meet the goals set out in that IEP; and

(ii) include services and modifications designed to address the behavior described in paragraph (1) or paragraph (2) so that it does not recur.

(4) Manifestation determination review

(A) In general

If a disciplinary action is contemplated as described in paragraph (1) or paragraph (2) for a behavior of a child with a disability described in either of those paragraphs, or if a disciplinary action involving a change of placement for more than 10 days is contemplated for a child with a disability who has engaged in other behavior that violated any rule or code of conduct of the local educational agency that applies to all children—

(i) not later than the date on which the decision to take that action is made, the parents shall be notified of that decision and of all procedural safeguards accorded under this section; and

(ii) immediately, if possible, but in no case later than 10 school days after the date on which the decision to take that action is made, a review shall be conducted of the relationship between the child's disability and the behavior subject to the disciplinary action.

(B) Individuals to carry out review

A review described in subparagraph (A) shall be conducted by the IEP Team and other qualified personnel.

(C) Conduct of review

In carrying out a review described in subparagraph (A), the IEP Team may determine that the behavior of the child was not a manifestation of such child's disability only if the IEP Team—

(i) first considers, in terms of the behavior subject to disciplinary action, all relevant information, including—

(I) evaluation and diagnostic results, including such results or other relevant information supplied by the parents of the child;

(II) observations of the child; and

(III) the child's IEP and placement; and

(ii) then determines that—

(I) in relationship to the behavior subject to disciplinary action, the child's IEP and placement were appropriate and the special education services, supplementary aids and services, and behavior intervention strategies were provided consistent with the child's IEP and placement;

(II) the child's disability did not impair the ability of the child to understand the impact and consequences of the behavior subject to disciplinary action; and

(III) the child's disability did not impair the ability of the child to control the behavior subject to disciplinary action.

(5) Determination that behavior was not manifestation of disability

(A) In general

If the result of the review described in paragraph (4) is a determination, consistent with paragraph (4)(C), that the behavior of the child with a disability was not a manifestation of the child's disability, the relevant disciplinary procedure applicable to children without disabilities may e applied to the child in the same manner in which they would be applied to children without disabilities, except as provided in Sec. 1412(a)(1).

(B) Additional requirement

If the public agency initiates disciplinary procedures applicable to all children, the agency shall ensure that the special education and disciplinary records of the child with a disability are transmitted for consideration by the person or persons making the final determination regarding the disciplinary action.

(6) Parent appeal

(A) In general

(i) If the child's parent disagrees with a determination that the child's behavior was not a manifestation of the child's disability or with any decision regarding placement, the parent may request a hearing.

(ii) The State or local educational agency shall arrange for an expedited hearing in any case described in this subsection when requested by a parent.

(B) Review of decision

(i) In reviewing a decision with respect to the manifestation determination, the hearing officer shall determine whether the public agency has demonstrated that the child's behavior was not a manifestation of such child's disability consistent with the requirements of paragraph (4)(C).

(ii) In reviewing a decision under paragraph (1)(A)(ii) to place the child in an interim alternative educational setting, the hearing officer shall apply the standards set out in paragraph (2).

(7) Placement during appeals

(A) In general

When a parent request a hearing regarding a disciplinary action described in paragraph (1)(A)(ii) or paragraph (2) to challenge the interim alternative educational setting pending the decision of the hearing officer or until the expiration of the time period provided for in paragraph (1)(A)(ii) or paragraph (2), whichever occurs first, unless the parent and the State or local educational agency agree otherwise.

(B) Current placement

If a child is placed in an interim alternative educational setting pursuant to paragraph (1)(A)(ii) or paragraph (2) and school personnel propose to change the child's placement after expiration of the interim alternative placement, during the pendency of any proceeding to challenge the proposed change in placement, the child shall remain in the current placement (the child's placement prior to the interim alternative educational setting), except as provided in subparagraph (C).

(C) Expedited hearing

(i) If school personnel maintain that it is dangerous for the child to be in the current placement (placement prior to removal to the interim alternative education setting) during the pendency of the due process proceedings, the local educational agency may request an expedited hearing.

(ii) In determining whether the child may be placed in the alternative educational setting or in another appropriate placement ordered by the hearing officer, the hearing officer shall apply the standards set out in paragraph (2).

(8) Protections for children not yet eligible for special education and related services.

(A) In general

A child who has not been determined to be eligible for special education and related services under this part and who has engaged in behavior that violated any rule or code of conduct of the local educational agency, including any behavior described in paragraph (1), may assert any of the protections provided for in this part if the local educational agency had knowledge (as determined in accordance with this paragraph) that the child was a child with a disability before the behavior that precipitated the disciplinary action occurred.

(B) Basis of knowledge

A local educational agency shall be deemed to have knowledge that a child is a child with a disability if—

(i) the parent of the child has expressed concern in writing (unless the parent is illiterate or has a disability that prevents compliance with the requirements contained in this clause) to personnel of the appropriate educational agency that the child is in need of special education and related services;

(ii) the behavior or performance of the child demonstrates the need for such services;

(iii) the parent of the child has requested an evaluation of the child pursuant to Sec. 1414; or

(iv) the teacher of the child, or other personnel of the local educational agency, has expressed concern about the behavior or performance of the child to the director of special education of such agency or to other personnel of the agency.

(C) Conditions that apply if no basis of knowledge

(i) In general

If a local educational agency does not have knowledge that a child is a child with a disability (in accordance with subparagraph (B)) prior to taking disciplinary measures against the child, the child may be subjected to the same disciplinary measures as measures applied to children with disabilities who engaged in comparable behaviors consistent with clause (ii).

(ii) Limitations

If a request is made for an evaluation of a child during the time period in which the child is subjected to disciplinary measures under paragraph (1) or (2), the evaluation shall be conducted in an expedited manner. If the child is determined to be a child with a disability, taking into consideration information from the evaluation conducted by the agency and information provided by the parents, the agency shall provide special education and related services in accordance with the provisions of this part, except that, pending the results of the evaluation, the child shall remain in the educational placement determined by school authorities.

(9) Referral to and action by law enforcement and judicial authorities

(A) Nothing in this part shall be construed to prohibit an agency from reporting a crime committed by a child with a disability to appropriate authorities or to prevent State law enforcement and judicial authorities from exercising their responsibilities with regard to the application of Federal and State law to crimes committed by a child with a disability.

(B) An agency reporting a crime committed by a child with a disability shall ensure that copies of the special education and disciplinary records of the child are transmitted for consideration by the appropriate authorities to whom it reports the crime.

(10) Definitions

For purposes of this subsection, the following definitions apply:

(A) Controlled substance

The term 'controlled substance' means a drug or other substance identified under schedules I, II, III, IV, or V in Sec. 202(c) of the Controlled Substances Act (21 U.S.C. 812(c)).

(B) Illegal drug

The 'illegal drug'—

(i) means a controlled substance; but

(ii) does not include such a substance that is legally possessed or used under the supervision of a licensed health-care professional or that is legally possessed or used under any other authority under that Act or under any other provision of Federal law.

(C) Substantial evidence

The term 'substantial evidence' means beyond a preponderance of the evidence.

(D) Weapon

The term 'weapon' has the meaning given the term 'dangerous weapon' under paragraph (2) of the first subsection (g) of Sec. 930 of title 18, United States Code.

(l) Rule of construction

Nothing in this part shall be construed to restrict or limit the rights, procedures, and remedies available under the Constitution, the Americans with Disabilities Act of 1990, title V of the Rehabilitation Act of 1973, or other Federal laws protecting the rights of children with disabilities, except that before the filing of a civil action under such laws seeking relief that is also available under this part, the procedures under subsections (f) and (g) shall be exhausted to the same extent as would be required had the action been brought under this part.

(m) Transfer of parental rights at age of majority

(1) In general

A State that receives amounts from a grant under this part may provide that, when a child with a disability reaches the age of majority under State law (except for a child with a disability who has been determined to be incompetent under State law)—

(A) the public agency shall provide any notice required by this section to both the individual and the parents;

(B) all other rights accorded to parents under this part transfer to the child;

(C) the agency shall notify the individual and the parents of the transfer of rights; and

(D) all rights accorded to parents under this part transfer to children who are incarcerated in an adult or juvenile Federal, State, or local correctional institution.

(2) Special rule

If, under State law, a child with a disability who has reached the age of majority under State law, who has not been determined to be incompetent, but who is determined not to have the ability to provide informed consent with respect to the educational program of the child, the State shall establish procedures for appointing the parent of the child, or if the parent is not available, another appropriate individual, to represent the educational interests of the child throughout the period of eligibility of the child under this part. [Apr. 13, 1970, Pub. I, 91-230, Title VI, part B, Sec. 615, as added, June 4, 1997, Pub. I, 105-17, Title I, Sec. 615, III Stat. 88.]

Sec. 1416   Withholding and judicial review

(a) Withholding of payments

(1) In general

Whenever the Secretary, after reasonable notice and opportunity for hearing to the State educational agency involved (and to any local educational agency or State agency affected by any failure described in subparagraph (B)), finds—

(A) that there has been a failure by the State to comply substantially with any provision of this part; or

(B) that there is a failure to comply with any condition of a local educational agency's or State agency's eligibility under this part, including the terms of any agreement to achieve compliance with this part within the timelines specified in the agreement; the Secretary shall, after notifying the State educational agency, withhold, in whole or in part, any further payments to the State under this part, or refer the matter for appropriate enforcement action, which may include referral to the Department of Justice.

(2) Nature of withholding

If the Secretary withholds further payments under paragraph (1), the Secretary may determine that such withholding will be limited to programs or projects, or portions thereof, affected by the failure, or under this part to specified local educational agencies or State agencies affected by the failure. Until the Secretary is satisfied that there is no longer any failure to comply with the provisions of this part, as specified in subparagraph (A) or (B) of paragraph (1), payments to the State under this part shall be withheld in whole or in part, or payments by the State educational agency under this part shall be limited to local educational agencies and State agencies whose actions did not cause or were not involved in the failure, as the case may be. Any State educational agency, State agency, or local educational agency that has received notice under paragraph (1) shall, by means of a public notice, take such measures as may be necessary to bring the pendency of an action pursuant to this subsection to the attention of the public within the jurisdiction of such agency.

(b) Judicial review

(1) In general

If any State is dissatisfied with the Secretary's final action with respect to the eligibility of the State under Sec. 1412, such State may, not later than 60 days after notice of such action, file with the United States court of appeals for the circuit in which such State is located a petition for review of that action. A copy of the petition shall be forthwith transmitted by the clerk of the court to the Secretary. The Secretary thereupon shall file in the court the record of the proceedings upon which the Secretary's action was based, as provided in Sec. 2112 of title 28, United States Code.

(2) Jurisdiction; review by United States Supreme Court

Upon the filing of such petition, the court shall have jurisdiction to affirm the action of the Secretary or to set it aside, in whole or in part. The judgement of the court shall be subject to review b the Supreme Court upon certiorari or certification as provided in Sec. 1254 of title 28, United States Code.

(3) Standards of review

The findings of fact by the Secretary, if supported by substantial evidence, shall be conclusive, but the court, for good cause shown, may remand the case to the Secretary to take further evidence, and the Secretary may thereupon make new or modified findings of fact and may modify the Secretary's previous action, and shall file in the court the record of the further proceedings. Such new or modified findings of fact shall likewise be conclusive if supported by substantial evidence.

(c) Divided state agency responsibility

For purposes of this section, where responsibility for ensuring that the requirements of this part are met with respect to children with disabilities who are convicted as adults under State law and incarcerated in adult prisons is assigned to a public agency other than the State educational agency pursuant to Sec. 1412(a)(11)(C), the Secretary, in instances where the Secretary finds that the failure to comply substantially with the provisions of this part are related to a failure by the public agency, shall take appropriate corrective action to ensure compliance with this part, except—

(1) any reduction or withholding of payments to the State is proportionate to the total funds allotted under Sec. 1411 to the State as the number of eligible children with disabilities in adult prisons under the supervision of the other public agency is proportionate to the number of eligible individuals with disabilities in the State under the supervision of the State educational agency; and

(2) any withholding of funds under paragraph (1) shall be limited to the specific agency responsible for the failure to comply with this part.

[Apr. 13, 1970, Pub. I, 91-230, Title VI, Part B, Sec. 616, as added, June 4, 1997, Pub. I, 105-17, Title I, Sec. 616, III, Stat. 99.]

Sec. 1417   Administration

(a) Responsibilities of Secretary

In carrying out this part, the Secretary shall—

(1) cooperate with, and (directly or by grant or contract) furnish technical assistance necessary to, the State in matters relating to—

(A) the education of children with disabilities; and

(B) carrying out this part; and

(2) provide short-term training programs and institutes.

(b) Rules and regulations

In carrying out the provisions of this part, the Secretary shall issue regulations under this Act only to the extent that such regulations are necessary to ensure that there is compliance with the specific requirements of this Act.

(c) Confidentiality

The Secretary shall take appropriate action, in accordance with the provisions of Sec. 444 of the General Education Provisions Act (20 U.S.C. 1232g), to ensure the protection of the confidentiality of any personally identifiable data, information, and records collected or maintained by the Secretary and by State and local educational agencies pursuant to the provisions of this part.

(d) Personnel

The Secretary is authorized to hire qualified personnel necessary to carry out the Secretary's duties under subsection (a) and under Secs. 1418, 1461, and 1473 (or their predecessor authorities through October 1, 1997) without regard to the provisions of title 5, United States Code, relating to appointments in the competitive service and without regard to chapter 51 and subchapter III of chapter 53 of such title relating to classification and general schedule pay rates, except that no more than twenty such personnel shall be employed at any time.

[20 USC 1417 will become effective on October 1, 1997. Consult former IDEA until this date.]

[Apr. 13, 1970, Pub. I, 91-230, Title VI, Part B, Sec. 617, as added, June 4, 1997, Pub. I, 105-17, Title I, Sec. 617, III Stat. 100.]

Sec. 1418   Program Information

(a) In general

Each State that receives assistance under this part, and the Secretary of the Interior, shall provide data each year to the Secretary—

(1)(A) on—

(i) the number of children with disabilities, by race, ethnicity, and disability category, who are receiving a free appropriate public education;

(ii) the number of children with disabilities, by race and ethnicity, who are receiving early intervention services;

(iii) the number of children with disabilities, by race, ethnicity, and disability category, who are participating in regular education;

(iv) the number of children with disabilities, by race, ethnicity, and disability category, who are in separate classes, separate schools or facilities, or public or private residential facilities;

(v) the number of children with disabilities, by race, ethnicity, and disability category, who, for each year of age from age 14 to 21, stopped receiving special education and related services because of program completion or other reasons and the reasons why those children stopped receiving special education and related services;

(vi) the number of children with disabilities, by race and ethnicity, who, from birth through age two, stopped receiving early intervention services because of program completion or for other reasons; and

(vii)(I) the number of children with disabilities, by race, ethnicity, and disability category, who under subparagraphs (A)(ii) and (B) of Sec. 1415(k)(1), are removed to an interim alternative educational setting;

(II) the acts or items precipitating those removals; and

(III) the number of children with disabilities who are subject to long-term suspensions or expulsions; and

(B) on the number of infants and toddlers, by race and ethnicity, who are at risk of having substantial developmental delays (as described in Sec. 1432), and who are receiving early intervention services under part C; and

(2) on any other information that may be required by the Secretary.

(b) Sampling

The Secretary may permit States and the Secretary of the Interior to obtain the data described in subsection (a) through sampling.

(c) Disproportionality

(1) In general

Each State that receives assistance under this part, and the Secretary of the Interior, shall provide for the collection and examination of data to determine if significant disproportionality based on race is occurring in the State with respect to—

(A) the identification of children as children with disabilities, including the identification of children as children with disabilities in accordance with a particular impairment described in Sec. 1401(3); and

(B) the placement in particular educational settings of such children.

(2) Review and revision of policies, practices, and procedures

In the case of a determination of significant disproportionality with respect to the identification of children as children with disabilities, or the placement in particular educational settings of such children, in accordance with paragraph (1), the State or the Secretary of the Interior, as the case may be, shall provide for the review and, if appropriate, revision of the policies, procedures, and practices used in such identification or placement to ensure that such policies, procedures, and practices comply with the requirements of this Act.

[20 USC 1418 becomes effective on July 1, 1998. Consult former IDEA until this date.]

[Apr. 13, 1970, Pub. I, 91-230, Title VI, Part B, Sec. 618, as added, June 4, 1997, Pub. I, 105-17, Title I, Sec. 618, III Stat. 101.]

Sec. 1419   Preschool grants

(a) In general

The Secretary shall provide grants under this section to assist States to provide special education and related services, in accordance with this part—

(1) to children with disabilities aged 3 to 5, inclusive; and

(2) at the State's discretion, to 2-year-old children with disabilities who will turn 3 during the school year.

(b) Eligibility

A State shall be eligible for a grant under this section if such State—

(1) is eligible under Sec. 1412 to receive a grant under this part; and

(2) makes a free appropriate public education available to all children with disabilities, aged 3 through 5, residing in the State.

(c) Allocations to states

(1) In general

After reserving funds for studies and evaluations under Sec. 1474(e), the Secretary shall allocate the remaining amount among the States in accordance with paragraph (2) or (3), as the case may be.

(2) Increase in funds

If the amount available for allocations to States under paragraph (1) is equal to or greater than the amount allocated to the States under this section for the preceding fiscal year, those allocations shall be calculated as follows:

(A)(i) Except as provided in subparagraph (B), the Secretary shall—

(I) allocate to each State the amount it received for fiscal year 1997;

(II) allocate 85 percent of any remaining funds to States on the basis of their relative populations of children aged 3 through 5; and

(III) allocate 15 percent of those remaining funds to States on the basis of their relative populations of all children aged 3 through 5 who are living in poverty.

(ii) For the purpose of making grants under this paragraph, the Secretary shall use the most recent population data, including data on children living in poverty, that are available and satisfactory to the Secretary.

(B) Notwithstanding subparagraph (A), allocations under this paragraph shall be subject to the following;

(i) No State's allocation shall be less than the greatest of—

(I) the sum of—

(aa) the amount it received for fiscal year 1997; and

(bb) one third of one percent of the amount by which the amount appropriated under subsection (j) exceeds the amount appropriated under this section for fiscal year 1997;

(II) the sum of—

(aa) the amount it received for the preceding fiscal year; and

(bb) that amount multiplied by the percentage by which the increase in the funds appropriated from the preceding fiscal year exceeds 1.5 percent; or

(III) the sum of—

(aa) the amount it received for the preceding fiscal year; and

(bb) that amount multiplied by 90 percent of the percentage increase in the amount appropriated from the preceding fiscal year.

(iii) Notwithstanding clause (ii), no State's allocation under this paragraph shall exceed the sum of—

(I) the amount it received for the preceding fiscal year; and

(II) that amount multiplied by the sum of 1.5 percent and the percentage increase in the amount appropriated.

(C) If the amount available for allocations under this paragraph is insufficient to pay those allocations in full, those allocations shall be ratably reduced, subject to subparagraph (B)(i).

(3) Decrease in funds

If the amount available for allocations to States under paragraph (1) is less than the amount allocated to the States under this section for the preceding fiscal year, those allocations shall be calculated as follows:

(A) If the amount available for allocations is greater than the amount allocated to the States for fiscal year 1997, each State shall be allocated the sum of—

(i) the amount it received for fiscal year 1997; and

(ii) an amount that bears the same relation to any remaining funds as the increase the State received for the preceding fiscal year over fiscal year 1997 bears to the total of all such increases for all States.

(B) If the amount available for allocations is equal to or less than the amount allocated to the States for fiscal year 1997, each State shall be allocated the amount it received for that year, ratably reduced, if necessary.

(4) Outlying areas

The Secretary shall increase the fiscal year 1998 allotment of each outlying area under Sec. 1411 by at least the amount that that area received under this section for fiscal year 1997.

(d) Reservations for state activities

(1) In general

Each State may retain not more than the amount described in paragraph (2) for administration and other State-level activities in accordance with subsections (e) and (f).

(2) Amount described

For each fiscal year, the Secretary shall determine and report to the State educational agency an amount that is 25 percent of the amount the State received under this section for fiscal year 1997, cumulatively adjusted by the Secretary for each succeeding fiscal year by the lesser of—

(A) the percentage increase, if any, from the preceding fiscal year in the State's allocation under this section; or

(B) the percentage increase, if any, from the preceding fiscal year in the Consumer Price Index For All Urban Consumers published by the Bureau of Labor Statistics of the Department of Labor.

(e) State administration

(1) In general

For the purpose of administering this section (including the coordination of activities under this part with, and providing technical assistance to, other programs that provide services to children with disabilities) a State may use not more than 20 percent of the maximum amount it may retain under subsection (d) for any fiscal year.

(2) Administration of part C

Funds described in paragraph (1) may also be used for the administration of part C of this Act, if the State educational agency is the lead agency for the State under that part.

(f) Other state-level activities

Each State shall use any funds it retains under subsection (d) and does not use for administration under subsection (e)—

(1) for support services (including establishing and implementing the mediation process required by Sec. 1415(e)), which may benefit children with disabilities younger than 3 or older than 5 as long as those services also benefit children with disabilities aged 3 through 5;

(2) for direct services for children eligible for services under this section;

(3) to develop a State improvement plan under subpart 1 of part D;

(4) for activities at the State and local levels to meet the performance goals established by the State under Sec. 1412(a)(16) and to support implementation of the State improvement plan under subpart 1 of part D if the State receives funds under that subpart; or

(5) to supplement other funds used to develop and implement a Statewide coordinated services system designed to improve results for children and families, including children with disabilities and their families, but not to exceed one percent of the amount received by the State under this section for a fiscal year.

(g) Subgrants to local educational agencies

(1) Subgrants required

Each State that receives a grant under this section for any fiscal year shall distribute any of the grant funds that it does not reserve under subsection (d) to local educational agencies in the State that have established their eligibility under Sec. 1413, as follows:

(A) Base payments

The State shall first award each agency described in paragraph (1) the amount that agency would have received under this section for fiscal year 1997 if the State had distributed 75 percent of its grant for that year under Sec. 1419(c)(3), as then in effect.

(B) Allocation of remaining funds

After making allocations under subparagraph (A), the State shall—

(i) allocate 85 percent of any remaining funds to those agencies on the basis of the relative numbers of children enrolled in public and private elementary and secondary schools within the agency's jurisdiction; and

(ii) allocate 15 percent of those remaining funds to those agencies in accordance with their relative numbers of children living in poverty, as determined by the State educational agency.

(2) Reallocation of funds

If a State educational agency determines that a local educational agency is adequately providing a free appropriate public education to all children with disabilities aged 3 through 5 residing in the area served by that agency with State and local funds, the State educational agency may reallocate any portion of the funds under this section that are not needed by that local agency to provide a free appropriate public education to other local educational agencies in the State that are not adequately providing special education and related services to all children with disabilities aged 3 through 5 residing in the areas they serve.

(h) Part C inapplicable

Part C of this Act does not apply to any child with a disability receiving a free appropriate public education, in accordance with this part, with funds received under this section.

(i) Definition

For the purpose of this section, the term 'State' means each of the 50 States, the District of Columbia, and the Commonwealth of Puerto Rico.

(j) Authorization of appropriations

For the purpose of carrying out this section, there are authorized to be appropriated to the Secretary $500,000,000 for fiscal year 1998 and such sums as may be necessary for each subsequent fiscal year.

[20 USC 1419 becomes effective beginning with funds appropriated for fiscal year 1998. Consult former IDEA until this date.]
[Apr. 13, 1970, Pub. I, 91-230, Title VI, Part B, Sec. 619, as added, June 4, 1997, Pub. I, 105-17, Title I, Sec. 619, III Stat. 102.]

Part C–Infants and Toddlers with Disabilities

[Publishers Note: The entirety of Part C of the IDEA will take effect on July 1, 1998. Consult part H of former IDEA until this date.]

Sec. 1431   Findings and policy

(a) Findings

The Congress finds that there is an urgent and substantial need—

(1) to enhance the development of infants and toddlers with disabilities and to minimize their potential for developmental delay;

(2) to reduce the educational costs to our society, including our Nation's schools, by minimizing the need for special education and related services after infants and toddlers with disabilities reach school age;

(3) to minimize the likelihood of institutionalization of individuals with disabilities and maximize the potential for their independently living in society;

(4) to enhance the capacity of families to meet the special needs of their infants and toddlers with disabilities; and

(5) to enhance the capacity of State and local agencies and service providers to identify, evaluate, and meet the needs of historically underrepresented populations, particularly minority, low-income, inner-city, and rural populations.

(b) Policy

It is therefore the policy of the United States to provide financial assistance to States—

(1) to develop and implement a statewide, comprehensive, coordinated, multidisciplinary, interagency system that provides early intervention services for infants and toddlers with disabilities and their families;

(2) to facilitate the coordination of payment for early intervention services from Federal, State, local, and private sources (including public and private insurance coverage);

(3) to enhance their capacity to provide quality early intervention services being provided to infants and toddlers with disabilities and their families; and

(4) to encourage States to expand opportunities for children under 3 years of age who would be at risk of having substantial developmental delay if they did not receive early intervention services.
[Apr. 13, 1970, Pub. I, 91-230, Title VI, Part C, Sec. 631, as added, June 4, 1997, Pub. I, 105-17, Title I, Sec. 631, III Stat. 106.]

Sec. 1432   Definitions

As used in this part:

(1) At-risk infant or toddler

The term 'at-risk infant or toddler' means an individual under 3 years of age who would be at risk of experiencing a substantial developmental delay if early intervention services were not provided to the individual.

(2) Council

The term 'council' means a State interagency coordinating council established under Sec. 1441.

(3) Developmental delay

The term 'developmental delay', when used with respect to an individual residing in a State, has the meaning given such term by the State under Sec. 1435(a)(1).

(4) Early intervention services

The term 'early intervention services' means developmental services that—

(A) are provided under public supervision;

(B) are provided at no cost except where Federal or State law provides for a system of payments by families, including a schedule of sliding fees;

(C) are designed to meet the developmental needs of an infant or toddler with a disability in any one or more of the following areas—

(i) physical development;

(ii) cognitive development;

(iii) communication development;

(iv) social or emotional development; or

(v) adaptive development;

(D) meet the standards of the State in which they are provided, including the requirements of this part;

(E) include—

(i) family training, counseling, and home visits;

(ii) special instruction;

(iii) speech-language pathology and audiology services;

(iv) occupational therapy;

(v) physical therapy;

(vi) psychological services;

(vii) service coordination services;

(viii) medical services only for diagnostic or evaluation purposes;

(ix) early identification, screening, and assessment services;

(x) health services necessary to enable the infant or toddler to benefit from the other early intervention services;

(xi) social work services;

(xii) vision services;

(xiii) assistive technology devices and assistive technology services; and

(xiv) transportation and related costs that are necessary to enable an infant or toddler and the infant's or toddler's family to receive another service described in this paragraph;

(F) are provided by qualified personnel, including—

(i) special educators;

(ii) speech-language pathologists and audiologists;

(iii) occupational therapists;

(iv) physical therapists;

(v) psychologists;

(vi) social workers;

(vii) nurses;

(viii) nutritionists;

(ix) family therapists;

(x) orientation and mobility specialists; and

(xi) pediatricians and other physicians;

(G) to the maximum extent appropriate, are provided in natural environments, including the home, and community settings in which children without disabilities participate; and

(H) are provided in conformity with an individualized family service plan adopted in accordance with Sec. 1436.

(5) Infant or toddler with a disability

The term 'infant or toddler with a disability'—

(A) means an individual under 3 years of age who needs early intervention services because the individual

(i) is experiencing developmental delays, as measured by appropriate diagnostic instruments and procedures in one or more of the areas of cognitive development, physical development, communication development, social or emotional development, and adaptive development; or

(ii) has a diagnosed physical or mental condition which has a high probability of resulting in developmental delay; and

(B) may also include, at a State's discretion, at-risk infants and toddlers.

[Apr. 13, 1970, Pub. I, 91-230, Title VI, Part C, Sec. 632, as added, June 4, 1997, Pub. I, 105-17, Title I, Sec. 632, III Stat. 106.]

Sec. 1433 General authority

The Secretary shall, in accordance with this part, make grants to States (from their allotments under Sec. 1443) to assist each State to maintain and implement a statewide, comprehensive, coordinated, multidisciplinary, interagency system to provide early intervention services for infants and toddlers with disabilities and their families.

[Apr. 13, 1970, Pub. I, 91-230, Title VI, Part C, Sec. 633, as added, June 4, 1997, Pub. I, 105-17, Title I, Sec. 633, III Stat. 108.]

Sec. 1434 Eligibility

In order to be eligible for a grant under Sec. 1433, a State shall demonstrate to the Secretary that the State—

(1) has adopted a policy that appropriate early intervention services are available to all infants and toddlers with disabilities in the State and their families, including Indian infants and toddlers with disabilities and their families residing on a reservation geographically located in the State; and

(2) has in effect a statewide system that meets the requirements of Sec. 1435.

[Apr. 13, 1970, Pub. I, 91-230, Title VI, Part C, Sec. 634, as added, June 4, 1997, Pub. I, 105-17, Title I, Sec. 634, III Stat. 108.]

Sec. 1435 Requirements for statewide system

(a) In general

A statewide system described in Sec. 1433 shall include, at a minimum, the following components:

(1) A definition of the term 'developmental delay' to be used

by the State in carrying out programs under this part.

(2) A State policy that is in effect and that ensures that appropriate early intervention services are available to all infants and toddlers with disabilities and their families, including Indian infants and toddlers and their families residing on a reservation geographically located in the State.

(3) A timely, comprehensive, multidisciplinary evaluation of the functioning of each infant or toddler with a disability in the State, and a family-directed identification of the needs of each family of such an infant or toddler, to appropriately assist in the development of the infant or toddler.

(4) For each infant or toddler with a disability in the State, an individualized family service plan in accordance with Sec. 1436, including service coordination services in accordance with such service plan.

(5) A comprehensive child find system, consistent with part B, including a system for making referrals to service providers that includes timelines and provides for participation by primary referral sources.

(6) A public awareness program focusing on early identification of infants and toddlers with disabilities, including the preparation and dissemination by the lead agency designated or established under paragraph (10) to all primary referral sources, especially hospitals and physicians, of information for parents on the availability of early intervention services, and procedures for determining the extent to which such sources disseminate such information to parents of infants and toddlers.

(7) A central directory which includes information on early intervention services, resources, and experts available in the State and research and demonstration projects being conducted in the State.

(8) A comprehensive system of personnel development, including the training of paraprofessionals and the training of primary referral sources respecting the basic components of early intervention services available in the State, that is consistent with the comprehensive system of personnel development described in Sec. 1412(a)(14) and may include—

(A) implementing innovative strategies and activities for the recruitment and retention of early education service providers;

(B) promoting the preparation of early intervention providers who are fully and appropriately qualified to provide early intervention services under this part;

(C) training personnel to work in rural and inner-city areas; and

(D) training personnel to coordinate transition services for infants and toddlers served under this part from an early intervention program under this part to preschool or other appropriate services.

(9) Subject to subsection (b), policies and procedures relating to the establishment and maintenance of standards to ensure that personnel necessary to carry out this part are appropriately and adequately prepared and trained, including—

(A) the establishment and maintenance of standards which are consistent with any State-approved or recognized certification, licensing, registration, or other comparable requirements which apply to the area in which such personnel are providing early intervention services; and

(B) to the extent such standards are not based on the highest requirements in the State applicable to a specific profession or discipline, the steps the State is taking to require the retraining or hiring of personnel that meet appropriate professional requirements in the State; except that nothing in this part, including this paragraph, prohibits the use of paraprofessionals and assistants who are appropriately trained and supervised, in accordance with State law, regulations, or written policy, to assist in the provision of early intervention services to infants and toddlers with disabilities under this part.

(10) A single line of responsibility in a lead agency designated or established by the Governor for carrying out—

(A) the general administration and supervision of programs and activities receiving assistance under Sec. 1433, and the monitoring of programs and activities used by the State to carry out this part, whether or not such programs or activities are receiving assistance made available under Sec. 1433, to ensure that the State complies with this part;

(B) the identification and coordination of all available resources within the State from Federal, State, local, and private sources;

(C) the assignment of financial responsibility in accordance with Sec. 1437(a)(2) to the appropriate agencies;

(D) the development of procedures to ensure that services are provided to infants and toddlers with disabilities and their families under this part in a timely manner pending the resolution of any disputes among public agencies or service providers;

(E) the resolution of intra- and interagency disputes; and

(F) the entry into formal interagency agreements that define the financial responsibility of each agency for paying for early intervention services (consistent with State law) and procedures for resolving disputes and that include all additional components necessary to ensure meaningful cooperation and coordination.

(11) A policy pertaining to the contracting or making of other arrangements with service providers to provide early intervention services in the State, consistent with the provisions of this part, including the contents of the application used and the conditions of the contract or other arrangements.

(12) A procedure for securing timely reimbursements of funds used under this part in accordance with Sec. 1440(a).

(13) Procedural safeguards with respect to programs under this part, as required by Sec. 1439.

(14) A system for compiling data requested by the Secretary under Sec. 1418 that relates to this part.

(15) A State interagency coordinating council that meets the requirements of Sec. 1441.

(16) Policies and procedures to ensure that, consistent with Sec. 1436(d)(5)—

(A) to the maximum extent appropriate, early intervention services are provided in natural environments; and

(B) the provision of early intervention services for any infant or toddler occurs in a setting other than a natural environment only when early intervention cannot be achieved satisfactorily for the infant or toddler in a natural environment.

(b) Policy

In implementing subsection (a)(9), a State may adopt a policy that includes making ongoing good-faith efforts to recruit and hire appropriately and adequately trained personnel to provide early intervention services to infants and toddlers with disabilities, including, in a geographic area of the State where there is a shortage of such personnel, the most qualified individuals available who are making satisfactory progress toward completing applicable course work necessary to meet the standards described in subsection (a)(9), consistent with State law within 3 years.

[Apr. 13, 1970, Pub. I, 91-230, Title VI, Part C, Sec. 635, as added, June 4, 1997, Pub. I, 105-17, Title I, Sec. 635, III Stat. 108.]

Sec. 1436   Individualized family service plan

(a) Assessment and program development

A statewide system described in Sec. 1433 shall provide, at a minimum, for each infant or toddler with a disability, and the infant's or toddler's family, to receive—

(1) a multidisciplinary assessment of the unique strengths and needs of the infant or toddler and the identification of services appropriate to meet such needs;

(2) a family-directed assessment of the resources, priorities, and concerns of the family and the identification of the supports and services necessary to enhance the family's capacity to meet the developmental needs of the infant or toddler; and

(3) a written individualized family service plan developed by a multidisciplinary team, including the parents, as required by subsection (e).

(b) Periodic review

The individualized family service plan shall be evaluated once a year and the family shall be provided a review of the plan at 6-month intervals (or more often where appropriate based on infant or toddler and family needs).

(c) Promptness after assessment

The individualized family service plan shall be developed within a reasonable time after the assessment required by subsection (a)(1) is completed. With the parents' consent, early intervention services may commence prior to the completion of the assessment.

(d) Content of plan

The individualized family service plan shall be in writing and contain—

(1) a statement of the infant's or toddler's present levels of physical development, cognitive development, communication development, social or emotional development, and adaptive development, based on objective criteria;

(2) a statement of the family's resources, priorities, and concerns relating to enhancing the development of the family's infant or toddler with a disability;

(3) a statement of the major outcomes expected to be achieved for the infant or toddler and the family, and the criteria, procedures, and timelines used to determine the degree to which progress toward achieving the outcomes is being made and whether modifications or revisions of the outcomes or services are necessary;

(4) a statement of specific early intervention services necessary to meet the unique needs of the infant or toddler and the family, including the frequency, intensity, and method of delivering services;

(5) a statement of the natural environments in which early intervention services shall appropriately be provided, including a justification of the extent, if any, to which the services will not be provided in a natural environment;

(6) the projected dates for initiation of services and the anticipated duration of the services;

(7) the identification of the service coordinator from the profession most immediately relevant to the infant's or toddler's or family's needs (or who is otherwise qualified to carry out all applicable responsibilities under this part) who will be responsible for the implementation of the plan and coordination with other agencies and persons; and

(8) steps to be taken to support transition of the toddler with a disability to preschool or other appropriate services.

(e) Parental consent

The contents of the individualized family service plan shall be fully explained to the parents and informed written consent from the parents shall be obtained prior to the provision of early intervention services described in such plan. If the parents do not provide consent with respect to a particular early intervention service, then the early intervention services to which consent is obtained shall be provided.

[Apr. 13, 1970, Pub. I, 91-230, Title VI, Part C, Sec. 636, as added, June 4, 1997, Pub. I, 105-17, Title I, Sec. 636, III Stat. 111.]

Sec. 1437   State application and assurances

(a) Application

A State desiring to receive a grant under Sec. 1433 shall submit an application to the Secretary at such time and in such manner as the Secretary may reasonably require. The application shall contain—

(1) a designation of the lead agency in the State that will be responsible for the administration of funds provided under Sec. 1433;

(2) a designation of an individual or entity responsible for assigning financial responsibility among appropriate agencies;

(3) information demonstrating eligibility of the State under Sec. 1434, including—

(A) information demonstrating to the Secretary's satisfaction that the State has in effect the statewide system required by Sec. 1433; and

(B) a description of services to be provided to infants and toddlers with disabilities and their families through the system;

(4) if the State provides services to at-risk infants and toddlers through the system, a description of such services;

(5) a description of the uses for which funds will be expended in accordance with this part;

(6) a description of the procedure used to ensure that resources are made available under this part for all geographic areas within the State;

(7) a description of State policies and procedures that ensure that, prior to the adoption by the State of any other policy or procedure necessary to meet the requirements of this part, there are public hearings, adequate notice of the hearings, and an opportunity for comment available to the general public, including individuals with disabilities and parents of infants and toddlers with disabilities;

(8) a description of the policies and procedures to be used—

(A) to ensure a smooth transition for toddlers receiving early intervention services under this part to preschool or other appropriate services, including a description of how—

(i) the families of such toddlers will be included in the transition plans required by subparagraph (C); and

(ii) the lead agency designated or established under Sec. 1435(a)(10) will—

(I) notify the local educational agency for the area in which such a child resides that the child will shortly reach the age of eligibility for preschool services under part B, as determined in accordance with State law;

(II) in the case of a child who may be eligible for such preschool services, with the approval of the family of the child, convene a conference among the lead agency, the family, and the local educational agency at least 90 days (and at the discretion of all such parties, up to 6 months) before the child is eligible for the preschool services, to discuss any such services that the child may receive; and

(III) in the case of a child who may not be eligible for such preschool services, with the approval of the family, make reasonable efforts to convene a conference among the lead agency, the family, and providers of other appropriate services for children who are not eligible for preschool services under part B, to discuss the appropriate services that the child may receive;

(B) to review the child's program options for the period from the child's third birthday through the remainder of the school year; and

(C) to establish a transition plan; and

(9) such other information and assurances as the Secretary may reasonably require.

(b) Assurances

The application described in subsection (a)—

(1) shall provide satisfactory assurance that Federal funds made available under Sec. 1443 to the State will be expended in accordance with this part;

(2) shall contain an assurance that the State will comply with the requirements of Sec. 1440;

(3) shall provide satisfactory assurance that the control of funds provided under Sec. 1443, and title to property derived from those funds, will be in a public agency for the uses and purposes provided in this part and that a public agency will administer such funds and property;

(4) shall provide for—

(A) making such reports in such form and containing such information as the Secretary may require to carry out the Secretary's functions under this part; and

(B) keeping such records and affording such access to them as the Secretary may find necessary to ensure the correctness and verification of those reports and proper disbursement of Federal funds under this part;

(5) provide satisfactory assurance that Federal funds made available under Sec. 1443 to the State—

(A) will not be commingled with State funds; and

(B) will be used so as to supplement the level of State and local funds expended for infants and toddlers with disabilities and their families and in no case to supplant those State and local funds;

(6) shall provide satisfactory assurance that fiscal control and fund accounting procedures will be adopted as may be necessary to ensure proper disbursement of, and accounting for, Federal funds paid under Sec. 1443 to the State;

(7) shall provide satisfactory assurance that policies and procedures have been adopted to ensure meaningful involvement of underserved groups, including minority, low-income, and rural families, in the planning and implementation of all the requirements of this part; and

(8) shall contain such other information and assurances as the Secretary may reasonably require by regulation.

(c) Standard for disapproval of application

The Secretary may not disapprove such an application unless the Secretary determines, after notice and opportunity for a hearing, that the application fails to comply with the requirements of this section.

(d) Subsequent state application

If a State has on file with the Secretary a policy, procedure, or assurance that demonstrates that the State meets a requirement of this section, including any policy or procedure filed under part H (as in effect before July 1, 1998), the Secretary shall consider the State to have met the requirement for purposes of receiving a grant under this part.

(e) Modification of application

An application submitted by a State in accordance with this section shall remain in effect until the State submits to the Secretary such modifications as the State determines necessary. This section shall apply to a modification of an application to the same extent and in the same manner as this section applies to the original application.

(f) Modifications required by the Secretary

The Secretary may require a State to modify its application under this section, but only to the extent necessary to ensure the State's compliance with this part, if—

(1) an amendment is made to this Act, or a Federal regulation issued under this Act;

(2) a new interpretation of this Act is made by a Federal court or the State's highest court; or

(3) an official finding of noncompliance with Federal law or regulations is made with respect to the State.

[Apr. 13, 1970, Pub. I, 91-230, Title VI, Part C, Sec. 637, as added, June 4, 1997, Pub. I, 105-17, Title I, Sec. 637, III, Stat. 112.]

Sec. 1438   Uses of funds

In addition to using funds provided under Sec. 1433 to maintain and implement the statewide system required by such section, a State may use such funds—

(1) for direct early intervention services for infants and toddlers with disabilities, and their families, under this part that are not otherwise funded through other public or private sources;

(2) to expand and improve on services for infants and toddlers and their families under this part that are otherwise available;

(3) to provide free appropriate public education, in accordance with part B, to children with disabilities from their 3rd birthday to the beginning of the next school year; and

(4) in any State that does not provide services for at-risk infants and toddlers under Sec. 1437(a)(4), to strengthen the statewide system by initiating, expanding, or improving collaborative efforts related to at-risk infants and toddlers, including establishing linkages with appropriate public or private community-based organizations, services, and personnel for the purposes of—

(A) identifying and evaluating at-risk infants and toddlers;

(B) making referrals of the infants and toddlers identified and evaluated under subparagraph (A); and

(C) conducting periodic follow-up on each such referral to determine if the status of the infant or toddler involved has changed with respect to the eligibility of the infant or toddler for services under this part.

[Apr. 13, 1970, Pub. I, 91-230, Title VI, Part C, Sec. 638, as added, June 4, 1997, Pub. I, 105-17, Title I, Sec. 638, III Stat. 114.]

Sec. 1439   Procedural safeguards

(A) Minimum procedures

The procedural safeguards required to be included in a statewide system under Sec. 1435(a)(13) shall provide, at a minimum, the following:

(1) The timely administrative resolution of complaints by parents. Any party aggrieved by the findings and decision regarding an administrative complaint shall have the right to bring a civil action with respect to the complaint in any State court of competent jurisdiction or in a district court of the United States without regard to the amount in controversy. In any action brought under this paragraph, the court shall receive the records of the administrative proceedings, shall hear additional evidence at the request of a party, and, basing its decision on the preponderance of the evidence, shall grant such relief as the court determines is appropriate.

(2) The right to confidentiality of personally identifiable information, including the right of parents to written notice of and written consent to the exchange of such information among agencies consistent with Federal and State law.

(3) The right of the parents to determine whether they, their infant or toddler, or other family members will accept or decline any early intervention service under this part in accordance with State law without jeopardizing other early intervention services under this part.

(4) The opportunity for parents to examine records relating to assessment, screening, eligibility determinations, and the development and implementation of the individualized family service plan.

(5) Procedures to protect the rights of the infant or toddler whenever the parents of the infant or toddler are not known or cannot be found or the infant or toddler is a ward of the State, including the assignment of an individual (who shall not be an employee of the State lead agency, or other State agency, and who shall not be any person, or any employee of a person, providing early intervention services to the infant or toddler or any family member of the infant or toddler) to act as a surrogate for the parents.

(6) Written prior notice to the parents of the infant or toddler with a disability whenever the State agency or service provider proposes to initiate or change or refuses to initiate or change the identification, evaluation, or placement of infant or toddler with a disability, or provision of appropriate early intervention services to infant or toddler.

(7) Procedures designed to ensure that the notice required by paragraph (6) fully informs the parents, in the parents' native language, unless it clearly is not feasible to do so, of all procedures available pursuant to this section.

(8) The right of parents to use mediation in accordance with Sec. 1415(e), except that—

(A) any reference in the section to a State educational agency shall be considered to be a reference to a State's lead agency established or designated under Sec. 1435(a)(10);

(B) any reference in the section to a local educational agency shall be considered to be a reference to a local service provider or the State's lead agency under this part, as the case may bee; and

(C) any reference in the section to the provision of free appropriate public education to children with disabilities shall be considered to be a reference to the provision of appropriate early intervention services to infants and toddlers with disabilities.

(b) Services during pendency of proceedings

During the pendency of any proceeding or action involving a complaint by the parents of an infant or toddler with a disability, unless the State agency and the parents otherwise agree, the infant or toddler shall continue to receive the appropriate early intervention services currently being provided or, if applying for initial services, shall receive the services not in dispute.

[Apr. 13, 1970, Pub. I, 91-230, Title VI, Part C, Sec. 639, as added, June 4, 1997,Pub. I, 105-17, Title I, Sec. 639, III Stat. 115.]

Sec. 1440 Payor of last resort

(a) Nonsubstitution

Funds provided under Sec. 1443 may not be used to satisfy a financial commitment for services that would have been paid for from another public or private source, including any medical program administered by the Secretary of Defense, but for the enactment of this part, except that whenever considered necessary to prevent a delay in the receipt of appropriate early intervention services by an infant, toddler, or family in a timely fashion, funds provided under Sec. 1443 may be used to pay the provider of services ending reimbursement from the agency that has ultimate responsibility for the payment.

(b) Reduction of other benefits

Nothing in this part shall be construed to permit the State to reduce medical or other assistance available or to alter eligibility under title V of the Social Security Act (relating to maternal and child health) or title XIX of the Social Security Act (relating to Medicaid for infants or toddlers with disabilities) within the State.

[Apr. 13, 1970, Pub. I, 91-230, Title VI, Part C, Sec. 640, as added, June 4, 1997,Pub. I, 105-17, Title I, Sec. 640, III Stat. 116.]

Sec. 1441 State Interagency Coordinating Council

(a) Establishment

(1) In general

A State that desires to receive financial assistance under this part shall establish a State interagency coordinating council.

(2) Appointment

The council shall be appointed by the Governor. In making appointments to the council, the Governor shall ensure that the membership of the council reasonably represents the population of the State.

(3) Chairperson

The Governor shall designate a member of the council to serve as the chairperson of the council, or shall require the council to so designate such a member. Any member of the council who is a representative of the lead agency designated under Sec. 1435(a)(10) may not serve as the chairperson of the council.

(b) Composition

(1) In general

The council shall be composed as follows:

(A) Parents

At least 20% of the members shall be parents of infants or toddlers with disabilities or children with disabilities aged 12 or younger, with knowledge of, or experience with, programs for infants and toddlers with disabilities. At least one such member shall be a parent of an infant or toddler with a disability or a child with a disability aged 6 or younger.

(B) Service providers

At least 20 percent of the members shall be public or private providers of early intervention services.

(C) State legislature

At least one member shall be from the State legislature.

(D) Personnel preparation

At least one member shall be involved in personnel preparation.

(E) Agency for early intervention services

At least one member shall be from each of the State agencies involved in the provision of, or payment for, early intervention services to infants and toddlers with disabilities and their families and shall have sufficient authority to engage in policy planning and implementation on behalf of such agencies.

(F) Agency for preschool services

At least one member shall be from the State educational agency responsible for preschool services to children with disabilities and shall have sufficient authority to engage in policy planning and implementation on behalf of such agency.

(G) Agency for health insurance

At least one member shall be from the agency responsible for the State governance of health insurance.

(H) Head Start agency

At least one representative from a Head Start agency or program in the State.

(I) Child care agency

At least one representative from a State agency responsible for child care.

(2) Other members

The council may include other members selected by the Governor, including a representative from the Bureau of Indian Affairs, or where there is no BIA-operated or BIA-funded school, from the Indian Health Service or the tribe or tribal council.

(c) Meeting

The council shall meet at least quarterly and in such places as it deems necessary. The meetings shall be publicly announced, and, to the extent appropriate, open and accessible to the general public.

(d) Management authority

Subject to the approval of the Governor, the council may prepare and approve a budget using funds under this part to conduct hearings and forums, to reimburse members of the council for reasonable and necessary expenses for attending council meetings and performing council duties (including child care for parent representatives), to pay compensation to a member of the council if the member is not employed or must forfeit wages from other employment when performing official council business, to hire staff, and to obtain the services of such professional, technical, and clerical personnel as may be necessary to carry out its functions under this part.

(e) Functions of council

(1) Duties

The council shall—

(A) advise and assist the lead agency designated or established under Sec. 1435(a)(10) in the performance of the responsibilities set forth in such section, particularly the identification of the sources of fiscal and other support for services for early intervention programs, assignment of financial responsibility to the appropriate agency, and the promotion of the interagency agreements;

(B) advise and assist the lead agency in the preparation of applications and amendments thereto;

(C) advise and assist the State educational agency regarding the transition of toddlers with disabilities to preschool and other appropriate services; and

(D) prepare and submit an annual report to the Governor and to the Secretary on the status of early intervention programs for infants and toddlers with disabilities and their families operated within the State.

(2) Authorized activity

The council may advise and assist the lead agency and the State educational agency regarding the provision of appropriate services for children from birth through age 5. The council may advise appropriate agencies in the State with respect to the integration of services for infants and toddlers with disabilities and at-risk infants and toddlers and their families, regardless of whether at-risk infants and toddlers are eligible for early intervention services in the State.

(f) Conflict of interests

No member of the council shall cast a vote on any matter that would provide direct financial benefit to that member or otherwise give the appearance of a conflict of interest under State law.
[Apr. 13, 1970, Pub. I, 91-230, Title VI, Part C, Sec. 641, as added, June 4, 1997, Pub. I, 105-17, Title I, Sec. 641, III Stat. 116.]

Sec. 1442   Federal administration

Secs. 1416, 1417, and 1418 shall, to the extent not inconsistent with this part, apply to the program authorized by this part, except that—

(1) any reference in such sections to a State educational agency shall be considered to be a reference to a State's lead agency established or designated under Sec. 1435(a)(10);

(2) any reference in such sections to a local educational agency, educational service agency, or a State agency shall be considered to be a reference to an early intervention service provider under this part; and

(3) any reference to the education of children with disabilities or the education of all children with disabilities shall be considered to be a reference to the provision of appropriate early intervention services to infants and toddlers with disabilities.
[Apr. 13, 1970, Pub. I, 91-230, Title VI, Part C, Sec. 642, as added, June 4, 1997, Pub. I, 105-17, Title I, Sec. 642, III Stat. 118.]

Sec. 1443   Allocation of funds

(a) Reservation of funds for outlying areas

(1) In general

From the sums appropriated to carry out this part for any fiscal year, the Secretary may reserve up to one percent for payments to Guam, American Samoa, the Virgin Islands, and the Commonwealth of the Northern Mariana Islands in accordance with their respective needs.

(2) Consolidation of funds

The provisions of Public Law 95-134, permitting the consolidation of grants to the outlying areas, shall not apply to funds those areas receive under this part.

(b) Payments to Indians

(1) In general

The Secretary shall, subject to this subsection, make payments to the Secretary of the Interior to be distributed to tribes, tribal organizations (as defined under Sec. 4 of the Indian Self-Determination and Education Assistance Act), or consortia of the above entities for the coordination of assistance in the provision of early intervention services by the States to infants and toddlers with disabilities and their families on reservations served by elementary and secondary schools for Indian children operated or funded by the Department of the Interior. The amount of such payment for any fiscal year shall be 1.25% of the aggregate of the amount available to all States under this part for such fiscal year.

(2) Allocation

For each fiscal year, the Secretary of the Interior shall distribute the entire payment received under paragraph (1) by providing to each tribe, tribal organization, or consortium an amount based on the number of infants and toddlers residing on the reservation, as determined annually, divided by the total of such children served by all tribes, tribal organizations, or consortia.

(3) Information

To receive a payment under this subsection, the tribe, tribal organization, or consortium shall submit such information to the Secretary of the Interior as is needed to determine the amounts to be distributed under paragraph (2).

(4) Use of funds

The funds received by a tribe, tribal organization, or consortium shall be used to assist States in child-find, screening, and other procedures for the early identification of Indian children under 3 years of age and for parent training. Such funds may also be used to provide early intervention services in accordance with this part. Such activities may be carried out directly or through contracts or cooperative agreements with the BIA, local educational agencies, and other public or private nonprofit organizations. The tribe, tribal organization, or consortium is encouraged to involve Indian parents in the development and implementation of these activities. The above entities shall, as appropriate, make referrals to local, State, or Federal entities for the provision of services or further diagnosis.

(5) Reports

To be eligible to receive a grant under paragraph (2), a tribe, tribal organization, or consortium shall make a biennial report to the Secretary of the Interior of activities undertaken under this subsection, including the number of contracts and cooperative agreements entered into, the number of children contacted and receiving services for each year, and the estimated number of children needing services during the 2 years following the year in which the report is made. The Secretary of the Interior shall include a summary of this information on a biennial basis to the Secretary of Education along with such other information as required under Sec. 1411(i)(3)(E). The Secretary of Education may require any additional information from the Secretary of the Interior.

(6) Prohibited uses of funds

None of the funds under this subsection may be used by the Secretary of the Interior for administrative purposes, including child count, and the provision of technical assistance.

(c) State allotments

(1) In general

Except as provided in paragraphs (2), (93), and (4), from the funds remaining for each fiscal year after the reservation and payments under subsections (a) and (b), the Secretary shall first allot to each State an amount that bears the same ratio to the amount of such remainder as the number of infants and toddlers in the State bears to the number of infants and toddlers in all States.

(2) Minimum allotments

Except as provided in paragraphs (3) and (4), no State shall receive an amount under this section for any fiscal year that is less than the greatest of—

(A) one-half of one percent of the remaining amount described in paragraph (1); or

(B) $500,000.

(3) Special rule for 1998 and 1999

(A) In general

Except as provided in paragraph (4), no State may receive an amount under this section for either fiscal year 1998 or 1999 that is less than the sum of the amounts such State received for fiscal year 1994 under—

(i) part H (as in effect for such fiscal year); and

(ii) subpart 2 of part D of chapter 1 of title I of the Elementary and Secondary Education Act of 1965 (as in effect on the day before the date of the enactment of the Improving America's Schools Act of 1994) for children with disabilities under 3 years of age.

(B) Exception

If, for fiscal year 1998 or 1999, the number of infants and toddlers in a State, as determined under paragraph (1), is less than the number of infants and toddlers so determined for fiscal year 1994, the amount determined under subparagraph (A) for the State shall be reduced by the same percentage by which the number of such infants and toddlers so declined.

(4) Ratable reduction

(A) In general

If the sums made available under this part for any fiscal year are insufficient to pay the full amounts that all States are eligible to receive under this subsection for such year, the Secretary shall ratably reduce the allotments to such States for such year.

(B) Additional funds

If additional funds become available for making payments under this subsection for a fiscal year, allotments that were reduced under subparagraph (A) shall be increased on the same basis they were reduced.

(5) Definitions

For the purpose of this subsection—

(A) the terms 'infants' and 'toddlers' mean children under 3 years of age; and

(B) the term 'State' means each of the 50 States, the District of Columbia, and the Commonwealth of Puerto Rico.

(d) Reallotment of funds

If a State elects not to receive its allotment under subsection (c), the Secretary shall reallot, among the remaining States, amounts from such State in accordance with such subsection.

[Apr. 13, 1970, Pub. I, 91-230, Title VI, Part C, Sec. 643, as added, June 4, 1997, Pub. I, 105-17, Title I, Sec. 643, III Stat. 118.]

Sec. 1444 Federal Interagency Coordinating Council

(a) Establishment and purpose

(1) In general

The Secretary shall establish a Federal Interagency Coordinating Council in order to—

(A) minimize duplication of programs and activities across Federal, State, and local agencies, relating to—

(i) early intervention services for infants and toddlers with disabilities (including at-risk infants and toddlers) and their families; and

(ii) preschool or other appropriate services for children with disabilities;

(B) ensure the effective coordination of Federal early intervention and preschool programs and policies across Federal agencies;

(C) coordinate the provision of Federal technical assistance and support activities to States;

(D) identify gaps in Federal agency programs and services; and

(E) identify barriers to Federal interagency cooperation.

(2) Appointments

The council established under paragraph (1) (hereafter in this section referred to as the 'Council') and the chairperson of the council shall be appointed by the Secretary in consultation with other appropriate Federal agencies. In making the appointments, the Secretary shall ensure that each member has sufficient authority to engage in policy planning and implementation on behalf of the department, agency, or program that the member represents.

(b) Composition

The Council shall be composed of—

(1) a representative of the Office of Special Education Programs;

(2) a representative of the National Institute on Disability and Rehabilitation Research and a representative of the Office of Educational Research and Improvement;

(3) a representative of the Maternal and Child Health Services Block Grant Program;

(4) a representative of programs administered under the Developmental Disabilities Assistance and Bill of Rights Act;

(5) a representative of the Health Care Financing Administration;

(6) a representative of the Division of Birth Defects and Developmental Disabilities of the Centers for Disease Control;

(7) a representative of the Social Security Administration;

(8) a representative of the special supplemental nutrition program for women, infants, and children of the Department of Agriculture;

(9) a representative of the National Institute of Mental Health;

(10) a representative of the National Institute of Child Health and Human Development;

(11) a representative of the Bureau of Indian Affairs of the Department of the Interior;

(12) a representative of the Indian Health Service;

(13) a representative of the Surgeon General;

(14) a representative of the Department of Defense;

(15) a representative of the Children's Bureau, and a representative of the Head Start Bureau, of the Administration for Children and Families;

(16) a representative of the Substance Abuse and Mental Health Services Administration;

(17) a representative of the Pediatric AIDS Health Care Demonstration Program in the Public Health Service;

(18) parents of children with disabilities age 12 or under (who shall constitute at least 20 percent of the members of the Council), of whom at least one must have a child with a disability under the age of 6;

(19) at least 2 representatives of State lead agencies for early intervention services to infants and toddlers, one of whom must be a representative of a State educational agency and the other a representative of a non-educational agency;

(20) other members representing appropriate agencies involved in the provision of, or payment for, early intervention services and special education and related services to infants and toddlers with disabilities and their families and preschool children with disabilities; and

(21) other persons appointed by the Secretary.

(c) Meetings

The Council shall meet at least quarterly and in such places as the Council deems necessary. The meetings shall be publicly announced, and, to the extent appropriate, open and accessible to the general public.

(d) Functions of the Council

The Council shall—

(1) advise and assist the Secretary of Education, the Secretary of Health and Human Services, the Secretary of Defense, the Secretary of the Interior, the Secretary of Agriculture, and the Commissioner of Social Security in the performance of their responsibilities related to serving children from birth through age 5 who are eligible for services under this part or under part B;

(2) conduct policy analyses of Federal programs related to the provision of early intervention services and special educational and related services to infants and toddlers with disabilities and their families and preschool children with disabilities, in order to determine areas of conflict, overlap, duplication, or inappropriate omission;

(3) identify strategies to address issues described in paragraph (2);

(4) develop and recommend joint policy memoranda concerning effective interagency collaboration, including modifications to regulations, and the elimination of barriers to interagency programs and activities;

(5) coordinate technical assistance and disseminate information on best practices, effective program coordination strategies, and recommendations for improved early intervention programming for infants and toddlers with disabilities and their families and preschool children with disabilities; and

(6) facilitate activities in support of States' interagency coordination efforts.

(e) Conflict of interest

No member of the Council shall cast a vote on any matter that would provide direct financial benefit to that member or otherwise give the appearance of a conflict of interest under Federal law.

(f) Federal Advisory Committee Act

The Federal Advisory Committee Act (5 U.S.C. App.) shall not apply to the establishment or operation of the Council.
[Apr. 13, 1970, pub. I, 91-230, Title VI, Part C, Sec. 644, as added, June 4, 1997, Pub. I, 105-17, Title I, Sec. 644, III Stat. 121.]

Sec. 1445 Authorization of appropriations

For the purpose of carrying out this part, there are authorized to be appropriated $400,000,000 for fiscal year 1998 and such sums as may be necessary for each of the fiscal years 1999 through 2002. [Apr. 13, 1970, Pub. I, 91-230, Title VI, Part C, Sec. 645, as added, June 4, 1997, Pub. I, 105-17, Title I, Sec. 645, III Stat. 123.]

Part D–National Activities to Improve Education of Children with Disabilities

[Publishers Note: Except as otherwise indicated, Part D will take effect on October 1, 1997. Consult former IDEA until that date.]

Subpart 1–State Program Improvement Grants for Children with Disabilities

Sec. 1451 Findings and purpose

(a) Findings

The Congress finds the following:

(1) States are responding with some success to multiple pressures to improve educational and transitional services and results for children with disabilities in response to growing demands imposed by ever-changing factors, such as demographics, social policies, and labor and economic markets.

(2) In order for States to address such demands and to facilitate lasting systemic change that is of benefit to all students, including children with disabilities. States must involve local educational agencies, parents, individuals with disabilities and their families, teachers and other service providers, and other interested individuals and organizations in carrying out comprehensive strategies to improve educational results for children with disabilities.

(3) Targeted Federal financial resources are needed to assist States, working in partnership with others, to identify and make needed changes to address the needs of children with disabilities into the next century.

(4) State educational agencies, in partnership with local educational agencies and other individuals and organizations, are in the best position to identify and design ways to meet emerging and expanding demands to improve education for children with disabilities and to address their special needs.

(5) Research, demonstration, and practice over the past 20 years in special education and related disciplines have built a foundation of knowledge on which State and local systemic-change activities can now be based.

(6) Such research, demonstration, and practice in special education and related disciplines have demonstrated that an effective educational system now and in the future must—

(A) maintain high academic standards and clear performance goals for children with disabilities, consistent with the standards and expectations for all students in the educational system, and provide for appropriate and effective strategies and methods to ensure that students who are children with disabilities have maximum opportunities to achieve those standards and goals;

(B) create a system that fully addresses the needs of all students, including children with disabilities, by addressing the needs of children with disabilities in carrying out educational reform activities;

(C) clearly define, in measurable terms, the school and post-school results that children with disabilities are expected to achieve;

(D) promote service integration, and the coordination of State and local education, social, health, mental health, and other services, in addressing the full range of student needs, particularly the needs of children with disabilities who require significant levels of support to maximize their participation and learning in school and the community;

(E) ensure that children with disabilities are provided assistance and support in making transitions as described in Sec. 1474(b)(3)(C);

(F) promote comprehensive programs of professional development to ensure that the persons responsible for the education or a transition of children with disabilities possess the skills and knowledge necessary to address the educational and related needs of those children;

(G) disseminate to teachers and other personnel serving children with disabilities research-based knowledge about successful teaching practices and models and provide technical assistance to local educational agencies and schools on how to improve results for children with disabilities;

(H) create school-based disciplinary strategies that will be used to reduce or eliminate the need to use suspension and expulsion as disciplinary options for children with disabilities;

(I) establish placement-neutral funding formulas and cost-effective strategies for meeting the needs of children with disabilities; and

(J) involve individuals with disabilities and parents of children with disabilities in planning, implementing, and evaluating systemic-change activities and educational reforms.

(b) Purpose

The purpose of this subpart is to assist State educational agencies, and their partners referred to in Sec. 1452(b), in reforming and improving their systems for providing educational, early intervention, and transitional services, including their systems for professional development, technical assistance, and dissemination of knowledge about best practices, to improve results for children with disabilities.

[Apr. 13, 1970, Pub. I, 91-230, Title VI, Part C, Subpart 1, Sec. 651, as added, June 4, 1997, Pub. I, 105-17, Title I, Sec. 651, III Stat. 123.]

Sec. 1452   Eligibility and collaborative process

(a) Eligible applicants

A State educational agency may apply for a grant under this subpart for a grant period of not less than 1 year and not more than 5 years.

(b) Partners

(1) Required partners

(A) Contractual partners

In order to be considered for a grant under this subpart, a State educational agency shall establish a partnership with local educational agencies and other State agencies involved in, or concerned with, the education of children with disabilities.

(B) Other partners

In order to be considered for a grant under this subpart, a State educational agency shall work in partnership with other persons and organizations involved in, and concerned with, the education of children with disabilities, including—

(i) the Governor;

(ii) parents of children with disabilities;

(iii) parents of nondisabled children;

(iv) individuals with disabilities;

(v) organizations representing individuals with disabilities and their parents, such as parent training and information centers;

(vi) community-based and other nonprofit organizations involved in the education and employment of individuals with disabilities;

(vii) the lead State agency for part C;

(viii) general and special education teachers, and early intervention personnel;

(ix) the State advisory panel established under part C;

(x) the State interagency coordinating council established under part C; and

(xi) institutions of higher education within the State.

(2) Optional partners

A partnership under subparagraph (A) or (B) of paragraph (1) may also include—

(A) individuals knowledgeable about vocational education;

(B) the State agency for higher education;

(C) the State vocational rehabilitation agency;

(D) public agencies with jurisdiction in the areas of health, mental health, social services, and juvenile justice; and

(E) other individuals.

[Apr. 13, 1970, Pub. I, 91-230, Title VI, Part D, Subpart 1, Sec. 652, as added, June 4, 1997, Pub. I, 105-17, Title I, Sec. 652, III Stat. 124.]

Sec. 1453   Applications

(a) In general

(1) Submission

A State educational agency that desires to receive a grant under this subpart shall submit to the Secretary an application at such time, in such manner, and including such information as the Secretary may require.

(2) State improvement plan

The application shall include a State improvement plan that—

(A) is integrated, to the maximum extent possible, with State plans under the Elementary and Secondary Education Act of 1965 and the Rehabilitation Act of 1973, as appropriate; and

(B) meets the requirements of this section.

(b) Determining child and program needs

(1) In general

Each State improvement plan shall identify those critical aspects of early intervention, general education, and special education programs (including professional development, based on an assessment of State and local needs) that must be improved to enable children with disabilities to meet the goals established by the State under Sec. 1412(a)(16).

(2) Required analyses

To meet the requirement of paragraph (1), the State improvement plan shall include at least—

(A) an analysis of all information, reasonably available to the State educational agency, on the performance of children with disabilities in the State, including—

(i) their performance on State assessments and other performance indicators established for all children, including dropout rates and graduation rates;

(ii) their participation in postsecondary education and employment; and

(iii) how their performance on the assessments and indicators described in clause (i) compares to that of non-disabled children;

(B) an analysis of State and local needs for professional development for personnel to serve children with disabilities that includes, at a minimum—

(i) the number of personnel providing special education and related services; and

(ii) relevant information on current and anticipated personnel vacancies and shortages (including the number of individuals described in clause (i) with temporary certification), and on the extent of certification or retraining necessary to eliminate such shortages, that is based, to the maximum extent possible, on existing assessments of personnel needs;

(C) an analysis of the major findings of the Secretary's most recent review of State compliance, as they relate to improving results for children with disabilities; and

(D) an analysis of other information, reasonably available to the State, on the effectiveness of the State's systems of early intervention, special education, and general education in meeting the needs of children with disabilities.

(c) Improvement strategies

Each State improvement plan shall—

(1) describe a partnership agreement that—

(A) specifies—

(i) the nature and extent of the partnership among the State educational agency, local educational agencies, and other State agencies involved in, or concerned with, the education of children with disabilities, and the respective roles of each member of the partnership; and

(ii) how such agencies will work in partnership with other persons and organizations involved in, and concerned with, the education of children with disabilities, including the respective roles of each of these persons and organizations; and

(B) is in effect for the period of the grant;

(2) describe how grant funds will be used in undertaking the systemic-change activities, and the amount and nature of funds from any other sources, including part B funds retained for use at the State level under Secs. 1411(f) and 1419(d), that will be committed to the systemic-change activities;

(3) describe the strategies the State will use to address the needs identified under subsection (b), including—

(A) how the State will change State policies and procedures to address systemic barriers to improving results for children with disabilities;

(B) how the State will hold local educational agencies and schools accountable for educational progress of children with disabilities;

(C) how the State will provide technical assistance to local educational agencies and schools to improve results for children with disabilities;

(D) how the State will address the identified needs for in-service and pre-service preparation to ensure that all personnel who work with children with disabilities (including both professional and paraprofessional personnel who provide special education, general education, related services, or early intervention services) have the skills and knowledge necessary to meet the needs of children with disabilities, including a description of how—

(i) the State will prepare general and special education personnel with the content knowledge and collaborative skills needed to meet the needs of children with disabilities, including how the State will work with other States on common certification criteria;

(ii) the State will prepare professionals and paraprofessionals in the area of early intervention with the content knowledge and collaborative skills needed to meet the needs of infants and toddlers with disabilities;

(iii) the State will work with institutions of higher education and other entities that (on both a pre-service and an in-service basis) prepare personnel who work with children with disabilities to ensure that those institutions and entities develop the capacity to support quality professional development programs that meet State and local needs;

(iv) the State will develop collaborative agreements with other States for the joint support and development of programs to prepare personnel for which there is not sufficient demand within a single State to justify support or development of a program of preparation;

(v) the State will work in collaboration with other States, particularly neighboring States, to address the lack of uniformity and reciprocity in the credentialing of teachers and other personnel;

(vi) the State will enhance the ability of teachers and others to use strategies, such as behavioral interventions, to address the conduct of children with disabilities that impedes the learning of children with disabilities and others;

(vii) the State will acquire and disseminate, to teachers, administrators, school board members, and related services personnel, significant knowledge derived from educational research and other sources, and how the State will adopt promising practices, materials, and technology;

(viii) the State will recruit, prepare, and retain qualified personnel, including personnel with disabilities and personnel from groups that are underrepresented in the fields of regular education, special education, and related services;

(ix) the plan is integrated, to the maximum extent possible, with other professional development plans and activities, including plans and activities developed and carried out under other Federal and State laws that address personnel recruitment and training; and

(x) the State will provide for the joint training of parents and special education, related services, and general education personnel.

(E) strategies that will address systemic problems identified in Federal compliance reviews, including shortages of qualified personnel;

(F) how the State will disseminate results of the local capacity-building and improvement projects funded under Sec. 1411(f)(4);

(G) how the State will address improving results for children with disabilities in the geographic areas of greatest need; and

(H) how the State will assess, on a regular basis, the extent to which the strategies implemented under this subpart have been effective; and

(4) describe how the improvement strategies described in paragraph (3) will be coordinated with public and private sector resources.

(d) Competitive awards

(1) In general

The Secretary shall make Grants under this subpart on a competitive basis.

(2) Priority

The Secretary may give priority to applications on the basis of need, as indicated by such information as the findings of Federal compliance reviews.

(e) Peer review

(1) In general

The Secretary shall use a panel of experts who are competent, by virtue of their training, expertise, or experience, to evaluate applications under this subpart.

(2) Composition of panel

A majority of a panel described in paragraph (1) shall be composed of individuals who are not employees of the Federal Government.

(3) Payment of fees and expenses of certain members

The Secretary may use available funds appropriated to carry out this subpart to pay the expenses and fees of panel members who are not employees of the Federal Government.

(f) Reporting procedures

Each State educational agency that receives a grant under this subpart shall submit performance reports to the Secretary pursuant to a schedule to be determined by the Secretary, but not more frequently than annually. The reports shall describe the progress of the State in meeting the performance goals established under Sec. 1412(a)(16), analyze the effectiveness of the State's strategies in meeting those goals, and identify any changes in the strategies needed to improve its performance.

[Apr. 13, 1970, Pub. I, 91-230, Title VI, Part D, Subpart I, Sec. 653, as added, June 4, 1997, Pub. I, 105-17, Title I, Sec. 653, III Stat. 125.]

Sec. 1454 Use of Funds

(a) In general

(1) Activities

A State educational agency that receives a grant under this subpart may use the grant to carry out any activities that are described in the State's application and that are consistent with the purpose of this subpart.

(2) Contracts and subgrants

Each such State educational agency—

(A) shall, consistent with its partnership agreement under Sec. 1452(b), award contracts or subgrants to local educational agencies, institutions of higher education, and parent training and information centers, as appropriate, to carry out its State improvement plan under this subpart; and

(B) may award contracts and subgrants to other public and private entities, including the lead agency under part C, to carry out such plan.

(b) Use of funds for professional development

A State educational agency that receives a grant under this subpart—

(1) shall use not less than 75 percent of the funds it receives under the grant for any fiscal year—

(A) to ensure that there are sufficient regular education, special education, and related services personnel who have the skills and knowledge necessary to meet the needs of children with disabilities and developmental goals of young children; or

(B) to work with other States on common certification criteria; or

(2) shall use not less than 50 percent of such funds for such purposes, if the State demonstrates to the Secretary's satisfaction that it has the personnel described in paragraph (1)(A).

(c) Grants to outlying areas

Public Law 95-134, permitting the consolidation of grants to the outlying areas, shall not apply to funds received under this subpart.

[Apr. 13, 1970, Pub. I, 91-230, Title VI, Part D, Subpart I, Sec. 654, as added, June 4, 1997, Pub. I, 105-17, Title I, Sec. 654, III Stat. 128.]

Sec. 1455 Minimum state grant amounts

(a) In general

The Secretary shall make a grant to each State educational agency whose application the Secretary has selected for funding under this subpart in an amount for each fiscal year that is—

(1) not less than $500,000, nor more than $2,000,000 in the case of the 50 States, the District of Columbia, and the Commonwealth of Puerto Rico; and

(2) not less than $80,000, in the case of an outlying area.

(b) Inflation adjustment

Beginning with fiscal year 1999, the Secretary may increase the maximum amount described in subsection (a)(1) to account for inflation.

(c) Factors

The Secretary shall set the amount of each grant under subsection (a) after considering—

(1) the amount of funds available for making the grants;

(2) the relative population of the State or outlying area; and

(3) the types of activities proposed by the State or outlying area.

[Apr. 13, 1970, Pub. I, 91-230, Title VI, Part D, Subpart 1, Sec. 655, as added, June 4, 1997, Pub. I, 105-17, Title I, Sec. 655, III Stat. 129.]

Sec. 1456 Authorization of appropriations

There are authorized to be appropriated to carry out this subpart such sums as may be necessary for each of the fiscal years 1998 through 2002.

[Apr. 13, 1970, Pub. I, 91-230, Title VI, Part D, Subpart 1, Sec. 656, as added, June 4, 1997, Pub. I, 105-17, Title I, Sec. 656, III Stat. 129.]

Subpart 2–Coordinated Research, Personnel Preparation, Technical Assistance, Support, and Dissemination of Information

Sec. 1461 Administrative provisions

(a) Comprehensive plan

(1) In general

The Secretary shall develop and implement a comprehensive plan for activities carried out under this subpart in order to enhance the provision of educational, related, transitional, and early intervention services to children with disabilities under parts B and C. The plan shall include mechanisms to address educational, related services, transitional, and early intervention needs identified by State educational agencies in applications submitted for State program improvement grants under subpart 1.

(2) participants in plan development

In developing the plan described in paragraph (1), the Secretary shall consult with—

(A) individuals with disabilities;

(B) parents of children with disabilities;

(C) appropriate professionals; and

(D) representatives of State and local educational agencies, private schools, institutions of higher education, other Federal agencies, the National Council on Disability, and national organizations with an interest in, and expertise in, providing services to children with disabilities and their families.

(3) Public comment

The Secretary shall take public comment on the plan.

(4) Distribution of funds

In implementing the plan, the Secretary shall, to the extent appropriate, ensure that funds are awarded to recipients under this subpart to carry out activities that benefit, directly or indirectly, children with disabilities of all ages.

(5) Reports to Congress

The Secretary shall periodically report to the Congress on the Secretary's activities under this subsection, including an initial report not later than the date that is 18 months after the date of the enactment of the Individuals with Disabilities Act Amendments of 1997.

(b) Eligible applicants

(1) In general

Except as otherwise provided in this subpart, the following entities are eligible to apply for a grant, or cooperative agreement under this subpart:

(A) A State educational agency.

(B) A local educational agency.

(C) An institution of higher education.

(D) Any other public agency.

(E) A private nonprofit organization

(F) An outlying area.

(G) An Indian tribe or a tribal organization (as defined under Sec. 4 of the Indian Self-Determination and Education Assistance Act).

(H) A for-profit organization, if the Secretary finds it appropriate in light of the purposes of a particular competition for a grant, contract, or cooperative agreement under this subpart.

(2) Special rule

The Secretary may limit the entities eligible for an award of a grant, contract, or cooperative agreement to one or more categories of eligible entities described in paragraph (1).

(c) Use of funds by Secretary

Notwithstanding any other provision of law, and in addition to any authority granted the Secretary under chapter 1 or chapter 2, the Secretary may use up to 20 percent of the funds available under either chapter 1 or chapter 2 for any fiscal year to carry out any activity, or combination of activities, subject to such conditions as the Secretary determines are appropriate effectively to carry out the purposes of such chapters, that—

(1) is consistent with the purposes of chapter 1, chapter 2, or both; and

(2) involves—

(A) research;

(B) personnel preparation;

(C) parent training and information;

(D) technical assistance and dissemination;

(E) technology development, demonstration, and utilization; or

(F) media services.

(d) Special populations

(1) Application requirements

In making an award of a grant, contract, or cooperative agreement under this subpart, the Secretary shall, as appropriate, require an applicant to demonstrate how the applicant will address the needs of children with disabilities from minority backgrounds.

(2) Outreach and technical assistance

(A) Requirement

Notwithstanding any other provision of this Act, the Secretary shall ensure that at least one percent of the total amount of funds appropriated to carry out this subpart is used for either or both of the following activities:

(i) To provide outreach and technical assistance to Historically Black Colleges and Universities, and to institutions of higher education with minority enrollments of at least 25%, to promote the participation of such colleges, universities, and institutions in activities under this subpart.

(ii) To enable Historically Black Colleges and Universities, and the institutions described in clause (i), to assist other colleges, universities, institutions, and agencies in improving educational and transitional results for children with disabilities.

(B) Reservation of funds

The Secretary may reserve funds appropriated under this subpart to satisfy the requirement of subparagraph (A).

(e) Priorities

(1) In general

Except as otherwise explicitly authorized in this subpart, the Secretary shall ensure that a grant, contract, or cooperative agreement under chapter 1 or 2 is awarded only—

(A) for activities that are designed to benefit children with disabilities, their families, or the personnel employed to work with such children or their families; or

(B) to benefit other individuals with disabilities that such chapter is intended to benefit.

(2) Priority for particular activities

Subject to paragraph (1), the Secretary, in making an award of a grant, contract, or cooperative agreement under this subpart, may, without regard to the rule making procedures under Sec. 553 of title 5, United States Code, limit competitions to, or otherwise give priority to—

(A) projects that address one or more—

(i) age ranges;

(ii) disabilities;

(iii) school grades;

(iv) types of educational placements or early intervention environments;

(v) types of services;

(vi) content areas, such as reading; or

(vii) effective strategies for helping children with disabilities learn appropriate behavior in the school and other community-based educational settings;

(B) projects that address the needs of children based on the severity of their disability;

(C) projects that address the needs of—

(i) low-achieving students;

(ii) underserved populations;

(iii) children from low-income families;

(iv) children with limited English proficiency;

(v) unserved and underserved areas;

(vi) particular types of geographic areas; or

(vii) children whose behavior interferes with their learning and socialization;

(D) projects to reduce inappropriate identification of children as children with disabilities, particularly among minority children;

(E) projects that are carried out in particular areas of the country, to ensure broad geographic coverage; and

(F) any activity that is expressly authorized in chapter 1 or 2.

(f) Applicant and recipient responsibilities

(1) Development and assessment of projects

The Secretary shall require that an applicant for, and a recipient of, a grant, contract, or cooperative agreement for a project under this subpart—

(A) involve individuals with disabilities or parents of individuals with disabilities in planning, implementing, and evaluating the project; and

(B) where appropriate, determine whether the project has any potential for replication and adoption by other entities.

(2) Additional responsibilities

The Secretary may require a recipient of a grant, contract, or cooperative agreement for a project under this subpart—

(A) to share in the cost of the project;

(B) to prepare the research and evaluation findings and products from the project in formats that are useful for specific audiences, including parents, administrators, teachers, early intervention personnel, related services personnel, and individuals with disabilities;

(C) to disseminate such findings and products; and

(D) to collaborate with other such recipients in carrying out subparagraphs (B) and (C).

(g) Application management

(1) Standing panel

(A) In general

The Secretary shall establish and use a standing panel of experts who are competent, by virtue of their training, expertise, or experience, to evaluate applications under this subpart that, individually, request more than $75,000 per year in Federal financial assistance.

(B) Membership

The standing panel shall include, at a minimum—

(i) individuals who are representatives of institutions of higher education that plan, develop, and carry out programs of personnel preparation;

(ii) individuals who design and carry out programs of research targeted to the improvement of special education programs and services;

(iii) individuals who have recognized experience and knowledge necessary to integrate and apply research findings to improve educational and transitional results for children with disabilities;

(iv) individuals who administer programs at the State or local level in which children with disabilities participate;

(v) individuals who prepare parents of children with disabilities to participate in making decisions about the education of their children;

(vi) individuals who establish policies that affect the delivery of services to children with disabilities;

(vii) individuals who are parents of children with disabilities who are benefiting, or have benefited, from coordinated research, personnel preparation, and technical assistance; and

(viii) individuals with disabilities.

(C) Training

The Secretary shall provide training to the individuals who are selected as members of the standing panel under this paragraph.

(D) Term

No individual shall serve on the standing panel for more than 3 consecutive years, unless the Secretary determines that the individual's continued participation is necessary for the sound administration of this subpart.

(2) Peer-review panels for particular competitions

(A) Composition

The Secretary shall ensure that each sub-panel selected from the standing panel that reviews applications under this subpart includes—

(i) individuals with knowledge and expertise on the issues addressed by the activities authorized by the subpart; and

(ii) to the extent practicable, parents of children with disabilities, individuals with disabilities, and persons from diverse backgrounds.

(B) Federal employment limitation

A majority of the individuals on each sub-panel that reviews an application under this subpart shall be individuals who are not employees of the Federal Government.

[20 USC 1461(g)(1) and 20 USC 1461(g)(2) will take effect on January 1, 1998. Consult former IDEA until that date.]

(3) Use of discretionary funds for administrative purposes

(A) Expenses and fees of non-federal panel members

The Secretary may use funds available under this subpart to pay the expenses and fees of the panel members who are not officers or employees of the Federal Government.

(B) Administrative support

The Secretary may use not more than 1 percent of the funds appropriated to carry out this subpart to pay non-Federal entities for administrative support related to management of applications submitted under this subpart.

(C) Monitoring

The Secretary may use funds available under this subpart to pay the expenses of Federal employees to conduct on-site monitoring of projects receiving $500,000 or more for any fiscal year under this subpart.

(h) Program evaluation

The Secretary may use funds appropriated to carry out this subpart to evaluate activities carried out under this subpart.

(i) Minimum funding required

(1) In general

Subject to paragraph (2), the Secretary shall ensure that, for each fiscal year, at least the following amounts are provided under this subpart to address the following needs:

(A) $12,832,000 to address the educational, related services, transitional, and early intervention needs of children with deaf-blindness.

(B) $4,000,000 to address the postsecondary, vocational, technical, continuing, and adult education needs of individuals with deafness.

(C) $4,000,000 to address the educational, related services, and transitional needs of children with an emotional disturbance and those who are at risk of developing an emotional disturbance.

(2) Ratable reduction

If the total mount appropriated to carry out Secs. 1472, 1473, and 1485 for any fiscal year is less than $130,000,000, the amounts listed in paragraph (1) shall be ratably reduced.

(j) Eligibility for financial assistance

Effective for fiscal years for which the Secretary may make grants under Sec. 1419(b), no State or local educational agency or educational service agency or other public institution or agency may receive a grant under this subpart which relates exclusively to programs, projects, and activities pertaining to children aged three to five, inclusive, unless the State is eligible to receive a grant under Sec. 1419(b).

[Apr. 13, 1970, Pub. I, 91-230, Title VI, Part D, Subpart 2, Ch. 1, Sec. 661, as added, June 4, 1997, Pub. I, 105-17, Title I, Sec. 661, III Stat. 130.]

Chapter 1–Improving Early Intervention, Educational, and Transitional Services and Results for Children with Disabilities through Coordinated Research and Personnel Preparation

Sec. 1471   Findings and purpose

(a) Findings

The Congress finds the following:

(1) The Federal Government has an ongoing obligation to support programs, projects, and activities that contribute to positive results for children with disabilities, enabling them—

(A) to meet their early intervention, educational, and transitional goals and, to the maximum extent possible, educational standards that have been established for all children; and

(B) to acquire the skills that will empower them to lead productive and independent adult lives.

(2)(A) As a result of more than 20 years of Federal support for research, demonstration projects, and personnel preparation, there is an important knowledge base for improving results for children with disabilities.

(B) Such knowledge should be used by States and local educational agencies to design and implement state-of-the-art educational systems that consider the needs of, and include, children with disabilities, especially in environments in which they can learn along with their peers and achieve results measured by the same standards as the results of their peers.

(3)(A) Continued Federal support is essential for the development and maintenance of a coordinated and high-quality program of research, demonstration projects, dissemination of information, and personnel preparation.

(B) Such support

(i) enables State educational agencies and local educational agencies to improve their educational systems and results for children with disabilities;

(ii) enables State and local agencies to improve early intervention services and results for infants and toddlers with disabilities and their families; and

(iii) enhances the opportunities for general and special education personnel, related services personnel, parents, and paraprofessionals to participate in pre-service and in-service training, to collaborate, and to improve results for children with disabilities and their families.

(4) The Federal Government plays a critical role in facilitating the availability of an adequate number of qualified personnel—

(A) to serve effectively over 5,000,000 children with disabilities;

(B) to assume leadership positions in administrative and direct-service capacities related to teacher training and research concerning the provision of early intervention services, special education, and related services; and

(C) to work with children with low-incidence disabilities and their families.

(5) The Federal Government performs the role described in paragraph (4)—

(A) by supporting models of personnel development that reflect successful practice including strategies for recruiting, preparing, and retaining personnel;

(B) by promoting the coordination and integration of—

(i) personnel-development activities for teachers of children with disabilities; and

(ii) other personnel-development activities supported under Federal law, including this chapter;

(C) by supporting the development and dissemination of information about teaching standards; and

(D) by promoting the coordination and integration of personnel-development activities through linkage with systemic-change activities within States and nationally.

(b) Purpose

The purpose of this chapter is to provide Federal funding for coordinated research, demonstration projects, outreach, and personnel-preparation activities that—

(1) are described in Secs. 1472 through 1474;

(2) are linked with, and promote, systemic change; and

(3) improve early intervention, educational, and transitional results for children with disabilities.

[Apr. 13, 1970, Pub. I, 91-230, Title VI, Part D, Subpart 2, Ch. 1, Sec. 671, as added, June 4, 1997, Pub. I, 105-17, Title I, Sec. 671, III Stat. 135.]

Sec. 1472 Research and innovation to improve services and results for children with disabilities

(a) In general

The Secretary shall make competitive grants to, or enter into contracts or cooperative agreements with, eligible entities to produce, and advance the use of, knowledge—

(1) to improve—

(A) services provided under this Act, including the practices of professionals and others involved in providing such services to children with disabilities; and

(B) educational results for children with disabilities;

(2) to address the special needs of preschool-aged children and infants and toddlers with disabilities, including infants and toddlers who would be at risk of having substantial developmental delays if early intervention services were not provided to them;

(3) to address the specific problems of over-identification and under-identification of children with disabilities;

(4) to develop and implement effective strategies for addressing inappropriate behavior of students with disabilities in schools, including strategies to prevent children with emotional and behavioral problems from developing emotional disturbances that require the provision of special education and related services;

(5) to improve secondary and postsecondary education and transitional services for children with disabilities; and

(6) to address the range of special education, related services, and early intervention needs of children with disabilities who need significant levels of support to maximize their participation and learning in school and in the community.

(b) New knowledge production; authorized activities

(1) In general

In carrying out this section, the Secretary shall support activities, consistent with the objectives described in subsection (a), that lead to the production of new knowledge.

(2) Authorized activities

Activities that may be carried out under this subsection include activities such as the following:

(A) Expanding understanding of the relationships between learning characteristics of children with disabilities and the diverse ethnic, cultural, linguistic, social, and economic backgrounds of children with disabilities and their families.

(B) Developing or identifying innovative, effective, and efficient curricula designs, instructional approaches, and strategies, and developing or identifying positive academic and social learning opportunities, that—

(i) enable children with disabilities to make effective transitions described in Sec. 1474(b)(3)(C) or transitions between educational settings; and

(ii) improve educational and transitional results for children with disabilities at all levels of the educational system in which the activities are carried out and, in particular, that improve the progress of the children, as measured by assessments within the general education curriculum involved.

(C) Advancing the design of assessment tools and procedures that will accurately and efficiently determine the special instructional, learning, and behavioral needs of children with disabilities, especially within the context of general education.

(D) Studying and promoting improved alignment and compatibility of general and special education reforms concerned with curricular and instructional reform, evaluation and accountability of such reforms, and administrative procedures.

(E) Advancing the design, development, and integration of technology, assistive technology devices, media, and materials, to improve early intervention, educational, and transitional services and results for children with disabilities.

(F) Improving designs, processes, and results of personnel preparation for personnel who provide services to children with disabilities through the acquisition of information on, and implementation of, research-based practices.

(G) Advancing knowledge about the coordination of education with health and social services.

(H) Producing information on the long-term impact of early intervention and education on results for individuals with disabilities through large-scale longitudinal studies.

(c) Integration of research and practice; authorized activities
(1) In general

In carrying out this section, the Secretary shall support activities, consistent with the objectives described in subsection (a), that integrate research and practice, including activities that support State systemic-change and local capacity-building and improvement efforts.

(2) Authorized activities

Activities that may be carried out under this subsection include activities such as the following:

(A) Model demonstration projects to apply and test research findings in typical service settings to determine the usability, effectiveness, and general applicability of such research findings in such areas as improving instructional methods, curricula, and tools, such as text books and media.

(B) Demonstrating and applying research-based findings to facilitate systemic changes, related to the provision of services to children with disabilities, in policy, procedure, practice, and the training and use of personnel.

(C) Promoting and demonstrating the coordination of early intervention and educational services for children with disabilities with services provided by health, rehabilitation, and social service agencies.

(D) Identifying and disseminating solutions that overcome systemic barriers to the effective and efficient delivery of early intervention, educational, and transitional services to children with disabilities.

(d) Improving the use of professional knowledge; authorized activities
(1) In general

In carrying out this section, the Secretary shall support activities, consistent with the objectives described in subsection (a), that improve the use of professional knowledge, including activi-

ties that support State systemic-change and local capacity-building and improvement efforts.

(2) Authorized activities

Activities that may be carried out under this subsection include activities such as the following:

(A) Synthesizing useful research and other information relating to the provision of services to children with disabilities, including effective practices.

(B) Analyzing professional knowledge bases to advance an understanding of the relationships, and the effectiveness of practices, relating to the provision of services to children with disabilities.

(C) Ensuring that research and related products are in appropriate formats for distribution to teachers, parents, and individuals with disabilities.

(D) Enabling professionals, parents of children with disabilities, and other persons, to learn about, and implement, the findings of research, and successful practices developed in model demonstration projects, relating to the provision of services to children with disabilities.

(E) Conducting outreach, and disseminating information relating to successful approaches to overcoming systemic barriers to the effective and efficient delivery of early intervention, educational, and transitional services, to personnel who provide services to children with disabilities.

(e) Balance among activities and age ranges

In carrying out this section, the Secretary shall ensure that there is an appropriate balance—

(1) among knowledge production, integration of research and practice, and use of professional knowledge; and

(2) across all age ranges of children with disabilities.

(f) Applications

An eligible entity that wishes to receive a grant, or enter into a contract or cooperative agreement, under this section shall submit an application to the Secretary at such time, in such manner, and containing such information as the Secretary may require.

(g) Authorization of appropriations

There are authorized to be appropriated to carry out this section such sums as may be necessary for each of the fiscal years 1998 through 2002.

[Apr. 13, 1970, Pub. I, 91-230, Title VI, Part D, Subpart 2, Ch. 1, Sec. 672, as added, June 4, 1997, Pub. I, 105-17, Title I, Sec. 672, III Stat 136.]

Sec. 1473 Personnel preparation to improve services and results for children with disabilities

(a) In general

The Secretary shall, on a competitive basis, make grants to, or enter into contracts or cooperative agreements with, eligible entities—

(1) to help address State-identified needs for qualified personnel in special education, related services, early intervention, and regular education, to work with children with disabilities; and

(2) to ensure that those personnel have the skills and knowledge, derived from practices that have been determined, through research and experience, to be successful, that are needed to serve those children.

(b) Low-incidence disabilities; authorized activities

(1) In general

In carrying out this section, the Secretary shall support activities, consistent with the objectives described in subsection (a), that benefit children with low-incidence disabilities.

(2) Authorized activities

Activities that may be carried out under this subsection include activities such as the following:

(A) Preparing persons who—

(i) have prior training in educational and other related service fields; and

(ii) are studying to obtain degrees, certificates, or licensure that will enable them to assist children with disabilities to achieve the objectives set out in their individualized education programs described in Sec. 1414(d), or to assist infants and toddlers with disabilities to achieve the outcomes described in their individualized family service plans described in Sec. 1436.

(B) Providing personnel from various disciplines with interdisciplinary training that will contribute to improvement in early intervention, educational, and transitional results for children with disabilities.

(C) Preparing personnel in the innovative uses and application of technology to enhance learning by children with disabilities through early intervention, educational, and transitional services.

(D) Preparing personnel who provide services to visually impaired or blind children to teach and use Braille in the provision of services to such children.

(E) Preparing personnel to be qualified educational interpreters, to assist children with disabilities, particularly deaf and hard-of-hearing children in school and school-related activities and deaf and hard-of-hearing infants and toddlers and preschool children in early intervention and preschool programs.

(F) Preparing personnel who provide services to children with significant cognitive disabilities and children with multiple disabilities.

(3) Definition

As used in this section, the term 'low-incidence disability' means—

(A) a visual or hearing impairment, or simultaneous visual and hearing impairments;

(B) a significant cognitive impairment; or

(C) any impairment for which a small number of personnel with highly specialized skills and knowledge are needed in order for children with that impairment to receive early intervention services or a free appropriate public education.

(4) Selection of recipients

In selecting recipients under this subsection, the Secretary may give preference to applications that propose to prepare personnel in more than one low-incidence disability, such as deafness and blindness.

(5) Preparation in use of Braille

The Secretary shall ensure that all recipients of assistance under this subsection who will use that assistance to prepare personnel to provide services to visually impaired or blind children that can appropriately be provided in Braille will prepare those individuals to provide those services in Braille.

(c) Leadership preparation; authorized activities

(1) In general

In carrying out this section, the Secretary shall support leadership preparation activities that are consistent with the objectives described in subsection (a).

(2) Authorized activities

Activities that may be carried out under this subsection include activities such as the following:

(A) Preparing personnel at the advanced graduate, doctoral, and post-doctoral levels of training to administer, enhance, or provide services for children with disabilities.

(B) Providing interdisciplinary training for various types of leadership personnel, including teacher preparation faculty, administrators, researchers, supervisors, principals, and other persons whose work affects early intervention, educational, and transitional services for children with disabilities.

(d) Projects of national significance; authorized activities

(1) In general

In carrying out this section, the Secretary shall support activities, consistent with the objectives described in subsection (a), that are of national significance and have broad applicability.

(2) Authorized activities

Activities that may be carried out under this subsection include activities such as the following:

(A) Developing and demonstrating effective and efficient practices for preparing personnel to provide services to children with disabilities, including practices that address any needs identified in the State's improvement plan under part C;

(B) Demonstrating the application of significant knowledge derived from research and other sources in the development of programs to prepare personnel to provide services to children with disabilities.

(C) Demonstrating models for the preparation of, and interdisciplinary training of, early intervention, special education, and general education personnel, to enable the personnel—

(i) to acquire the collaboration skills necessary to work within teams to assist children with disabilities; and

(ii) to achieve results that meet challenging standards, particularly within the general education curriculum.

(D) Demonstrating models that reduce shortages of teachers, and personnel from other relevant disciplines, who serve children with disabilities, through reciprocity arrangements between States that are related to licensure and certification.

(E) Developing, evaluating, and disseminating model teaching standards for persons working with children with disabilities.

(F) Promoting the transferability, across State and local jurisdictions, of licensure and certification of teachers and administrators working with such children.

(G) Developing and disseminating models that prepare teachers with strategies, including behavioral interventions, for addressing the conduct of children with disabilities that impedes their learning and that of others in the classroom.

(H) Institutes that provide professional development that addresses the needs of children with disabilities to teachers or teams of teachers, and where appropriate, to school board members, administrators, principals, pupil-service personnel, and other staff from individual schools.

(I) Projects to improve the ability of general education teachers, principals, and other administrators to meet the needs of children with disabilities.

(J) Developing, evaluating, and disseminating innovative models for the recruitment, induction, retention, and assessment of new, qualified teachers, especially from groups that are underrepresented in the teaching profession, including individuals with disabilities.

(K) Supporting institutions of higher education with minority enrollments of at least 25% for the purpose of preparing personnel to work with children with disabilities.

(e) High-incidence disabilities; authorized activities

(1) In general

In carrying out this section, the Secretary shall support activities, consistent with the objectives described in subsection (a), to benefit children with high-incidence disabilities, such as children with specific learning disabilities, speech or language impairment, or mental retardation.

(2) Authorized activities

Activities that may be carried out under this subsection include the following:

(A) Activities undertaken by institutions of higher education, local educational agencies, and other local entities—

(i) to improve and reform their existing programs to prepare teachers and related services personnel—

(I) to meet the diverse needs of children with disabilities for early intervention, educational, and transitional services; and

(II) to work collaboratively in regular classroom settings; and

(ii) to incorporate best practices and research-based knowledge about preparing personnel so they will have the knowledge and skills to improve educational results for children with disabilities.

(B) Activities incorporating innovative strategies to recruit and prepare teachers and other personnel to meet the needs of areas in which there are acute and persistent shortages of personnel.

(C) Developing career opportunities for paraprofessionals to receive training as special education teachers, related services personnel, and early intervention personnel, including interdisciplinary training to enable them to improve early intervention, educational, and transitional results for children with disabilities.

(f) Applications

(1) In general

Any eligible entity that wishes to receive a grant, or enter into a contract or cooperative agreement, under this section shall submit an application to the Secretary at such time, in such manner, and containing such information as the Secretary may require.

(2) Identified state needs

(A) Requirement to address identified needs

Any application under subsection (b), (c), or (e) shall include information demonstrating to the satisfaction of the Secretary that the activities described in the application will address needs identified by the State or States the applicant proposes to serve.

(B) Cooperation with state educational agencies

Any applicant that is not a local educational agency or a State educational agency shall include information demonstrating to the satisfaction of the Secretary that the applicant and one or more State educational agencies have engaged in a cooperative effort to plan the project to which the application pertains, and will cooperate in carrying out and monitoring the project.

(3) Acceptance by states of personnel preparation requirements

The Secretary may require applicants to provide letters from one or more States stating that the States—

(A) intend to accept successful completion of the proposed personnel preparation program as meeting State personnel standards for serving children with disabilities or serving infants and toddlers with disabilities; and

(B) need personnel in the area or areas in which the applicant proposes to provide preparation, as identified in the States'

comprehensive systems of personnel development under parts B and C.

(g) Selection of recipients

(1) Impact of project

In selecting recipients under this section, the Secretary may consider the impact of the project proposed in the application in meeting the need for personnel identified by the States.

(2) Requirement on applicants to meet state and professional standards

The Secretary shall make grants under this section only to eligible applicants that meet State and professionally-recognized standards for the preparation of special education and related services personnel, if the purpose of the project is to assist personnel in obtaining degrees.

(3) Preferences

In selecting recipients under this section, the Secretary may—

(A) give preference to institutions of higher education that are educating regular education personnel to meet the needs of children with disabilities in integrated settings and educating special education personnel to work in collaboration with regular educators in integrated settings; and

(B) give preference to institutions of higher education that are successfully recruiting and preparing individuals with disabilities and individuals from groups that are underrepresented in the profession for which they are preparing individuals.

(h) Service obligation

(1) In general

Each application for funds under subsections (b) and (e), and to the extent appropriate subsection (d), shall include an assurance that the applicant will ensure that individuals who receive a scholarship under the proposed project will subsequently provide special education and related services to children with disabilities for a period of 2 years for every year for which assistance was received or repay all or part of the cost of that assistance, in accordance with regulations issued by the Secretary.

(2) Leadership preparation

Each application for funds under subsection (c) shall include an assurance that the applicant will ensure that individuals who receive a scholarship under the proposed project will subsequently perform work related to their preparation for a period of 2 years for every year for which assistance was received or repay all or part of such costs, in accordance with regulations issued by the Secretary.

(i) Scholarships

The Secretary may include funds for scholarships, with necessary stipends and allowances, in awards under subsections (b), (c), (d), and (e).

(j) Authorization of appropriations

There are authorized to be appropriated to carry out this section such sums as may be necessary for each of the fiscal years 1998 through 2002.

[Apr. 13, 1970, Pub. I, 91-230, Title VI, Part D, Subpart 2, Ch. 1, Sec. 673, as added, June 4, 1997, Pub. I, 105-17, Title I, Sec. 673, III Stat. 139.]

Sec. 1474   Studies and evaluations

(a) Studies and evaluations

(1) In general

The Secretary shall, directly or through grants, contracts, or cooperative agreements, assess progress in the implementation of this Act, including effectiveness of State and local efforts to provide—

(A) a free appropriate public education to children with disabilities; and

(B) early intervention services to infants and toddlers with disabilities and infants and toddlers who would be at risk of having substantial developmental delays if early intervention services were not provided to them.

(2) Authorized activities

In carrying out this subsection, the Secretary may support studies, evaluations, and assessments, including studies that—

(A) analyze measurable impact, outcomes, and results achieved by State educational agencies and local educational agencies through their activities to reform policies, procedures, and practices designed to improve educational and transitional services and results for children with disabilities;

(B) analyze State and local needs for professional development, parent training, and other appropriate activities that can reduce the need for disciplinary actions involving children with disabilities;

(C) assess educational and transitional services and results for children with disabilities from minority backgrounds, including—

(i) data on—

(I) the number of minority children who are referred for special education evaluation;

(II) the number of minority children who are receiving special education and related services and their educational or other service placement; and

(III) the number of minority children who graduated from secondary and postsecondary education programs; and

(ii) the performance of children with disabilities from minority backgrounds on State assessments and other performance indicators established for all students;

(D) measure educational and transitional services and results of children with disabilities under this Act, including longitudinal studies that—

(i) examine educational and transitional services and results for children with disabilities who are 3 through 17 years of age and are receiving special education and related services under this Act, using a national, representative sample of distinct age cohorts and disability categories; and

(ii) examine educational results, postsecondary placement, and employment status of individuals with disabilities, 18 through 21 years of age, who are receiving or have received special education and related services under this Act; and

(E) identify and report on the placement of children with disabilities by disability category.

(b) National assessment

(1) In general

The Secretary shall carry out a national assessment of activities carried out with Federal funds under this Act in order—

(A) to determine the effectiveness of this Act in achieving its purposes;

(B) to provide information to the President, the Congress, the States, local educational agencies, and the public on how to implement the Act more effectively; and

(C) to provide the President and the Congress with information that will be useful in developing legislation to achieve the purposes of this Act more effectively.

(2) Consultation

The Secretary shall plan, review, and conduct the national assessment under this subsection in consultation with researchers, State practitioners, local practitioners, parents of children with disabilities, individuals with disabilities, and other appropriate individuals.

(3) Scope of assessment

The national assessment shall examine how well schools, local educational agencies, States, other recipients of assistance under this Act, and the Secretary are achieving the purposes of this Act, including—

(A) improving the performance of children with disabilities in general scholastic activities and assessments as compared to nondisabled children;

(B) providing for the participation of children with disabilities in the general curriculum;

(C) helping children with disabilities make successful transitions from—

(i) early intervention services to preschool education;

(ii) preschool education to elementary school; and

(iii) secondary school to adult life;

(D) placing and serving children with disabilities, including minority children, in the least restrictive environment appropriate;

(E) preventing children with disabilities, especially children with emotional disturbances and specific learning disabilities, from dropping out of school;

(F) addressing behavioral problems of children with disabilities as compared to nondisabled children;

(G) coordinating services provided under this Act with each other, with other educational and pupil services (including preschool services), and with health and social services funded from other sources;

(H) providing for the participation of parents of children with disabilities in the education of their children; and

(I) resolving disagreements between education personnel and parents through activities such as mediation.

(4) Interim and final reports

The Secretary shall submit to the President and the Congress—

(A) an interim report that summarizes the preliminary findings of the assessment not later than October 1, 1999; and

(B) a final report of the findings of the assessment not later than October 1, 2001.

(c) Annual report

The Secretary shall report annually to the Congress on—

(1) an analysis and summary of the data reported by the States and the Secretary of the Interior under Sec. 1418;

(2) the results of activities conducted under subsection (a);

(3) the findings and determinations resulting from reviews of State implementation of this Act.

(d) Technical assistance to LEAs

The Secretary shall provide directly, or through grants, contracts, or cooperative agreements, technical assistance to local educational agencies to assist them in carrying out local capacity-building and improvement projects under Sec. 1411(f)(4) and other LEA systemic improvement activities under this Act.

(e) Reservation for studies and technical assistance

(1) In general

Except as provided in paragraph (2) and notwithstanding any other provision of this Act, the Secretary may reserve up to one-half of one percent of the amount appropriated under parts B and C for each fiscal year to carry out this section.

(2) Maximum amount

For the first fiscal year in which the amount described in paragraph (1) is at least $20,000,000, the maximum amount the Secretary may reserve under paragraph (1) is $20,000,000. For each subsequent fiscal year, the maximum amount the Secretary may reserve under paragraph (1) is $20,000,000, increased by the cumulative rate of inflation since the fiscal year described in the previous sentence.

(3) Use of maximum amount

In any fiscal year described in paragraph (2) for which the Secretary reserves the maximum amount described in that paragraph, the Secretary shall use at least half of the reserved amount for activities under subsection (d).

[Apr. 13, 1970, Pub. I, 91-230, Title VI, Part D, Subpart 2, Ch. 1, Sec. 674, as added, June 4, 1997, Pub. I, 105-17, Title I, Sec. 674, III, Stat. 143.]

Chapter 2–Improving Early Intervention Educational, and Transitional Services and Results for Children with Disabilities through Coordinated Technical Assistance, Support, and Dissemination of Information

Sec. 1481 Findings and purposes

(a) In general

The Congress finds as follows:

(1) National technical assistance, support, and dissemination activities are necessary to ensure that parts B and C are fully implemented and achieve quality early intervention, educational, and transitional results for children with disabilities and their families.

(2) Parents, teachers, administrators, and related services personnel need technical assistance and information in a timely, coordinated, and accessible manner in order to improve early intervention, educational, and transitional services and results at the State and local levels for children with disabilities and their families.

(3) Parent training and information activities have taken on increased importance in efforts to assist parents of a child with a disability in dealing with the multiple pressures of rearing such a child and are of particular importance in—

(A) ensuring the involvement of such parents in planning and decision making with respect to early intervention, educational, and transitional services;

(B) achieving quality early intervention, educational, and transitional results for children with disabilities;

(C) providing such parents information on their rights and protections under this Act to ensure improved early intervention, educational, and transitional results for children with disabilities;

(D) assisting such parents in the development of skills to participate effectively in the education and development of their children and in the transitions described in Sec. 1474(b)(3)(C); and

(E) supporting the roles of such parents as participants within partnerships seeking to improve early intervention, educational, and transitional services and results for children with disabilities and their families.

(4) Providers of parent training and information activities need to ensure that such parents who have limited access to serv-ices and supports, due to economic, cultural, or linguistic barriers, are provided with access to appropriate parent training and information activities.

(5) Parents of children with disabilities need information that helps the parents to understand the rights and responsibilities of their children under part B.

(6) The provision of coordinated technical assistance and dissemination of information to State and local agencies, institutions of higher education, and other providers of services to children with disabilities is essential in—

(A) supporting the process of achieving systemic change;

(B) supporting actions in areas of priority specific to the improvement of early intervention, educational, and transitional results for children with disabilities;

(C) conveying information and assistance that are—

(i) based on current research (as of the date the information and assistance are conveyed);

(ii) accessible and meaningful for use in supporting systemic-change activities of State and local partnerships; and

(iii) linked directly to improving early intervention, educational, and transitional services and results for children with disabilities and their families; and

(D) organizing systems and information networks for such information, based on modern technology related to—

(i) storing and gaining access to information; and

(ii) distributing information in a systematic manner to parents, students, professionals, and policymakers.

(7) Federal support for carrying out technology research, technology development, and educational media services and activities has resulted in major innovations that have significantly improved early intervention, educational, and transitional services and results for children with disabilities and their families.

(8) Such Federal support is needed—

(A) to stimulate the development of software, interactive learning tools, and devices to address early intervention, educational, and transitional needs of children with disabilities who have certain disabilities;

(B) to make information available on technology research, technology development, and educational media services and activities to individuals involved in the provision of early intervention, educational, and transitional services to children with disabilities;

(C) to promote the integration of technology into curricula to improve early intervention, educational, and transitional results for children with disabilities;

(D) to provide incentives for the development of technology and media devices and tools that are not readily found or available because of the small size of potential markets;

(E) to make resources available to pay for such devices and tools and educational media services and activities;

(F) to promote the training of personnel—

(i) to provide such devices, tools, services, and activities in a competent manner; and

(ii) to assist children with disabilities and their families in using such devices, tools, services, and activities; and

(G) to coordinate the provision of such devices, tools, services, and activities—

(i) among State human services programs; and

(ii) between such programs and private agencies.

(b) Purposes

The purposes of this chapter are to ensure that—

(1) children with disabilities, and their parents, receive training and information on their rights and protections under this Act, in order to develop the skills necessary to effectively participate in planning and decision making relating to early intervention, educational, and transitional services and in systemic-change activities;

(2) parents, teachers, administrators, early intervention personnel, related services, personnel, and transition personnel receive coordinated and accessible technical assistance and information to assist such persons, through systemic-change activities and other efforts, to improve early intervention, educational, and transitional services and results for children with disabilities and their families;

(3) appropriate technology and media are researched, developed, demonstrated, and made available in timely and accessible formats to parents, teachers, and all types of personnel providing services to children with disabilities to support their roles as partners in the improvement and implementation of early intervention, educational, and transitional services and results for children with disabilities and families;

(4) on reaching the age of majority under State law, children with disabilities understand their rights and responsibilities under part B, if the State provides for the transfer of parental rights under Sec. 1415(m); and

(5) the general welfare of deaf and hard-of-hearing individuals is promoted by—

(A) bringing to such individuals understanding and appreciation of the films and television programs that play an important part in the general and cultural advancement of hearing individuals;

(B) providing, through those films and television programs, enriched educational and cultural experiences through which deaf and hard-of-hearing individuals can better understand the realities of their environment; and

(C) providing wholesome and rewarding experiences that deaf and hard-of-hearing individuals may share.

[Apr. 13, 1970, Pub. I, 91-230, Title VI, Part D, Subpart 2, Ch. 2, Sec. 681, as added, June 4, 1997, Pub. I, 105-17, Title I, Sec. 681, III Stat. 146.]

Sec. 1482   Parent training and information centers

(a) Program authorized

The Secretary may make grants to, and enter into contracts and cooperative agreements with, parent organizations to support parent training and information centers to carry out activities under this section.

(b) Required activities

Each parent training and information center that receives assistance under this section shall—

(1) provide training and information that meets the training and information needs of parents of children with disabilities living in the area served by the center, particularly underserved parents and parents of children who may be inappropriately identified;

(2) assist parents to understand the availability of, and how to effectively use, procedural safeguards under this Act, including encouraging the use, and explaining the benefits, of alternative methods of dispute resolution, such as the mediation process described in Sec. 1415(e);

(3) serve the parents of infants, toddlers, and children with the full range of disabilities;

(4) assist parents to—

(A) better understand the nature of their children's disabilities and their educational and developmental needs;

(B) communicate effectively with personnel responsible for providing special education, early intervention, and related services;

(C) participate in decision-making processes and the development of individualized education programs under part B and individualized family service plans under part C;

(D) obtain appropriate information about the range of options, programs, services, and resources available to assist children with disabilities and their families;

(E) understand the provisions of this Act for the education of, and the provision of early intervention services to, children with disabilities; and

(F) participate in school reform activities;

(5) in States where the State elects to contract with the parent training and information center, contract with State educational agencies to provide, consistent with subparagraphs (B) and (D) of Sec. 1415(e)(2), individuals who meet with parents to explain the mediation process to them;

(6) network with appropriate clearinghouses, including organizations conducting national dissemination activities under Sec. 1485(d), and with other national, State, and local organizations and agencies, such as protection and advocacy agencies, that serve parents and families of children with the full range of disabilities; and

(7) annually report to the Secretary on—

(A) the number of parents to whom it provided information and training in the most recently concluded fiscal year; and

(B) the effectiveness of strategies used to reach and serve parents, including underserved parents of children with disabilities.

(c) Optional activities

A parent training and information center that receives assistance under this section may—

(1) provide information to teachers and other professionals who provide special education and related services to children with disabilities;

(2) assist students with disabilities to understand their rights and responsibilities under Sec. 1415(m) on reaching the age of majority; and

(3) assist parents of children with disabilities to be informed participants in the development and implementation of the State's State improvement plan under subpart 1.

(d) Application requirements

Each application for assistance under this section shall identify with specificity the special efforts that the applicant will undertake—

(1) to ensure that the needs for training and information of underserved parents of children with disabilities in the area to be served are effectively met; and

(2) to work with community-based organizations.

(e) Distribution of funds

(1) In general

The Secretary shall make at least 1 award to a parent organization in each State, unless the Secretary does not receive an application from such an organization in each State of sufficient quality to warrant approval.

(2) Selection requirement

The Secretary shall select among applications submitted by parent organizations in a State in a manner that ensures the most effective assistance to parents, including parents in urban and rural areas, in the State.

(f) Quarterly review

(1) Requirements

(A) Meetings

The board of directors or special governing committee of each organization that receives an award under this section shall meet at least once in each calendar quarter to review the activities for which the award was made.

(B) Advising board

Each special governing committee shall directly advise the organization's governing board of its views and recommendations.

(2) Continuation award

When an organization requests a continuation award under this section, the board of directors or special governing committee shall submit to the Secretary a written review of the parent training and information program conducted by the organization during the preceding fiscal year.

(g) Definition of parent organization

As used in this section, the term 'parent organization' means a private nonprofit organization (other than an institution of higher education) that—

(1) has a board of directors—

(A) the majority of whom are parents of children with disabilities;

(B) that includes—

(i) individuals working in the fields of special education, related services, and early intervention; and

(ii) individuals with disabilities; and

(C) the parent and professional members of which are broadly representative of the population to be served; or

(2) has—

(A) a membership that represents the interests of individuals with disabilities and has established a special governing committee that meets the requirements of paragraph (1); and

(B) a memorandum of understanding between the special governing committee and the board of directors of the organization that clearly outlines the relationship between the board and the committee and the decision making responsibilities and authority of each.

[Apr. 13, 1970, Pub. I, 91-230, Title VI, Part D, Subpart 2, Ch. 2, Sec. 682, as added, June 4, 1997, Pub. I, 105-17, Title I, Sec. 682, III Stat. 149.]

Sec. 1483   Community parent resource centers

(a) In general

The Secretary may make grants to, and enter into contracts and cooperative agreements with, local parent organizations to support parent training and information centers that will help ensure that underserved parents of children with disabilities, including low-income parents, parents of children with limited English proficiency, and parents with disabilities, have the training and information they need to enable them to participate effectively in helping their children with disabilities—

(1) to meet developmental goals and, to the maximum extent possible, those challenging standards that have been established for all children; and

(2) to be prepared to lead productive independent adult lives, to the maximum extent possible.

(b) Required activities

Each parent training and information center assisted under this section shall—

(1) provide training and information that meets the training and information needs of parents of children with disabilities proposed to be served by the grant, contract, or cooperative agreement;

(2) carry out the activities required of parent training and information centers under paragraphs (2) through (7) of Sec. 1482(b);

(3) establish cooperative partnerships with the parent training and information centers funded under Sec. 1482; and

(4) be designed to meet the specific needs of families who experience significant isolation from available sources of information and support.

(c) Definition

As used in this section, the term 'local parent organization' means a parent organization, as defined in Sec. 1482(g), that either—

(1) has a board of directors the majority of whom are from the community to be served; or

(2) has—

(A) as part of its mission, serving the interests of individuals with disabilities from such community; and

(B) a special governing committee to administer the grant, contract, or cooperative agreement, a majority of the members of which are individuals from such community.

[Apr. 13, 1970, Pub. I, 91-230, Title VI, Part D, Subpart 2,Ch. 2, Sec. 683, as added, June 4, 1997, Pub. I, 105-17, Title I, Sec. 683, III Stat. 151.]

Sec. 1484   Technical assistance for parent training and information centers

(a) In general

The Secretary may, directly or through awards to eligible entities, provide technical assistance for developing, assisting, and coordinating parent training and information programs carried out by parent training and information centers receiving assistance under Secs. 1482 and 1483.

(b) Authorized activities

The Secretary may provide technical assistance to a parent training and information center under this section in areas such as—

(1) effective coordination of parent training efforts;

(2) dissemination of information

(3) evaluation by the center of itself;

(4) promotion of the use of technology, including assistive technology devices and assistive technology services;

(5) reaching underserved populations;

(6) including children with disabilities in general education programs;

(7) facilitation of transitions from—

(A) early intervention services to preschool;

(B) preschool to school; and

(C) secondary school to postsecondary environments; and

(8) promotion of alternative methods of dispute resolution.

[Apr. 13, 1970, Pub. I, 91-230, Title VI, Part D, Subpart 2, Ch. 2, Sec. 684, as added, June 4, 1997, Pub. I, 105-17, Title I, Sec. 684, III Stat. 152.]

Sec. 1485   Coordinated technical assistance and dissemination

(a) In general

The Secretary shall, by competitively making grants or

entering into contracts and cooperative agreements with eligible entities, provide technical assistance and information, through such mechanisms as institutes, Regional Resource Centers, clearinghouses, and programs that support States and local entities in building capacity, to improve early intervention, educational, and transitional services, and results for children with disabilities and their families, and address systemic-change goals and priorities.

(b) Systemic technical assistance; authorized activities

(1) In general

In carrying out this section, the Secretary shall carry out or support technical assistance activities, consistent with the objectives described in subsection (a), relating to systemic change.

(2) Authorized activities

Activities that may be carried out under this subsection include activities such as the following:

(A) Assisting States, local educational agencies, and other participants in partnerships established under subpart 1 with the process of planning systemic changes that will promote improved early intervention, educational, and transitional results for children with disabilities.

(B) Promoting change through a multistate or regional framework that benefits States, local educational agencies, and other participants in partnerships that are in the process of achieving systemic-change outcomes.

(C) Increasing the depth and utility of information in ongoing and emerging areas of priority need identified by States, local educational agencies, and other participants in partnerships that are in the process of achieving systemic-change outcomes.

(D) Promoting communication and information exchange among States, local educational agencies, and other participants in partnerships, based on the needs and concerns identified by the participants in the partnerships, rather than on externally imposed criteria or topics, regarding—

(i) the practices, procedures, and policies of the States, local educational agencies, and other participants in partnerships; and

(ii) accountability of the States, local educational agencies, and other participants in partnerships for improved early intervention, educational, and transitional results for children with disabilities.

(c) Specialized technical assistance; authorized activities

(1) In general

In carrying out this section, the Secretary shall carry out or support activities, consistent with the objectives described in subsection (a), relating to areas of priority or specific populations.

(2) Authorized activities

Examples of activities that may be carried out under this subsection include activities that—

(A) focus on specific areas of high-priority need that—

(i) are identified by States, local educational agencies, and other participants in partnerships;

(ii) require the development of new knowledge, or the analysis and synthesis of substantial bodies of information not readily available to the States, agencies, and other participants in partnerships; and

(iii) will contribute significantly to the improvement of early intervention, educational, and transitional services and results for children with disabilities and their families;

(B) focus on needs and issues that are specific to a population of children with disabilities, such as the provision of single-State and multi-State technical assistance and in-service training—

(i) to schools and agencies serving deaf-blind children and their families; and

(ii) to programs and agencies serving other groups of children with low-incidence disabilities and their families; or

(C) address the postsecondary education needs of individuals who are deaf or hard of hearing.

(d) National information dissemination; authorized activities

(1) In general

In carrying out this section, the Secretary shall carry out or support information dissemination activities that are consistent with the objectives described in subsection (a), including activities that address national needs for the preparation and dissemination of information relating to eliminating barriers to systemic-change and improving early intervention, educational, and transitional results for children with disabilities.

(2) Authorized activities

Examples of activities that may be carried out under this subsection include activities relating to—

(A) infants and toddlers with disabilities and their families, and children with disabilities and their families;

(B) services for populations of children with low-incidence disabilities, including deaf-blind children, and targeted age groupings;

(C) the provision of postsecondary services to individuals with disabilities;

(D) the need for and use of personnel to provide services to children with disabilities, and personnel recruitment, retention, and preparation;

(E) issues that are of critical interest to State educational agencies and local educational agencies, other agency personnel, parents of children with disabilities, and individuals with disabilities;

(F) educational reform and systemic change within States; and

(G) promoting schools that are safe and conducive to learning.

(3) Linking States to information sources

In carrying out this subsection, the Secretary may support projects that link States to technical assistance resources, including special education and general education resources, and may make research and related products available through libraries, electronic networks, parent training projects, and other information sources.

(e) Applications

An eligible entity that wishes to receive a grant, or enter into a contract or cooperative agreement, under this section shall submit an application to the Secretary at such time, in such manner, and containing such information as the Secretary may require.

[Apr. 13, 1970, Pub. I, 91-230, Title VI, Part D, Subpart 2, Ch. 2, Sec. 686, as added, June 4, 1997, Pub. I, 105-17, Title I, Sec. 685, III Stat. 152.]

Sec. 1486   Authorization of appropriations

There are authorized to be appropriated to carry out Secs. 1481 through 1485 such sums as may be necessary for each of the fiscal years 1998 through 2002.

[Apr. 13, 1970, Pub. I, 91-230, Title VI, Part D, Subpart 2, Ch. 2, Sec. 671, as added, June 4, 1997, Pub. I, 105-17, Title I, Sec. 686, III Stat. 154.]

Sec. 1487   Technology development, demonstration, and utilization, and media services

(a) In general

The Secretary shall competitively make grants to, and enter into contracts and cooperative agreements with, eligible entities to support activities described in subsections (b) and (c)

(b) Technology development, demonstration, and utilization; authorized activities

(1) In general

In carrying out this section, the Secretary shall support activities to promote the development, demonstration, and utilization of technology.

(2) Authorized activities

Activities that may be carried out under this subsection include activities such as the following:

(A) Conducting research and development activities on the use of innovative and emerging technologies for children with disabilities.

(B) Promoting the demonstration and use of innovative and emerging technologies for children with disabilities by improving and expanding the transfer of technology from research and development to practice.

(C) Proving technical assistance to recipients of other assistance under this section, concerning the development of accessible, effective, and usable products.

(D) Communicating information on available technology and the uses of such technology to assist children with disabilities.

(E) Supporting the implementation of research programs on captioning or video description.

(F) Supporting research, development, and dissemination of technology with universal-design features, so that the technology is accessible to individuals with disabilities without further modifications or adaptation.

(G) Demonstrating the use of publicly-funded telecommunications systems to provide parents and teachers with information and training concerning early diagnosis of, intervention for, and effective teaching strategies for, young children with reading disabilities.

(c) Educational media services; authorized activities

In carrying out this section, the Secretary shall support—

(1) educational media activities that are designed to be of educational value to children with disabilities;

(2) providing video description, open captioning, or closed captioning of television programs, videos, or educational materials through September 30, 2001; and after fiscal year 2001, providing video description, open captioning, or closed captioning of educational, news, and informational television, videos, or materials;

(3) distributing captioned and described videos or educational materials through such mechanisms as a loan service;

(4) providing free educational materials, including textbooks, in accessible media for visually impaired and print-disabled students in elementary, secondary, postsecondary, and graduate schools;

(5) providing cultural experiences through appropriate non-profit organizations, such as the National Theater of the Deaf, that—

(A) enrich the lives of deaf and hard-of-hearing children and adults;

(B) increase public awareness and understanding of deafness and of the artistic and intellectual achievements of deaf and hard-of-hearing persons; or

(C) promote the integration of hearing, deaf, and hard-of-

hearing persons through shared cultural, educational, and social experiences; and

(6) compiling and analyzing appropriate data relating to the activities described in paragraphs (1) through (5).

(d) Applications

Any eligible entity that wishes to receive a grant, or enter into a contract or cooperative agreement, under this section shall submit an application to the Secretary at such time, in such manner, and containing such information as the Secretary may require.

(e) Authorization of appropriations

There are authorized to be appropriated to carry out this section such sums as may be necessary for each of the fiscal years 1998 through 2002.

[Apr. 13, 1970, Pub. I, 91-230, Title VI, Part D, Subpart 2, Ch. 2, Sec. 671, as added, June 4, 1997, Pub. I, 105-17, Title I, Sec. 687, III Stat. 154.]

Miscellaneous Provisions

Effective Dates

(a) Parts A and B

(1) In general

Except as provided in paragraph (2), parts A and B of the Individuals with Disabilities Education Act, as amended by title I, shall take effect upon the enactment of this Act.

(2) Exceptions

(A) In general

Secs. 1412(a)(4), 1412(a)(14), 1412(a)(16), 1414(d) (except for paragraph (6)), and 1418 of the Individuals with Disabilities Education Act, as amended by title I, shall take effect on July 1, 1998.

(B) Sec. 1417

Sec. 1417 of the Individuals with Disabilities Education Act, as amended by title I, shall take effect on October 1, 1997.

(C) Individualized education programs and comprehensive system of personnel development

Sec. 1418 of the Individuals with Disabilities Education Act, as in effect on the day before the date of the enactment of this Act, and the provisions of parts A and B of the Individuals with Disabilities Education Act relating to individualized education programs and the State's comprehensive system of personnel development, as so in effect, shall remain in effect until July 1, 1998.

(D) Secs. 1411 and 1419

Secs. 1411 and 1419, as amended by title I, shall take effect beginning with funds appropriated for fiscal year 1998.

(b) Part C

Part C of the Individuals with Disabilities Education Act, as amended by title I, shall take effect on July 1, 1998.

(c) Part D

(1) In general

Except as provided in paragraph (2), part D of the Individuals with Disabilities Education Act, as amended by title I, shall take effect on October 1, 1997.

(2) Exception

Paragraphs (1) and (2) of Sec. 1461(g) of the Individuals with Disabilities Education Act, as amended by title I, shall take effect on January 1, 1998.

Transition

Notwithstanding any other provision of law, beginning on October 1, 1997, the Secretary of Education may use funds appropriated under part D of the Individuals with Disabilities Education Act to make continuation awards for projects that were funded under Sec. 1418 and parts C through G of such Act (as in effect on September 30, 1997).

Repealers

(a) Part 1

Effective October 1, 1998, part I of the Individuals with Disabilities Education Act is hereby repealed.

(b) Part H

Effective July 1, 1998, part H of such Act is hereby repealed.

(c) Parts C, E, F, and G

Effective October 1, 1997, parts C, E, F, and G of such Act are hereby repealed.

F

Rehabilitation Act of 1973

NONDISCRIMINATION UNDER
FEDERAL GRANTS AND PROGRAMS

Sec. 504 (a) No otherwise qualified individual with a disability in the United States, as defined in section 7(20), shall, solely by reason of her or his disability, be excluded from the participation in, be denied the benefits of, or be subjected to discrimination under any program or activity receiving Federal financial assistance or under any program or activity program or activity receiving Federal financial assistance or under any program or activity conducted by any Executive agency or by the United States Postal Service. The head of each such agency shall promulgate such regulations as may be necessary to carry out the amendments to this section made by the Rehabilitation, Comprehensive Services, and Developmental Disabilities Act of 1978. Copies of any proposed regulation shall be submitted to appropriate authorizing committees of Congress, and such regulations may take effect no earlier than the thirtieth day after the date on which such regulation is so submitted to such committees.

(b) For the purposes of this section, the term "program or activity" means all of the operations of—

(1)(A) a department, agency, special purpose district, or other instrumentality of a State or of a local government; or

(B) the entity of such a State or local government that distributes such assistance and each such department or agency (and each other State or local government entity) to which the assistance is extended, in the case of assistance to a State or local government;

(2)(A) a college, university, or other postsecondary institution, or a public system of higher education; or

(B) a local educational agency (as defined in section 14101 of the Elementary and Secondary Education Act of 1965), system of vocational education, or other school system;

(3)(A) an entire corporation, partnership, or other private organization, or an entire sole proprietorship—

(i) if assistance is extended to such corporation, partnership, private organization, or sole proprietorship as a whole; or

(ii) which is principally engaged in the business of providing education, health care, housing, social services, or parks and recreation; or

(B) the entire plant or other comparable, geographically separate facility to which Federal financial assistance is extended, in the case of any corporation, partnership, private organization, or sole proprietorship; or

(4) any other entity which is established by two or more of the entities described in paragraph (1), (2), or (3); any part of which is extended Federal financial assistance.

(c) Small providers are not required by subsection (a) to make significant structural alterations to their existing facilities for the purpose of assuring program accessibility, if alternative means of providing the services are available. The terms used in this subsection shall be construed with reference to the regulations existing on the date of the enactment of this subsection.

(d) The standards used to determine whether this section has been violated in a complaint alleging employment discrimination under this section shall be the standards applied under title I of the Americans with Disabilities Act of 1990 (42 U.S.C. 12111 et seq.) and the provisions of sections 501 through 504, and 510, of the Americans with Disabilities Act of 1990 (42 U.S.C. 12201-12204 and 12210), as such sections relate to employment.

From http://www.nfb.org/rehabact.htm

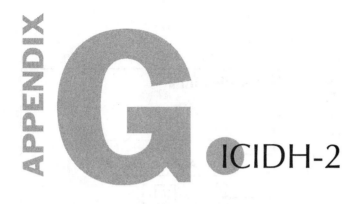

World Health Organization
Geneva, 2000
(Reprinted with permission.)

TOWARDS A COMMON LANGUAGE FOR FUNCTIONING AND DISABILITY: ICIDH–2
The International Classification of Functioning and Disability World Health Organization

Introduction

In 1980, the World Health Organization published the first trial version of the ICIDH *(International Classification of Impairments, Disabilities, and Handicaps)* as a tool for the classification of the *"consequences of disease".* Since classifications of diseases fail to capture the variety of experiences of people with health problems, the ICIDH was designed to fill that gap.

After two decades of use, it has become clear that the classification requires revision in the light of *changes in health care* and a *new social understanding of disability.*

At a Glance

What's New?
- Operational definitions given for all categories
- Neutral terminology
- Includes environmental factors
- Social model orientation
- 'Participation' rather than 'Handicap'
- 'Activity' instead of 'Disability'
- Structural and functional impairments separated

In accordance with the WHO mandate to develop a *global common language* in the field of health, broadly understood to include physical, mental and social well-being, WHO has now revised the ICIDH by a process of wide consultation to reach an international consensus. The new version, known as the ICIDH-2 Beta-2 draft, is now being field tested.

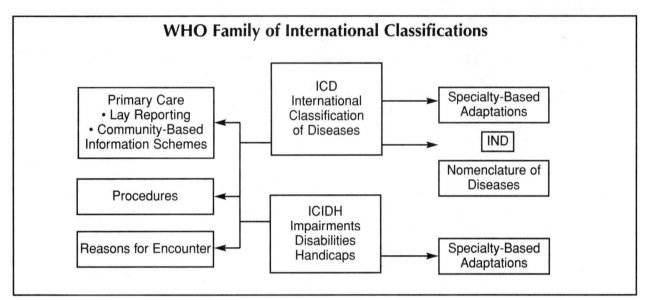

Figure G-1. WHO family of international classifications.

The ICIDH-2 is a multi-purpose classification designed for use in different settings and provides a common framework for understanding the dimensions of disability and functioning at three different levels: the body, the person, and society.

ICIDH-2 and the WHO Family of International Classifications

The ICIDH-2 belongs to the WHO family of international classifications, the best known member of which is the *International Statistical Classification of Diseases and Related Health Problems (ICD)*. The ICD classifies "diseases" and has evolved from a list of *"causes of death"*. It has a medical orientation and has given rise to a number of applications and adaptations. The *ICIDH-2*, by contrast, classifies *human functioning* at the level of the body, the whole person, and the person within the complete social and physical environmental context. These classifications can then be used to identify a variety of consequences of health conditions including diseases, disorders, injuries and other conditions. Thus, the ICIDH-2 complements the ICD and its applications and adaptations (Figure G-1).

Why Is There a Need for the ICIDH-2?

- To better define the *need for health services* and related interventions;
- To define *health outcomes* in terms of body, person and social functioning;
- To provide a *common framework* for research, clinical work, and social policy;
- To ensure the *cost-effective* provision and management of health care and related services;
- To characterize *physical, mental, social, economic or environmental interventions* that will improve the lives and levels of human functioning.

Studies have shown that in the health services sector, diagnosis alone does not predict service needs, length of hospitalization, level of care or outcomes. We also know that a medical condition is not an accurate predictor of receipt of disability benefits, work performance, return to work potential, or the likelihood of social integration. So, a purely medical classification of diagnoses does not provide us with the information we require for planning and management purposes. However, when data on functioning are taken into account, the predictive power and understanding of needs and outcomes are increased.

The health care sector is also shifting its focus from hospital-based care of acute conditions to long-term services for chronic conditions in the communities where people live and work. Social welfare agencies are looking for ways to provide better and more cost-efficient disability benefits. In the public and private sectors around the world there is a need for an international "common language" to describe and classify the consequences of disease, disorders, injuries and other health conditions.

There is also an increased recognition among social planners and service agencies that reducing the incidence and severity of disability in a population involves modifying the social and physical environment as well as enhancing the level of functioning of the person.

Designed to meet these growing needs, the ICIDH-2 has potential uses in many different sectors:

- Health services
- Insurance
- Social security and pensions
- Employment
- Human rights
- Research
- Planning and policy formulation
- Education and training
- Economics and human development

Thus, the ICIDH-2, in addition to providing a scientific model for the study of functioning and disability, meets the urgent need for a common, international language for globalized data collection, research, health care resource allocation and management, and social welfare programming.

How Can the ICIDH-2 Be Used?

The ICIDH-2 provides a model of human functioning and disability, as well as a classification system that is useful at all levels of service provision and policy development, scientific research, intervention strategies and economic analyses.

Service Provision and Policy Development

Individual level: Personal evaluation
- For the assessment of individuals: *What is the condition or level of functioning?*
- For individual treatment planning: *What treatments or interventions can maximize functioning?*
- For the evaluation of treatment and other interventions: *What are the outcomes? How useful were the interventions?*
- For communication among different categories of health care workers and community agencies (e.g., physicians, nurses, physiotherapists, occupational therapists, social workers) and coordination of different types of care: *Who says what? What do they actually mean? Can one understand the other? Can data between users and sectors be compared?*
- For self-evaluation by consumers: *How will people evaluate their functioning themselves?*

Institutional level: Services
- For educational and training purposes: *Educating staff and clients*
- For resource planning and development: *What services will be needed?*
- For quality improvement: *How well do we serve? What are the basic indicators for quality assurance?*
- *For management and outcome evaluation: How useful is the service?*
- For managed care models of health care delivery: *How effective is the service? Is it effective? Is the service worth the cost? How can it be improved in terms of quality or cost?*

Societal level: Social Needs
- For research: local, regional, national and international data collection
    How many people have a problem with functioning?
    Who are these people?

> *What are their needs?*
> *Which services do they use?*
> *How much better do they get?*

- For eligibility criteria for state entitlements C social security benefits, disability pensions, workers= compensation and insurance: *What are the criteria for eligibility for disability benefits?*
- For social policy development, including legislative reviews, model legislation, regulations and guidelines, and definitions for anti-discrimination legislation: *What are the rights of individuals and the duties of the society towards its members?*
- For needs assessments: *What are the needs of persons with various levels of disability C impairments, activity limitations and participation restrictions?*
- For environmental assessment for universal design, implementation of mandated accessibility, identification of environmental facilitators and barriers, and changes to social policy: *How can we make the social and built environment more accessible for all persons with disabilities?*

Scientific Research

Traditionally, scientists have measured the *outcomes* of health conditions by relying on mortality data. More recently, the international concern about health care outcomes has shifted to the assessment of functioning at the level of the whole human being, in day-to-day life. The need here is for universally applicable classification and *assessment tools,* both for activity levels and for overall levels of participation, by the individual in the basic areas and roles of social life. This is what the ICIDH-2 provides and makes possible.

Intervention Strategies

The conceptual model of the ICIDH-2 helps to characterize the kind and level of intervention that is appropriate to the actual disability needs of the individual:

> *Impairment interventions:* Medical interventions to deal with the impairment, and preventive interventions to avoid activity limitation.
>
> *Activity limitation interventions:* Rehabilitative interventions and provision of assistive devices and personal assistance to mitigate the activity limitation, and preventive interventions to avoid participation restrictions.
>
> *Participation restriction interventions:* Public education, equalization of opportunities, social reform and legislation, architectural "universal design" applications and other ways of accommodating activity limitations in major life areas.

Economic Analyses

The effective use of resources for health care and other social services requires a consistent and standard classification of health outcomes that can be costed and compared internationally. To prevent restrictions on participation, it is important to cost the economic impact of functional deficits as compared to the costs of modifying the built and social environment. The ICIDH-2 makes both of these tasks possible.

The Model of the ICIDH-2

The ICIDH-2 has been constructed to reflect a specific model of disability, the biopsychosocial model. In that model, human functioning and disability are viewed as outcomes of an interaction between a person's physical or mental condition and the social and physical environment. The so-called 'medical' model of disability, which locates disability entirely within the person, and views medical interventions as the only possible response to disability, has long been criticized and rejected by experts. Yet, there are appropriate medical responses to some aspects of disability, so the underlying message of the medical model cannot be wholly abandoned. What is needed instead is a *synthesis of the social and the medical models,* and this is what has been attempted in the ICIDH-2 (Figure G-2).

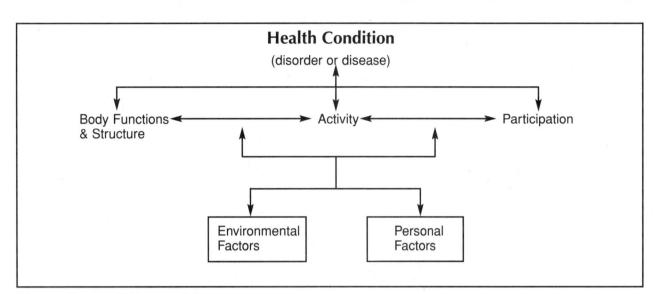

Figure G-2. ICIDH-2 model.

The precise extent to which the resulting level of functioning in a particular instance has been influenced by intrinsic features of the individual, or features of the external world is a matter for scientific research. Whether people with specific health conditions typically have predictable activity limitations or encounter the same kinds of environmental barriers are also questions that need to be empirically discovered. In short, the process of disability is open to scientific inquiry. The ICIDH-2 is a classification system which, for the first time, incorporates the social model of disability, thereby opening the way to explore multiple determinants of disability.

Concepts of Disability and Functioning

The fundamental structural components of the ICIDH-2 are classifications of human functioning conceptualized at three levels: the body or body part, the whole person, and the whole person in a social context. Functioning is understood to occur in a context, characterized by all aspects of the physical and social environment, as well as other features of the individual, such as their sex, age, educational background and so on. In the ICIDH-2 these factors are listed in the Contextual Factors. Disabilities are therefore the dimensions of dysfunctioning that may result for an individual at three levels:
- Losses or abnormalities of bodily function and structure
- Limitations of activities
- Restrictions of participation

As Figure G-2 indicates, in the ICIDH-2 model, disability and functioning are viewed as outcomes of interactions between *health conditions* and *contextual factors*. The interaction is complex, bi-directional, and dynamic. The model does not posit a causal linkage between the three dimensions of disability; rather, at each level, disability occurs within and by means of contextual factors.

Two sorts of contextual factors are identified *environmental factors* (for example, social attitudes, architectural characteristics, legal and social structures, as well as climate, terrain, and so forth); and *personal factors,* which include gender, age, coping styles, social background, education, profession, past and current experience, overall behaviour pattern, character and other factors that influence how disability is experienced by the individual.

It is possible to conceive the dimensions of functioning and disability as a continuum (Figure G-3)

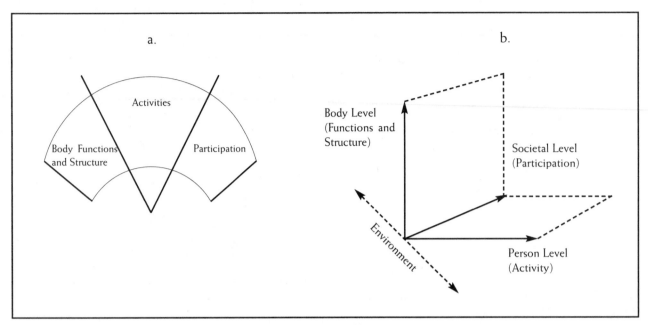

Figure G-3. Different conceptualizations of the dimensions of functioning and disability.

In a continuum approach, boundaries need to be drawn between Body Functions (B), Activities (A), and Participation (P). For example, a function should only be in one dimension. A multidimensional approach, however, allows various functions be viewed in different dimensions at the same time. For example, a state can be seen as a composite of body functions, activities and participation at the same time. Since the nature of functions within each dimension of B, A, P are different, multidimensional approach is preferred in ICIDH-2. For example, an individual may have difficulties with memory, experience activity limitations in learning new things, and have limited participation in areas of life that require learning.

The Definitions of the Levels of Functioning in the ICIDH-2

The ICIDH-2 sets out three levels of functioning – Impairments, Activities, and Participation – and the three levels form distinct but parallel classifications. Limitations of activities and restrictions of participation constitute, along with impairments, the three dimensions of disability. The conceptual definitions of the dimensions, set out below, provide the key to applying the new model.

In the Context of a Health Condition:

Body Functions are the physiological or psychological functions of body systems.

Body Structures are anatomic parts of the body such as organs, limbs and their components.

Impairments are problems in body function or structure such as a significant deviation or loss.

Activity is the performance of a task or action by an individual.

Activity Limitations are difficulties an individual may have in the performance of activities.

Participation is an individual's involvement in life situations in relation to Health Conditions, Body Functions and Structure, Activities, and Contextual factors.

Participation Restrictions are problems an individual may have in the manner or extent of involvement in life situations.

Thus, there are four dimensions represented in the ICIDH-2, three levels of functioning and contextual factors. The three levels of functioning (at the body, person, and social levels), in interaction with contextual factors yield as outcomes either positive or negative levels of functioning, and both can be classified in the ICIDH-2. The negative levels of functioning are the three kinds of disabilities impairments, activity limitations and participation restrictions.

	Body Functions and Structures	**Activities**	**Participation**	**Contextual Factors**[1]
Level of Functioning	Body (body parts)	Individual (person as a whole)	Society (life situations)	Environmental Factors (external influence on functioning) + Personal Factors (internal influence on functioning)
Characteristics	Body function Body structure	Performance of individual's activities	Involvement in life situations	Features of the physical, social, and attitudinal world + Attributes of the person
Positive aspect (Functioning)	Functional and structural integrity	Activity	Participation	Facilitators
Negative aspect (Disability)	Impairment	Activity limitation	Participation restriction	Barriers/hindrances
Qualifiers: First Qualifier	*Uniform Qualifier: Extent or Magnitude*			
Second Qualifier	Localization	Assistance	Subjective satisfaction (under development)	(under development)
1. Contextual Factors are an essential component of the classification and interact with all three dimensions.				

Figure G-4. Overview of the ICIDH-2 components.

Figure G-4 presents an overview of the components of the ICIDH-2.

The three dimensions and the environmental factors in ICIDH-2 are presented in two versions in order to meet the needs of different users for varying levels of detail. The first version is a *short (concise) version* that gives two levels of categories for each dimension or component. The second version is a *long (detailed) version* (Figure G-5) that provides all levels of classification and allows for 9999 categories per component. The long-version categories can be aggregated into the short version when summary information is required.

Figure G-6 gives some possible examples of disabilities that may be associated with the three levels of functioning, linked to a health condition.

Figure G-7 indicates how the different levels of disability are linked to three different levels of intervention.

Body

Function:

Mental Functions
Sensory Functions
Voice and Speech Functions
Functions of the Cardiovascular, Hematological,
    Immunological, and Respiratory Systems
Functions of the Digestive, Metabolic, Endocrine
    Systems
Genitourinary and Reproductive Functions
Neuromusculoskeletal and Movement-Related
    Functions
Functions of the Skin and Related Structures

Structure:

Structure of the Nervous System
The Eye, Ear, and Related Structures
Structures Involved in Voice and Speech
Structure of the Cardiovascular, Immunological,
    and Respiratory Systems
Structures Related to the Digestive, Metabolism,
    and Endocrine Systems
Structure Related to Genitourinary System
Structure Related to Movement
Skin and Related Structures

Activities

Activities of Learning and Applying Knowledge
Communication Activities
Movement Activities
Activities of Moving Around
Self-Care Activities
Domestic Activities
Interpersonal Activities
Performing Tasks and Major Life Activities

Participation

Participation in Personal Maintenance
Participation in Mobility
Participation in Exchange of Information
Participation in Social Relationships
Participation in Home Life and Assistance to Others
Participation in Education
Participation in Work and Employment
Participation in Economic Life
Participation in Community, Social, and Civic Life

Environmental Factors

Products and Technology
Natural Environment and Human-Made Changes to Environment
Support and Relationships
Attitudes, Values, and Beliefs
Services
Systems and Policies

Figure G-5. The content of the long version.

Health Condition	Impairment	Activity Limitation	Participation Restriction
Leprosy	Loss of sensation of extremities	Difficulties in grasping objects	Denied employment because of the stigma of leprosy
Panic Disorder	Anxiety	Limitations in going out alone	Restricted involvement in social relationships because of fears of the impairments
Spinal Injury	Paralysis	Limitations in using public transportation	Restricted participation in religious activities
Juvenile diabetes	Pancreatic dysfunction	None (controlled by medication)	Restricted participation in food consumption
Vitiligo	Facial disfigurement	None	Restrictions in participation in social relations due to fears of contagion
Person who formally had a mental health problem and was treated for a psychotic disorder	None	None	Denied employment because of employer's prejudice

Figure G-6. Possible examples of disabilities that may be associated with the three levels of functioning linked to a health condition.

	Intervention	Prevention
Health Condition	Medical treatment/care Medication	Health promotion Nutrition
Impairment	Medical treatment/care Medication Surgery	Prevention of the development of further activity limitations
Activity Limitation	Assistive devices Personal assistance Rehabilitation therapy	Preventive rehabilitation Prevention of the development of participation restrictions
Participation Restriction	Accommodations Public education Anti-discrimination law Universal design	Environmental change Employment strategies Accessible services Universal design Lobbying for change

Figure G-7. How the different levels of disability are linked to three different levels of intervention.

New Features and Improvements in the ICIDH-2

The revision of the ICIDH-2 has arisen from a consensus among experts and persons with disabilities about the essential features of a classification of functioning and disability. The biopsychosocial model of disability, already described, provided the conceptual framework for the ICIDH-2. Linked to this model are important principles that have guided every step of the revision process:

Universality

Classifications of disability are applicable to all people irrespective of health condition. Therefore, the ICIDH-2 is about all people. It concerns everyone's functioning. Thus, it should not become a tool for labeling persons with disabilities as a separate group.

Parity

Underlying the classifications is the principle that there is no distinction, at the level of impairment, activity limitation or participation restriction, between different health conditions (e.g., mental and physical). In other words, disability is not differentiated by etiology.

Definitions

All categories and individual items in the four dimensions are operationally defined; their basic attributes, boundaries, and measurement characteristics are provided and in most instances concrete examples are given.

Neutrality

As many category and item terms as possible are worded in neutral language so that the classifications can express both positive and negative aspects of each dimension.

Structure and Function

Impairments of structure and impairments of function are separately classified in order to capture all aspects of body-level functioning.

Activities

Instead of classifying disabilities, the ICIDH-2 classifies the full range of human activities that a person actually performs, so that, by means of a severity qualifier, limitations of these activities can be recorded.

Participation

Instead of classifying the handicaps that a person may face, the ICIDH-2 classifies the full range of areas of social life in which people participate, and this classification of Participation can be used, in conjunction with the list of environmental factors to identify degrees of a person's participation in various areas of life.

Environmental Factors

In order to complete the social model of disability, the ICIDH-2 includes Contextual Factors, in which environmental factors are listed. These factors range from physical factors such as climate and terrain, to social attitudes, institutions, and laws. These factors can be employed to identify environmental barriers and facilitators that affect Participation levels.

The Revision Process

The ICIDH-2 is being revised by means of an international, consensual process in which experts and persons with disabilities around the world contribute to the aim of ensuring that the ICIDH-2 is translatable into several languages and is applicable in many cultures. Beginning from 1995, two successive revisions/drafts (Alpha Draft 1996 and Beta-1 Draft 1997) have been published, translated into some 20 languages, and tested according to standard protocols to obtain feedback on the the concepts, feasibility, and utility of the classification. With the publication of the Beta-2 Draft in 1999 and the start of Beta-2 field trials, the revision process has entered its last stage before finalization of the classification.

The Beta-2 Field Trial Protocols

In over 45 countires worldwide the Beta-2 Draft of ICIDH-2 is currently undergoing extensive field testing. While the Beta-1 field trials focused on the development of the conceptual framework and used an approach of international consensus building, the Beta-2 field trials aim to test the practical uses of ICIDH-2 in terms of feasibility and ease of use. Therefore, an evidence-based revision process has been adopted using formal testing procedures to assess coding.

To elicit systematic information on the properties and utility of the ICIDH-2, the following protocols are being carried out:

The Core Studies:

Study One: Translation and Linguistic Evaluation

Study Two: Basic Questions

Study Three: Feasibility and Reliability for Cases and Case Summaries

Additional Studies:

Study Four: Feasibility and Reliability in Evaluating Health Records

Study Five: Feasibility and Reliability in a Survey

Study Six: Face Validity and Predictive Validity

Study Seven: Utility for Intervention Planning and Evaluation

Study Eight: Individual Centre and Task Force Recommended Studies

The current phase of the field trials will continue until July 2000. Therafter, data gathered will be analysed and the draft revised. The ICIDH-2 is scheduled to be placed before the Governing Bodies of the World health Organization for final approval in 2001.

The international activity that has gone into the revision of the ICIDH-2, and the work yet to be done, has been coordinated by the following centers, task forces, and non-governmental organizations:

Collaborating Centers:

Australia: Australian Institute of Health and Welfare, GPO Box 570, Canberra ACT 2601, Australia
Contact: Ros Madden.

Canada: Canadian Institute for Health Information, 377 Dalhousie Street, Suite 200, Ottawa Ontario KIN9N8, Canada
Contact: Janice Miller.

France: Centre technique national d'études et de recherches sur les handicaps et les inadaptations (TNERHI), 236 bis, rue de Tolbiac, 75013 Paris, France
Contact: Marc Maudinet.

Japan: Japan College of Social Work, 3-1-30 Takeoka, Kiyosehi, Tokyo 204, Japan
Contact: Hisao Sato.

The Netherlands: Center for Standardization of Informatics in Health Care (CSIZ), Driebergseweg 3, 3708 JA Zeist, The Netherlands,
Contacts: Willem Hirs and Marijke W. de Kleijn de Vrankrijker.

Nordic countries: Department of Public Health and Caring Sciences, Uppsala Science Park, SE Uppsala Sweden
Contact: Björn Smedby.

United Kingdom: NHS Information Authority, Coding and Classification, Woodgate, Loughborough, Leics LE11 2TG, United Kingdom.
Contact: Ann Harding, Jane Millar

USA: National Center for Health Statistics, Room 850, 6525, Belcrest Road, Hyattsville MD 20782, USA
Contact: Paul Placek.

Task Forces:

The International Task Force on Mental Health and Addictive, Behavioural, Cognitive, and Developmental Aspects of ICIDH, Chair: Cille Kennedy, Assistant Director for Disability Research, NIMH Division of Services and Intervention Research, 6001 Executive Blvd., Room 7138, Bethesda MD 20892-9631, USA. Co-Chair: Karen Ritchie.

Children and Youth Task Force, Chair: Rune J. Simeonsson, Professor of Education, Frank Porter Graham Child Development Center, CB # 8185, University of North Carolina, Chapel Hill, NC 27599-8185, USA. Co-Chair: Matilde Leonardi.

Environmental Factors Task Force, Chair: Rachel Hurst, 11 Belgrave Road, London SW1V 1RB, United Kingdom. Co-Chair: Janice Miller.

Networks:

La Red de Habla Hispana en Discapacidades (The Spanish Network). Co-ordinator: Jose Luis Vazquez-Barquero, Unidad de Investigacion en Psiquiatria Clinical y Social Hospital Universitario "Marques de Valdecilla", Avda. Valdecilla s/n, Santander 39008 Spain.

The Council of Europe Committee of Experts for the Application of ICIDH, Council of Europe, F-67075, Strasbourg, France. Contact: Lauri Sivonen.

Non Governmental Organizations:

Disabled Peoples International, 11 Belgrave Road, London SW1V 1RB, United Kingdom. Contact: Rachel Hurst.

European Disability Forum, Square Ambiorix, 32 Bte 2/A, B-1000, Bruxelles, Belgium. Contact: Frank Mulcahy.

European Regional Council for the World Federation of Mental Health (ERCWFM), Blvd Clovis N.7, 1000 Brussels, Belgium. Contact: John Henderson.

Inclusion International, 13D Chemin de Levant, F-01210, Ferney-Voltaire, France. Contact: Nancy Breitenbach

Rehabilitation International, 25 E. 21st Street, New York, NY 10010, USA. Contact: Judith Hollenweger, Chairman RI Education Commission, Institute of Special Education, University of Zurich, Hirschengraben 48, 8001 Zurich, Switzerland.

Participants in the revision process are being continuously updated on the webpage <www.who.ch/icidh>

Conclusion

The ICIDH-2 offers an international, scientific tool for the paradigm shift from the purely medical model to an integrated biopsychosocial model of human functioning and disability. It is a valuable tool in research into disability, in all its dimensions—impairments at the body and body part level, person level activity limitations, and societal level restrictions of participation. The ICIDH-2 also provides the conceptual model and classification required for instruments to assess the social and built environment.

The ICIDH-2 will be an essential basis for the standardization of data concerning all aspects of human functioning and disability around the world. The ICIDH-2 will be used by persons with disabilities and professionals alike to evaluate health care settings that deal with chronic illness and disability, such as rehabilitation centers, nursing homes, psychiatric institutions, and community services.

The ICIDH-2 will be useful for persons with all forms of disabilities, not only for identifying their health care and rehabilitative needs, but also in identifying and measuring the effect of the physical and social environment on the disadvantages that they experience in their lives.

From the viewpoint of health economics, the ICIDH-2 will help monitor and explain health care and other disability costs. Measuring functioning and disabilities will make it possible to quantify the productivity loss and its impact on the lives of the people in each society. The classification will also be of great use in the evaluation of intervention programs.

In some of the developed countries, the ICIDH and its model of disability have been introduced into legislation and social policy. As the ICIDH-2 becomes the world standard for disability data and social policy modelling, it will be introduced in the legislation of many more countries around the globe.

In sum, the ICIDH-2 will continue to be an indispensable classification tool for international use for scientific research, data collection, service management, legislation, and social policy. It meets the essential requirement for a common language with which to communicate the consequences of health conditions, and to describe and measure human functioning.

For further information contact:
Dr. T.B. Üstün
World Health Organization
Group Leader, Assessment, Classification and Epidemiology
20 Avenue Appia
CH-1211 Geneva 27
Switzerland
Tel: 41 22 791.36.09
Fax: 41 22 791.48.85
E-mail: Ustunt@who.ch

Tap the potential of the ICIDH-2 home page
What can you find on http://www.who.ch/icidh?

- Read the introduction to the ICIDH-2 Beta-2 draft
- Review the ICIDH-2 Beta-2 draft in hypertext form. (This will include the translated versions when they are ready)
- While browsing the classification you may send your comments on ICIDH items, which will be automatically stored in our database.
- Download the ICIDH-2 Beta-2 draft in PDF format for printing.
- Download the order form for the ICIDH-2 Beta-2 draft
- Consult the training materials
- Download the field trial protocols
- Keep up with the latest developments in the ICIDH-2
- Use the Beginner's Guide
- Register yourself for receiving news or information via e-mail.

H

Public Law Number 101-336: Americans with Disabilities Act

OVERVIEW OF THE AMERICANS WITH DISABILITIES ACT

Over 43 million Americans with physical or mental impairments that substantially limit daily activities are protected under the ADA. These activities include working, walking, talking, seeing, hearing, or caring for oneself. People who have a record of such an impairment and those regarded as having an impairment are also protected.

The ADA has the following five titles:

- Title I – Employment (all Title II employers and private employers with 15 or more employees)
- Title II – Public Services (state and local government including public school districts and public transportation)
- Title III – Public Accommodations and Services Operated by Private Entities
- Title IV – Telecommunications
- Title V – Miscellaneous Provisions

The following is a brief summary of some of the major requirements contained in the ADA statute.

To determine all of the requirements that a covered entity must satisfy, it is necessary to refer to the regulations, guidelines, and/or technical assistance materials that have been developed by the Department of Justice (DOJ), the Equal Employment Opportunity Commission (EEOC), the Department of Transportation (DOT), the Federal Communications Commission (FCC), and the Architectural and Transportation Barriers Compliance Board (the Access Board). In addition, the Internal Revenue Service (IRS) has developed regulations on the tax relief available for certain costs of complying with the ADA, such as small business tax credits.

Title I – Employment

Title I of the ADA prohibits discrimination in employment against people with disabilities. It requires employers to make reasonable accommodations to the known physical or mental limitations of a qualified applicant or employee, unless such accommodation would impose an undue hardship on the employer. Reasonable accommodations include such actions as making worksites accessible, modifying existing equipment, providing new devices, modifying work schedules, restructuring jobs, and providing readers or interpreters.

Title I also prohibits the use of employment tests and other selection criteria that screen out, or tend to screen out, individuals with disabilities, unless such tests or criteria are shown to be job-related and consistent with business necessity. It also bans the use of pre-employment medical examinations or inquiries to determine if an applicant has a disability. It does, however, permit the use of a medical examination after a job offer has been made if the results are kept confidential; all persons offered employment in the same job category are required to take them; and the results are not used to discriminate.

Employers are permitted, at any time. To inquire about the ability of a job applicant or employee to perform job-related functions. The EEOC is the enforcement agency for Title I.

Title II – Public Services

Title II of the ADA requires that the services and programs of local and State governments, as well as other non-Federal government agencies, shall operate their programs so that when viewed in their entirety are readily accessible to and usable by individuals with disabilities.

Title II entities:

• Do not need to remove physical barriers, such as stairs, in all existing buildings, as long as they make their programs accessible to individuals who are unable to use an inaccessible existing facility.

• Must provide appropriate auxiliary aids to ensure that communications with individuals with hearing, vision, or speech impairments are as effective as communications with others, unless an undue burden or fundamental alteration would result.

• May impose safety requirements that are necessary for the safe operation of a Title II program if they are based on actual risks and not on mere speculation, stereotypes, or generalizations about individuals with disabilities.

In addition, Title II seeks to ensure that people with disabilities have access to existing public transportation services. All new buses must be accessible. Transit authorities must provide supplementary paratransit services or other special transportation services for individuals with disabilities who cannot use fixed-route bus services, unless this would present an undue burden.

Title III – Public Accommodations

Public accommodations include the broad range of privately-owned entities that affect commerce, including sales, rental, and service establishments; private educational institutions; recreational facilities; and social service centers. In providing goods and services, a public accommodation may not use eligibility requirements that exclude or segregate individuals with disabilities, unless the requirements are "necessary" for the operation of the public accommodation. As an example, restricting people with Down's Syndrome to a certain area of a restaurant would violate Title III. It also requires public accommodations to make reasonable modifications to policies, practices, and procedures, unless those modifications would fundamentally alter the nature of the services provided by the public accommodation.

Title III also requires that public accommodations provide auxiliary aids necessary to enable persons who have visual, hearing, or sensory impairments to participate in the program, but only if their provision will not result in an undue burden on the business. Thus, for example, a restaurant would not be required to provide menus in Braille for blind patrons if it requires its waitpersons to read the menu. The auxiliary aid requirement is flexible. A public accommodation may choose among various alternatives as long as the result is effective communication.

With respect to existing facilities of public accommodations, physical barriers must be removed when it is "readily achievable" to do so (i.e., when it can be accomplished easily and without much expense). Tax write-offs are available to minimize the costs associated with the removal of barriers in existing buildings or in providing auxiliary aids, including interpreters for the deaf. Modifications that would be readily achievable in most cases include the ramping of a few steps. However, all construction of new building facilities and alterations of existing facilities in public accommodations, as well as in commercial facilities such as office buildings, must comply with the ADA Accessibility Guidelines (ADAAG) so they are accessible to people with disabilities. New privately owned buildings are not required to install elevators if they are less than three stories high or have less than 3,000 square feet per story, unless the building is a shopping center, mall, or a professional office of a health care provider.

Title III also addressees transportation provided by private entities.

Title IV – Telecommunications

Title IV of the ADA amends the Communications Act of 1934 to require that telephone companies provide telecommunication relay services. The relay services must provide speech-impaired or hearing-impaired individuals who use TTYs or other non-voice terminal devices opportunities for communication that are equivalent to those provided to other customers.

Title V – Miscellaneous Provisions

This title addresses such issues as the ADA's relationship to other laws including the Rehabilitation Act of 1973, requirements relating to the provision of insurance, regulations by the Access Board, prohibition of State immunity, inclusion of Congress as a covered entity, implementation of each title, promotion of alternative means of dispute resolution, and provision of technical assistance.

Additional Information

For additional information and answers to your questions, call 1-800-949-4232.

Index

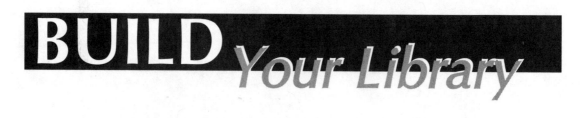

BUILD *Your Library*

This book and many others on numerous different topics are available from SLACK Incorporated. For further information or a copy of our latest catalog, contact us at:

Professional Book Division
SLACK Incorporated
6900 Grove Road
Thorofare, NJ 08086 USA
Telephone: 1-856-848-1000
1-800-257-8290
Fax: 1-856-853-5991
E-mail: orders@slackinc.com
www.slackbooks.com

We accept most major credit cards and checks or money orders in US dollars drawn on a US bank. Most orders are shipped within 72 hours.

Contact us for information on recent releases, forthcoming titles, and bestsellers. If you have a comment about this title or see a need for a new book, direct your correspondence to the Editorial Director at the above address.

Thank you for your interest and we hope you found this work beneficial.